Diabetes and its Management

D0239541

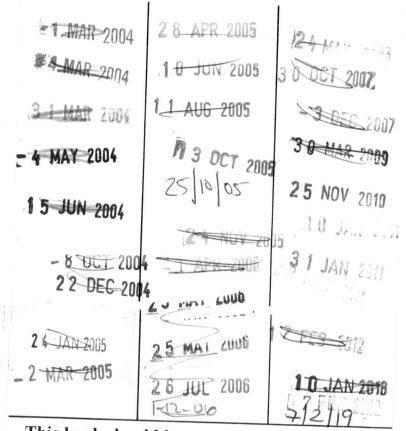

This book should be returned by the last date stamped above. You may renew the loan personally, by post or telephone for a further period if the book is not required by another reader.

Diabetes and its Management

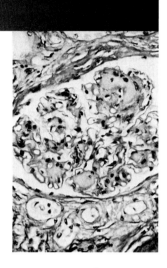

Peter J. Watkins
King's College Hospital, London

Stephanie A. Amiel
King's College, London

Simon L. Howell
King's College, London

Eileen Turner
King's College Hospital, London

SIXTH EDITION

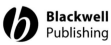

Blackwell
Publishing

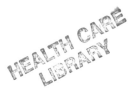

Blackwell Publishing, Inc., 350 Main Street, Malden, Massachusetts 02148-5020, USA
Blackwell Publishing Ltd, 9600 Garsington Road, Oxford OX4 2DQ, UK
Blackwell Publishing Asia Pty Ltd, 550 Swanston Street, Carlton, Victoria 3053, Australia

First published 1973
Second edition 1975
Third edition 1978
Fourth edition 1990
Fifth edition 1996
Reprinted 1997
Sixth edition 2003

ISBN 1-4051-0725-1

Library of Congress Cataloging-in-Publication Data

Diabetes and its management. – 6th ed. / Peter J. Watkins . . . [et al.].
      p.   ;   cm.
Rev. ed. of: Diabetes and its management / Peter J. Watkins, Paul L. Drury, Simon L. Howell. 5th ed. 1996.
Includes bibliographical references and index.
      ISBN 1-4051-0725-1 (alk. paper)
   1. Diabetes.   2. Diabetes in children.
      [DNLM: 1. Diabetes Mellitus.   2. Diabetes Mellitus – therapy. WK 810 D53722 2003]   I. Watkins, Peter J.

   RC660.W34   2003
   616.4′62 – dc21   2003009081

A catalogue record for this title is available from the British Library

Set in 10/12pt Minion by SNP Best-set Typesetter Ltd., Hong Kong
Printed and bound in Great Britain at Ashford Colour Press, Gosport

Commissioning Editor: Alison Brown
Editorial Assistant: Elizabeth Callaghan
Production Editor: Julie Elliott
Production Controller: Kate Charman

For further information on Blackwell Publishing, visit our website:
http://www.blackwellpublishing.com

Contents

SECTION 5: **Diabetic Care**

Preface to the Sixth Edition

A new energy and commitment to treatment entered the field of diabetes at the beginning of the 21st century. The introduction of new technologies and new medications raise expectations for better outcomes. They bring potential for improvements to the health of diabetic patients and diminish the impact of its complications. New standards of care have been established as a result of the two hugely influential trials of the 1990s, the North American Diabetes Control and Complications Trial (DCCT) and the UK Prospective Diabetes Study (UKPDS), each demonstrating the effectiveness of tight blood glucose (and, for UKPDS, blood pressure) control in retarding complications in Type 1 and Type 2 diabetes respectively. Prospects of cell therapy for Type 1 diabetes, and of prevention strategies for Type 2 diabetes are tantalizing prospects for the future.

Government now acknowledges the impact of diabetes as a major public health problem, perhaps especially because of the projected increase in the prevalence of Type 2 diabetes. The UK's National Service Framework for diabetes, announced in 2002, sets out in detail the requirements for modern diabetes care and following this important statement it is to be hoped that appropriate resources for its implementation will follow. Already a national eye screening scheme has been established in Wales, providing a model for its extension to the rest of the UK.

In many ways, the field of diabetes care has led the way for modern management of chronic diseases by early establishing the teams of professionals needed to offer complex programmes for the optimal care of those with diabetes and starting the integration of primary and secondary care. The role of specialist nurses remains one of the linchpins of diabetes care and the recent establishment of consultant nurses gives them a new impetus.

It is appropriate in this sixth edition to introduce new authors for this book, namely Professor Stephanie Amiel, R.D. Lawrence Professor of Diabetic Medicine, and Mrs Eileen Turner, Nurse Consultant, both at King's. At the same time we acknowledge the earlier contribution of Dr Paul Drury who now heads diabetes services in Auckland, New Zealand.

The book has been extensively rewritten. Our aims remain those of the original authors, namely that it should be of practical help for doctors caring for patients both in hospital and in general practice and to the growing number of diabetes specialist nurses who have committed themselves to this work. It is intended as an aide-memoire for the experienced and as a guide for those in training, including those preparing for higher examinations. It is also intended that it should help interested students who would like to expand their knowledge of diabetes beyond that of standard textbooks. We hope that many other specialists—obstetricians, ophthalmologists, renal physicians and cardiovascular physicians and surgeons, involved in the care of diabetic patients—will also find helpful information in this book.

Throughout, our inspiration has come from those who first conceived and delivered this book. We hope that the thoughtfulness and wisdom of the late Drs Wilfrid Oakley, David Pyke and Professor Keith Taylor, all of whom made immense contributions to the study of diabetes and to the care of their many patients, will live permanently in its pages.

King's Diabetes Centre
King's College Hospital
London SE5 9RS

Peter Watkins
Stephanie Amiel
Simon Howell
Eileen Turner

Preface to the First Edition

This book has been written as a practical guide to the management of diabetes for the benefit, we hope, of clinicians. It is based on our larger book, *Clinical Diabetes and its Biochemical Basis,* but whereas that was a detailed review of the present state of knowledge concerning all aspects of diabetes, this book is an expression of our own clinical practice. We hope it will be helpful to those with charge of diabetics and also that it will be valuable, either in general practice or in hospital. We hope also that it will be valuable for students who want to know rather more about diabetes than is usually found in general medical textbooks.

Since diabetes affects so many systems, it is the concern of various specialists, for example obstetricians, ophthalmologists, and orthopaedic surgeons, and we trust that they too will find the information they need in this book.

If it is also useful to those taking higher examinations, so much the better.

Diabetic Department
King's College Hospital
London SE5 9RS

W.G. Oakley
D.A. Pyke
K.W. Taylor

Acknowledgements

Close collaboration with colleagues at King's both past and present has made possible many of the joint ventures described here, and we are grateful to them all. We wish to pay special tribute to Miss Maggie Blott (obstetrician), Dr Charles Buchanan (paediatrician), Mr Dominic McHugh (ophthalmologist), Dr Phin Kon (renal physician), Drs Stephen Thomas and Michael Edmonds (physicians), Mrs Ali Foster (podiatrist), Pauline Weir (dietitian), and Pat Gillard, Karen Jones, Helen Reid and Val Watkins (diabetes specialist nurses), all of whom have formed the team which has shaped the Diabetes Centre at King's. Dr Tyrrell Evans (GP) helped to forge the community links. Dr Paul Drury, co-author of the previous edition, has left King's and moved to New Zealand. The work of our registrars and research fellows and above all our patients has been a constant source of inspiration.

Basic Principles of Diabetes and its Biochemistry

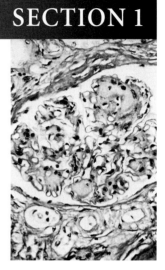

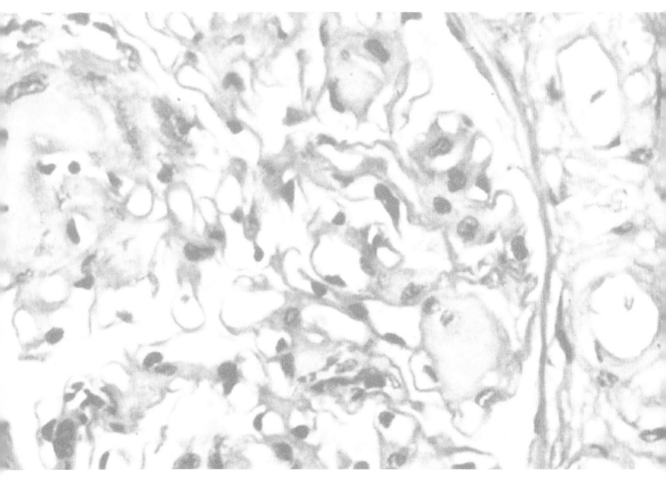

Diagnosis and Classification

Summary

- Diabetes is an ancient disease transformed by the introduction of insulin in 1922 and oral hypoglycaemic agents in the 1950s

- Diagnosis must be established by laboratory measurement of blood glucose or in some cases where doubt exists by a glucose tolerance test

- The majority of patients have either Type 1 (insulin dependent) diabetes or Type 2 (non-insulin dependent) diabetes

- There are numerous other causes of both primary and secondary diabetes and a classification is presented

Background

Diabetes mellitus was known in antiquity and remains today a worldwide and increasing health problem with a high cost from associated premature coronary artery disease, blindness, renal failure and amputations. The scientific basis of diabetes has evolved over centuries; it was long thought to be caused by kidney disease, a theory not altered by the discovery of the sweetness of the urine (Thomas Willis, 1621–79) or of glycosuria itself (Matthew Dobson, 1776). The concepts of glucose production by the liver (Claude Bernard, 1813–78) and the discovery that pancreatectomy causes diabetes (O. von Mering and J. Minkowski, Strasbourg, 1889) led to the true scientific understanding of diabetes. After several abortive attempts, N. Paulesco in Romania extracted insulin (1921), but it was in Canada, also in 1921, that Frederick Banting and Charles Best, together with J.J.R. Macleod and the biochemist James Collip, successfully extracted and organized the manufacture and distribution of insulin, sharing the Nobel prize for this great discovery. A 14-year-old boy, Leonard Thompson, was the first patient to be treated in 1922. The major impetus to diabetes treatment and care stems from that date.

The impact of insulin treatment is shown in Fig. 1.1 and is best recorded from Dr Banting's accounts of his patient, Elizabeth Hughes, aged 14 years. He wrote on 16 August 1922: 'weight 45 lb, height 5 ft, patient extremely emaciated, slight oedema of ankles, skin dry and scaly, hair brittle and thin, abdomen prominent, shoulders dropped, muscles extremely wasted, subcutaneous tissues almost completely absorbed. She was scarcely able to walk on account of weakness.' She started insulin, and 5 weeks later wrote to her mother:

'I look entirely different everybody says, gaining every hour it seems to me in strength and weight . . . it is truly miraculous. Dr Banting considers my progress simply miraculous . . . he brings all these eminent doctors in from all over the world who come to Toronto to see for themselves the workings of this wonderful discovery, and I wish you could see the expression on their faces as they read my charts, they are so astounded in my unheard of progress.'

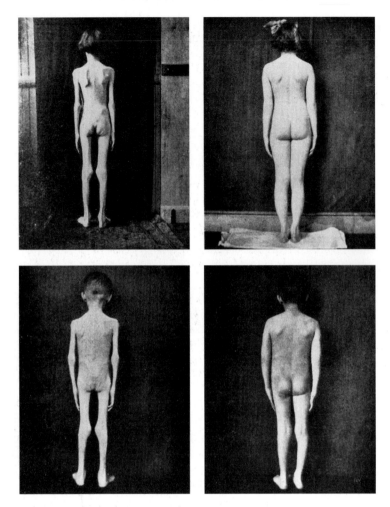

Figure 1.1 Insulin dependent diabetes: a view from 1922. Patients before and after starting insulin. (Geyelis, H.R. & Harrop, G. (1922) *Journal of Metabolism Research* **2**, 767–791).

The era of optimism through the 1920s was followed in subsequent decades by recognition of the major problems faced by patients with long-term diabetes as the specific complications of diabetes were established during the 1930s. P. Kimmelstiel and C. Wilson (1936) described the glomerular nodules which still bear their names; several authorities classified the specific retinal changes associated with diabetes; and the first comprehensive accounts of neuropathy were published (W.R. Jordan, 1936; R.W. Rundles, 1945). The disastrous situation of diabetic pregnancy was described in the 1940s by Sir John Peel and Dr Wilfred Oakley when they showed that more than one-third of babies died either *in utero* or in the neonatal period.

Physicians were, during the 1950s and 1960s, observers of these calamities; there is now a renewed optimism for diabetic patients, as this book shows. Retardation of the development of complications is now possible and the incidence of nephropathy is decreasing. When complications do develop, there are now ways to halt their progression or limit resulting damage so that amputation rates are halved and blindness brought about by retinopathy can be reduced by over 70%. Even when end-stage disease such as renal failure occurs, appropriate treatment is now available. Perhaps one of the most striking successes of all is the improvement of outlook in diabetic pregnancy, with a reduction in fetal mortality from more than 30% to its present level below 5%.

New technologies abound; there is a vast development in patient education, serious involvement of patients in making choices with regard to their treatment, and important developments in the delivery of care with strong new links in the community. This book describes these developments and their clinical application.

Definition

Diabetes mellitus is a disorder in which the level of blood glucose is persistently raised above the normal range. It occurs because of a lack of insulin, with or without factors that oppose the action of insulin. Hyperglycaemia results from insufficient insulin action. There are many associated metabolic abnormalities, notably the development of hyperketonaemia when there is a severe lack of insulin, together with alterations of fatty acid, lipid and protein turnover and there are also changes in haemorheological factors and oxidant status. Diabetes is a permanent condition in all but a few special situations in which it can be transient. For most patients, diabetes once diagnosed is for life. The perseverance and self-discipline needed to achieve control over a lifetime can tax even the most robust of people to the limit. Those caring for them also require patience and perseverance and an understanding of humanity combined with a cautious optimism to guide those with diabetes through the peaks and troughs of their lives.

Diagnosis of diabetes

Hyperglycaemia must be established in order to make a diagnosis of diabetes. The plasma glucose must be measured by a laboratory method; it is not adequate to use blood glucose strips read visually or with a meter (Box 1.1).

- The presence of symptoms with a single random venous plasma glucose value ≥ 11.1 mmol/L or fasting (no caloric intake for at least 8 h) venous plasma glucose ≥ 7.0 mmol/L are diagnostic of diabetes.
- If there are no symptoms, diagnosis requires at least two elevated plasma glucose readings on different days.

> ### Box 1.1 WHO diagnostic criteria for diabetes
>
> 1 Symptoms of diabetes plus casual venous plasma glucose ≥ 11.1 mmol/L. Casual is defined as anytime of day without regard to time of last meal. The classic symptoms of diabetes include polyuria, polydipsia and unexplained weight loss
> 2 Fasting plasma glucose ≥ 7.0 mmol/L or whole blood ≥ 6.1 mmol/L. Fasting is defined as no caloric intake for at least 8 h
> 3 2-h plasma glucose ≥ 11.1 mmol/L during oral glucose tolerance test using 75-g glucose load
>
> In the absence of symptoms, these criteria should be confirmed by repeat testing on a different day. If the fasting or random values are not diagnostic, the 2-h value post glucose load should be used
>
> *Note*
> Fasting plasma glucose < 6.1 mmol/L — normal
> Fasting plasma glucose ≥ 6.1 and < 7.0 mmol/L — impaired fasting blood glucose
> Fasting plasma glucose ≥ 7.0 mmol/L — provisional diagnosis of diabetes; the diagnosis must be confirmed (see above)

- Glycosuria *alone* is insufficient evidence on which to make a diagnosis of diabetes.

Glucose tolerance test

A glucose tolerance test is not normally needed in routine clinical practice, and then only if uncertainty exists, for example in younger patients or to establish an exact diagnosis in pregnancy.

The oral glucose tolerance test is performed using a 75-g glucose load in 250–300 mL of water (or in children 1.75 g/kg to a maximum of 75 g). It should be performed in the morning after at least 3 days of unrestricted diet, containing, for an adult, at least 250 g/day carbohydrate and a high carbohydrate meal the evening before the test, and usual physical activity. It is preceded by an overnight fast during which only water may be drunk. Smoking is not permitted. Intercurrent illness or medication may affect the results and the test should preferably not be performed under such adverse circumstances. Elevated fasting and 2-h blood glucose levels (Box 1.2) estab-

---

Box 1.2 Glucose tolerance test

	Glucose concentration (mmol/L)		
	Venous whole blood	Capillary whole blood	Venous plasma
*Diabetes mellitus**			
Fasting	≥6.1	≥6.1	≥7.0
2 h after glucose load	≥10.0	≥11.1	≥11.1
Impaired glucose tolerance			
Fasting	<6.1	<6.1	<7.0
2 h after glucose load	≥6.7–<10.0	≥7.8–<11.1	≥7.8–<11.1

*In the absence of symptoms at least one additional abnormal blood glucose concentration is needed to confirm clinical diagnosis; for example, 1-h value of 11 mmol/L or more.

---

lish the presence of diabetes, without the need for intermediate levels, although these will corroborate the diagnosis. The criteria for impaired glucose tolerance (IGT) are also shown in Box 1.2. In pregnancy, any form of IGT is diagnosed as diabetes.

Measurement of plasma glucose should be a routine part of medical consultation when the cause of presenting symptoms has not been established, otherwise cases of diabetes will be missed.

Glucose tolerance tests may also show the following.

1 *Renal glycosuria.* This occurs when there is glycosuria but normal plasma glucose concentrations. It is a benign condition, only rarely indicating unusual forms of renal disease. It is worth issuing these patients with a certificate to prevent them from being subjected to repeated glucose tolerance tests at every medical examination.

2 *Steeple or lag curve.* This is described when fasting and 2-h concentrations are normal but those between are high, causing glycosuria. This is also a benign condition, which most commonly occurs after gastrectomy but may occur in healthy people.

Classification

Clinical types of diabetes mellitus

The division of diabetes into two major types (Table 1.1) has long been known. Over a century ago

Bouchardat described patients as having 'diabète maigre' or 'diabète gras', roughly corresponding to today's Types 1 and 2. J. Bornstein and R.D. Lawrence (1951) were the first to show that types of diabetes could be distinguished by the presence or absence of plasma insulin. The distinction between Type 1 (previously described as insulin dependent) diabetes, and Type 2 (previously non-insulin dependent) diabetes is of fundamental importance. In practice, many Type 2 diabetic patients need insulin for their wellbeing but not for survival and the value of this simple and useful classification depends on the recognition of the mechanisms underlying the development of the two types. These mechanisms, the associated clinical features and appropriate therapies are described in the following chapters.

Diabetes has many causes. Most patients have 'primary diabetes', although even this results from several different underlying mechanisms and is clearly not a single entity. Many different conditions cause secondary diabetes and these are listed in Table 1.1 using the present World Health Organization (WHO) classification.

In practice, the important identification of diabetes as Type 1 is achieved by clinical observation and simple investigations although the condition can be further defined by genetic and immunological markers. Type 2 diabetes is present in patients who do not have Type 1 diabetes or any of the other specific causes. Insulin dependence, the hallmark of Type 1 diabetes, implies a need for insulin injections in

Table 1.1 World Health Organization (WHO) classification of diabetes.

I Type 1 diabetes (previously insulin dependent diabetes) is caused by B-cell destruction, usually leading to absolute insulin deficiency A Immune mediated B Idiopathic	*Endocrinopathies* Acromegaly or gigantism Cushing's disease Glucagonoma Phaeochromocytoma Somatostatinoma Conn's syndrome

II Type 2 diabetes (previously non-insulin dependent diabetes) ranges from those with predominant insulin resistance associated with relative insulin deficiency, to those with a predominantly insulin secretory defect with insulin resistance

Some other specific types

Genetic defects of beta cell function
MODY*
    chromosome 12 HNF-1alpha (formerly MODY 3)
    chromosome 7 glucokinase defect (formerly MODY 2)
    chromosome 20 HNF-4alpha (formerly MODY 1)
    insulin promoter factor 1 (formerly MODY 4)
Other
    mitochondrial DNA 3423 mutation
    Wolfram's syndrome (diabetes insipidus, diabetes mellitus, optic atrophy, deafness—DIDMOAD)

Genetic defects in insulin action
Type A insulin resistance (genetic defects in insulin receptor)
Lipoatrophic diabetes
Genetic defects in the PPAR gamma receptor
Rabson—Mendenhall syndrome
Leprechaunism

Diseases of the exocrine pancreas
Pancreatitis
Pancreatectomy
Carcinoma of pancreas
Cystic fibrosis
Fibrocalculous pancreatopathy
Haemochromatosis and haemosiderosis
Alpha$_1$-antitrypsin deficiency
Congential absence of pancreas or islets

Drug induced (these agents in particular exacerbate hyperglycaemia in established diabetics)
Corticosteroids
Diazoxide
Beta-adrenergic agonists (e.g. intravenous salbutamol)
Thiazides
Alpha interferon
Asparaginase

Infections
Congenital rubella
Cytomegalovirus

Uncommon forms of immune-mediated diabetes
Stiff man syndrome
Polyglandular syndromes
Anti-insulin receptor antibodies (Type B insulin resistance)

Some other genetic syndromes sometimes associated with diabetes
Down's syndrome
Turner's syndrome
Klinefelter's syndrome
Prader–Willi syndrome
Laurence–Moon–Biedl syndrome
Myotonic dystrophy
Ataxia telangiectasia
Porphyria

*The MODY classification is expanding as new genes are identified. MODY, maturity onset diabetes of the young.

order to survive. It is often easy to establish clinically because of ketosis and often the more acute onset of disease and the diagnosis may be confirmed by demonstrating severe depletion of circulating C-peptide. In Type 2 diabetes, there is a mixture of insulin resistance and insulin deficiency. Commonly, the insulin resistance is a major feature although, for hyperglycaemia to result, at least a degree of pancreatic insufficiency must be present (the 'healthy' response to insulin resistance is hyperinsulinaemia and hyperglycaemia occurs only when pancreatic insulin

reserve is unable to keep up). However, there are many middle-aged non-obese patients who need insulin to control symptoms of hyperglycaemia but may not be dependent on it for survival, at least initially; these people may just have reached the end of the decline in pancreatic reserve that happens at a variable rate over the lifetime of all patients with Type 2 diabetes. Alternatively, they may have a late onset and slowly progressive autoimmune pancreatic islet destruction which has been referred to as 'LADA' (late onset autoimmune diabetes of adults) and is true

Type 1 disease. All other types of diabetes are classified as 'other specific types' and the classification system continues to depend upon pathogenesis. Thus, single gene defects causing insulin deficiency or insulin resistance, diabetes secondary to pancreatic disease or infection or as a result of very high levels of anti-insulin hormones are all included.

In tropical countries, young people with diabetes may present with marked associated nutritional deficiency. One cause of the diabetes in these regions is fibrocalculous (calcific) pancreatopathy (page 9). The other forms of diabetes that, in earlier classification systems, were joined with fibrocalculous pancreatopathy as malnutrition-related diabetes, are now recognized as either Type 1 or Type 2 disease, occurring in the presence of malnutrition, commonly with high degrees of insulin resistance and an absence of fat perhaps preventing development of ketosis.

Gestational diabetes is diagnosed when glucose intolerance is first detected in pregnancy. Reclassification by glucose tolerance test is necessary post-partum.

People who have previously, during intercurrent illness, shown an abnormal glucose tolerance that has subsequently reverted to normal are at great risk of developing diabetes in later years, especially during periods of serious illness with or without the presence of infection. This phenomenon is most frequently observed when gestational diabetes returns in subsequent pregnancies. Hyperglycaemia in illness in children may indicate the presence of maturity onset diabetes of the young (MODY).

Impaired glucose tolerance is defined on page 6. These patients have a risk of cardiovascular disease little different from people with Type 2 diabetes and a high risk of developing Type 2 diabetes. Over 10 years, approximately half of those with IGT will develop diabetes, one-quarter will persist with IGT, and one-quarter will revert to normal. Lifestyle advice and management of cardiovascular risk factors is indicated and follow-up to ensure early diagnosis of diabetes if it occurs. IGT patients are not at risk of diabetic microvascular disease. IGT is characterized by insulin resistance and the progression to Type 2 diabetes is caused by loss of insulin secretory capacity over time. Associated with obesity, hyperlipi-

---

Box 1.3 World Health Organization definition of metabolic syndrome

One of
- Diabetes mellitus
- Impaired glucose tolerance
- Impaired fasting glucose (≥ 6.1 mmol/L)

Plus two or more of
- Insulin resistance (lowest quartile of insulin sensitivity)
- Blood pressure $\geq 140/90$ mmHg
- Triglyceride ≥ 1.7 mmol/L and/or high-density cholesterol < 0.9 mmol/L or 1.0 F
- Central obesity: weight : height ratio > 0.9 M > 0.85 F
- Microalbuminuria ≥ 20 µg/min or albumin : creatinine ratio ≥ 3

---

daemia, hypertension and microalbuminuria, IGT forms part of the metabolic syndrome (Box 1.3). Pregnant women with IGT must be treated as having diabetes.

The 1998 classifications used a fasting venous plasma glucose of ≥ 7 mmol/L as diagnostic of diabetes, is based on its association with retinopathy in epidemiological studies. However, it is recognized that levels ≥ 6 mmol/L are also not normal. These patients are defined as having impaired fasting glucose (IFG) and are at increased risk of developing diabetes and probably also cardiovascular risk, although equivalence between IGT and IFG has not been established and different people may have one or the other.

Secondary diabetes, special syndromes and related endocrine disease

The many disorders that cause or are associated with secondary diabetes account for a very small proportion of all cases. Diabetes may result from an excess of insulin-antagonistic hormones produced either by disease or administered therapeutically, or precipitated by the use of drugs. Several pancreatic disorders are also associated with diabetes and it is a feature of some rare hereditary syndromes. The causes are listed in Table 1.1.

Endocrine causes of diabetes

Corticosteroids and adrenocorticotrophic hormone (ACTH), growth hormone, glucagon and catecholamines all induce insulin resistance. Patients with tumours producing such hormones often have diabetes.

Cushing's syndrome

Most patients with Cushing's syndrome of either pituitary, adrenal or ectopic origin have either overt diabetes (25%) or glucose intolerance. It tends to be more common and severe in patients with the ectopic ACTH syndrome, often requiring insulin. Improvement, or cure, of the diabetes occurs when the causative tumour is removed or when satisfactory medical treatment is given.

Pituitary causes of diabetes

F.G. Young in the 1930s was able to produce permanent diabetes by giving extracts of growth hormone to dogs. Diabetes is common in patients with acromegaly and occurs in almost one-third of patients, sometimes with quite severe insulin resistance. The diabetes improves after the acromegaly is treated. Microvascular complications can occur.

Rather curiously, various growth hormone deficiency states are also associated with diabetes, notably in patients with isolated growth hormone deficiency, Laron dwarfism, hereditary panhypopituitary dwarfism and pituitary dwarfism.

Other adrenal causes

Phaeochromocytoma produces similar effects through catecholamine excess; glucose intolerance is common, perhaps as high as 75%, although typically intermittent.

Pancreatic diabetes

Diabetes results from surgical removal or destructive disease of the pancreas.

Pancreatectomy

Severe insulin dependent diabetes mellitus always occurs immediately following total pancreatectomy.

Because of the concomitant absence of glucagon in these cases, very small doses of insulin are needed and control is exquisitely sensitive to minor changes of dose, often with serious problems from hypoglycaemia.

Pancreatic disease

Acute pancreatitis causes diabetes in approximately half of the cases, the increase in plasma glucose being related to the severity of the pancreatitis and therefore most likely in those also suffering multiorgan failure. It is usually transient, resolving over a few days or up to 6 weeks, although it remains permanent in approximately 10% of cases. Hypoglycaemia can occur, albeit rarely, during the acute phase of pancreatitis. Subsequent development of diabetes following acute pancreatitis occurs infrequently. Pancreatitis in established diabetes temporarily increases the insulin requirement.

Fibrocalculous pancreatitis, better described as pancreatic lithiasis, is responsible for 95% of chronic pancreatitis cases. Pancreatic lithiasis is chiefly associated with a high alcohol intake or, in tropical countries, notably southern India, parts of Africa and Brazil. While alcohol appears to be by far the most common cause of chronic pancreatitis in Africa, other suggested mechanisms have included protein malnutrition and chronic cyanide poisoning from ingestion of cassava although this now seems unlikely. The common presenting features are abdominal pain, malabsorption and diabetes, and the diagnosis is readily made on a plain abdominal X-ray (Fig. 1.2) or by ultrasound examination. The condition is most common in males who develop diabetes characteristically between 15 and 35 years of age; the diabetes appears to be insulin resistant and without a tendency to ketosis.

Chronic calcific pancreatitis is a very rare cause of diabetes in the Western world and affects fewer than 10 patients in the entire diabetic clinic of several thousand patients at King's College Hospital.

Cystic fibrosis

With improved treatment for cystic fibrosis patients, the prognosis has improved and the median survival is now 31 years and rising. As prognosis improves, the

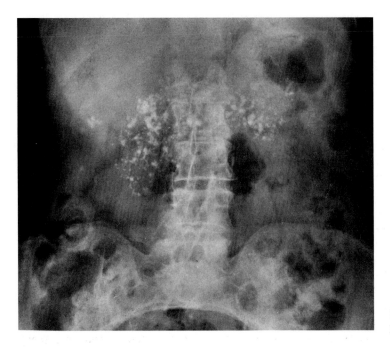

Figure 1.2 Extensive calcification of the pancreas.

development of diabetes increases and as many as 30–50% of adult patients with this disease will develop glucose intolerance and diabetes. This results chiefly from reduced production of insulin from the diseased pancreas. The development of cystic fibrosis-related diabetes is usually insidious and often symptomless. Awareness of the increasing risk of developing diabetes amongst the older age groups makes it important to screen for diabetes in these patients so that appropriate treatment can be delivered. The diagnosis is established in the usual ways although misleading results can sometimes be obtained from fasting or random plasma glucose levels in relation to the very high calorie feeding that is often necessary. Older teenagers and adults will have a routine oral glucose tolerance test during an admission for exacerbation of chest infection or if there are concerns regarding their weight.

The diabetes usually starts as non-insulin requiring and can be treated with oral hypoglycaemic agents. However, because a high fat, high carbohydrate diet, sometimes delivered by nasogastric tube or gastrostomy, is often required to reverse the malnutrition from which these patients suffer, together with the occasional need for corticosteroids, insulin is often essential. Handling the insulin administration in these cases requires considerable skill but is essential to give the insulin to match the high calorie diets prescribed. Trying to control the plasma glucose by dietary restriction is not an option, as the extra calories are necessary and leaving the patient hyperglycaemic by faulty or inadequate insulinization will waste much of the caloric replacement through glycosuria. Microvascular complications have been recorded in some patients with long-standing diabetes.

Carcinoma of the pancreas

Diabetes is common in patients with carcinoma of the pancreas and has been recorded in about onefifth of cases. The reason for this association is obscure: the tumour most commonly affects the head of the pancreas while most of the islets are in the tail. It is presumed that the tumour itself causes the diabetes although specific humoral factors have not been identified. The diabetes and the carcinoma are usually diagnosed within a few months of each other. When diabetes and jaundice develop in a patient within a few weeks, carcinoma of the pancreas is nearly always the cause. Some older patients who continue to lose weight soon after starting treatment for what appears to be routine Type 2 diabetes may also prove to have this condition or some other malignancy.

Haemochromatosis

Haemochromatosis is the most common inherited liver disease in the UK. It affects about one in 200 of the population and occurs 10 times more often than cystic fibrosis. It is characterized by a slate-grey skin pigmentation, hepatomegaly, absence of body hair, testicular atrophy, gynaecomastia, impotence, cardiac disease and is sometimes accompanied by arthritis from chondrocalcinosis. It is caused by iron overload leading to the accumulation of iron in the tissues resulting from excessive iron absorption, together with other defects of iron metabolism. The concentration of iron in the liver and pancreas is 50–100 times normal levels. Other endocrine glands also show heavy deposition of iron. Patients are predominantly male (M:F 9:1) and usually present between 40 and 60 years of age; about two-thirds have diabetes, mostly requiring insulin. Glomerulosclerosis and retinopathy may occur in those patients with long-standing diabetes. The hypogonadism results directly from iron overload or from hypopituitarism.

The genetic defect responsible for haemochromatosis is a single base change at the locus of the *HFE* gene on chromosome 6. Genetic analysis is now available for diagnosis and for screening family members. The serum ferritin is extremely high. Liver biopsy may be needed to determine the extent of hepatic damage. Patients who are homozygous for the mutation require regular venesection to prevent further tissue damage. Frequent venesection is needed perhaps for 2–3 years, followed by maintenance therapy removing about 2–6 units annually. Hepatic and cardiac failure occur much less commonly after treatment though many patients later succumb to hepatoma.

Transfusion-induced iron overload causing haemosidcrosis in some chronic refractory anaemias, such as thalassaemia or sickle cell disease, may also occasionally cause diabetes.

Box 1.4 Drugs provoking hyperglycaemia

Corticosteroids
Diazoxide
Thiazide diuretics (larger doses)
Non-selective beta-blockers
Dopexamine
Beta-adrenergic agonists (intravenous salbutamol, terbutaline, ritodrine)
Ciclosporin
Protease inhibitors
Clozapine

Drugs provoking hyperglycaemia (Box 1.4)

Corticosteroids

Corticosteroids have by far the most powerful effect on glucose tolerance and clinical diabetes of any group of drugs. They impair glucose tolerance chiefly by increasing gluconeogenesis and increasing insulin resistance. They almost always cause deterioration of diabetic control, often within a few hours of administration. They may precipitate diabetes although they do not normally cause diabetes by themselves unless massive doses are used, such as in transplant rejection episodes, when they become toxic to beta cells. Diabetes is thus most likely to occur in those who have had a previous abnormality of glucose tolerance or gestational diabetes and most cases do not remit when steroids are withdrawn. Most patients who develop diabetes in relation to steroid treatment can be managed with oral hypoglycaemic agents: patients with established diabetes often require an increase of their treatment and those on oral therapy quite often require insulin.

Thiazide diuretics

Thiazides reduce glucose tolerance by impairing insulin secretion. Diazoxide has a potent direct effect, opening the inwardly rectifying potassium channels on the beta cell and stopping insulin secretion. Except in Type 1 diabetes, diazoxide may cause severe hyperglycaemia, an effect that is sometimes used to advantage in the treatment of insulinoma. Other thiazide diuretics have a small but still significant hyperglycaemic effect in Type 2 diabetes, probably as a result of hypokalaemia, but this is really only a problem with older agents such as hydrochlorothiazide and larger doses of these and more modern agents. Bendrofluazide (bendroflumethiazide) 2.5 mg/day can be safely used in diabetic patients for hypertension. A recent epidemiological study of drug use for hypertension in elderly people found no association between diabetes and thiazide use. Loop diuretics do not significantly affect glucose tolerance.

Beta-blockers
Beta-blockers may impair glucose tolerance and exacerbate hyperglycaemia. In the epidemiological study mentioned above, use of beta-blockers was associated with an increased prevalence of diabetes. In contrast, when used in diabetic patients on insulin, beta-blockers may reduce some of the early warning symptoms of hypoglycaemia (page 86), while increasing sweating. Nevertheless, their use in diabetic patients can be very valuable and is described further in Chapter 19.

Others
Serious hyperglycaemia is also provoked by dopexamine (an inotropic support agent) and intravenous beta-adrenergic agents (salbutamol, terbutaline, ritodrine). The immunosuppressive drug ciclosporin can also exacerbate hyperglycaemia and some other immunosuppressive agents are toxic to beta cells, e.g. tacrolimus and high-dose steroids.

Protease inhibitors used in the treatment of patients with HIV can cause a syndrome of lipodystrophy, hyperlipidaemia and insulin resistance leading to severe exacerbation of hyperglycaemia or even causing diabetes.

Clozapine may provoke hyperglycaemia so that careful monitoring is needed if this drug is used in a diabetic patient and the drug may be associated with diabetes *de novo*.

Oral contraceptives have negligible effects on diabetes.

Islet-cell tumours

Glucagonoma
This very rare tumour of the islet glucagon-secreting A cells is accompanied by characteristic clinical features: diabetes, a skin rash (necrolytic migratory erythema), normochromic anaemia and thromboembolic disease. Excision of the tumour leads to a remission of these symptoms. The prognosis when there are hepatic metastases is poor, but improved by chemotherapy.

Somatostatinoma
Most reported cases of this exceptionally rare D cell tumour of the islets have been associated with diabetes. Insulin, glucagon, pancreatic polypeptide and growth hormone levels are all reduced. Diagnosis is usually made late in the course of the disease.

Insulinoma
B-cell tumours causing uncontrolled hyperinsulinaemia cause serious and spontaneous hypoglycaemia. This condition is not considered further in this book.

Insulin-resistant diabetic states

Severe insulin resistance is rare. It occurs in a range of rare genetic abnormalities, may be acquired in a group of patients with lipodystrophic syndromes, or following the development of autoantibodies.

Type A insulin resistance
Type A insulin resistance is brought about by genetic defects in the insulin receptor or in the post-receptor pathway. It occurs predominantly in women, and is accompanied by acanthosis nigricans and variable androgenism. Leprechaunism, Rabson–Mendenhall syndrome and congenital lipodystrophies are some examples. Genetic defects in the PPARγ receptors also result in insulin resistance.

Lipoatrophic diabetes
Absence of subcutaneous fat, either partial or total, is the hallmark of this very rare group of disorders,

originally described by R.D. Lawrence in 1946 who noted that the chief features were 'lipodystrophy and hepatomegaly with diabetes, lipidaemia and other metabolic disturbances'. There are two congenital types (one dominantly and one recessively inherited); and syndromes of acquired total (Lawrence's syndrome) or partial lipodystrophy. Absence of body fat results in a striking appearance and the face especially is characteristically emaciated. The main features of this group of disorders are of lipidaemia, sometimes with xanthomas, some have acanthosis nigricans, and the gross hepatomegaly is a result of lipid and glycogen storage. Death from premature cardiovascular disease is the main outcome.

Type B insulin resistance

Type B insulin resistance develops in the presence of immunoglobulin G (IgG) autoantibodies to the insulin receptor. Insulin resistance, hyperglycaemia or occasionally hypoglycaemia may occur. Most patients with Type B insulin resistance to insulin receptor autoantibodies are women, usually of African descent, who develop this syndrome in their late thirties or early forties in association with an autoimmune disease, notably systemic lupus erythematosus. Acanthosis nigricans is common in these patients. They may need hundreds or even thousands of units of insulin to lower the blood glucose. Corticosteroids and/or immunosuppressives, perhaps with plasmapheresis as well, may help.

Hereditary and other causes of diabetes

Type 2 diabetes in children and young people

Hitherto, childhood diabetes was witnessed in some ethnic minorities and in those with the rare inherited MODY syndromes described below. There is now growing recognition of a substantial increase of this disease in the prosperous industrialized nations. In the USA, between 8 and 45% of recently diagnosed cases of diabetes among children and adolescents are Type 2 diabetes, and the problem is increasing. It is most likely to occur at 12–14 years of age, more frequently in girls, and is strongly associated with obesity, physical inactivity and family history of Type 2 diabetes. When young people of lean physique are discovered to have Type 2 diabetes, it is important to attempt to establish whether they may represent those with LADA. There is also evidence that in approximately one-quarter of such patients diabetes is a result of a specific genetic defect including those of the MODY group described below or other rare genetic syndromes listed in Table 1.1.

Dominantly inherited Type 2 diabetes (MODY)

Seven genetic syndromes—three of which are shown in Table 1.1—cause MODY, defined as an early onset of dominantly inherited Type 2 diabetes. Two (or, at the very least, one) members of such families should have been diagnosed before 25 years of age, three generations (usually first-degree) should have diabetes, and they should not normally require insulin until they have had diabetes for more than 5 years. Each of the genetic types has characteristic clinical features.

HNF1alpha. This is the genetic group most commonly reported (69%). It is a progressive disease with a variable age of onset. Treatment is by insulin secretagogues initially, progressing to insulin over time. Diabetic complications can occur. Renal glycosuria caused by a renal tubule glucose transport defect is a feature in some of these cases.

Glucokinase gene defect. This defect accounts for approximately 14% of dominantly inherited MODY syndromes. Hyperglycaemia is caused by an islet glucose sensing defect. As a result, fasting blood glucose values lie in the range 6–8 mmol/L. This benign disorder is lifelong, non-progressive and diabetic complications do not develop. It is satisfactorily treated by diet alone although insulin may be needed in pregnancy.

Mitochondrial diabetes

Mitochondrial diabetes and deafness is a rare form of diabetes maternally transmitted, and is related to the A3243G mitochondrial DNA mutation. Hyperglycaemia results from a decrease of insulin secretion associated with diminishing numbers of B cells, although insulin sensitivity is normal. It may be found in families, sometimes presenting simply as young onset Type 2 diabetes. However, diabetes is usually diagnosed in the fourth or fifth decades, often in thin symptomatic patients. They respond better to sulphonylureas than diet alone. A form of retinal pigmentary degeneration occurs in some patients giving rise to a 'salt and pepper' retinal appearance (depigmented and pigmented spots). Diabetic microvascular complications may occur.

DIDMOAD (also Wolfram's) syndrome (diabetes insipidus, diabetes mellitus, optic atrophy, deafness)

This is a recessively inherited syndrome in which Type 1 diabetes is associated with the development of diabetes insipidus, optic atrophy leading to blindness, and gradual onset of high-tone deafness. Many of these patients also have distended bladders with hydroureter and hydronephrosis. Cerebral atrophy gradually develops and the prognosis is poor. Absence of the posterior pituitary has been demonstrated in this syndrome.

Other hereditary syndromes

There are numerous syndromes associated with impairment of glucose tolerance or clinical diabetes. These include pancreatic degenerative syndromes (including congenital absence of islets), haematological conditions, metabolic abnormalities, neurological syndromes and often chromosomal abnormalities. The better known syndromes are shown in Table 1.2. Even this list, although long, is incomplete. The genetic defect and chromosomal location for many of these disorders have been established.

Other autoimmune and endocrine diseases associated with diabetes

Associations of Type 1 diabetes with antibodies to several endocrine tissues are well described. Clinical associations with thyroid disease and pernicious anaemia are weak, although rather stronger with Addison's disease which is much more common in Type 1 diabetes patients than in the general population. There may also be a weak association with vitiligo which is said to be associated with Type 1 diabetes.

Thyroid disease

There is no clear evidence for an association between

Table 1.2 Some syndromes associated with diabetes mellitus.

Type of defect	Syndrome or description
Metabolic	Acute intermittent porphyria Glycogen storage disease Type 1 Hyperlipidaemias Lipoatrophic diabetic syndromes
Neuromuscular and neurological	Ataxia telangiectasia Laurence–Moon–Biedl syndrome (retinitis, paraplegia, hypogonadism, obesity, mental retardation, polydactyly) Friedreich's ataxia Huntington's chorea Myotonic dystrophy Refsum's syndrome Wolfram's syndrome (DIDMOAD)
Miscellaneous	Leprechaunism (prominent eyes, thick lips and phallus, hirsutism, intrauterine growth retardation, fasting hypoglycaemia) Mendenhall's syndrome (facies, large genitalia, hyper pigmentation)
Associated with premature ageing	Cockayne dwarfism (dwarf, mental retardation, deaf, blind) Werner's syndrome (cataracts, arteriosclerosis)
Genetic obesity syndromes	Prader–Willi (obesity, short stature, acromicria, mental retardation) Achondroplastic dwarfism
Cytogenetic disorders	Down's syndrome Klinefelter's syndrome Turner's syndrome

thyrotoxicosis and Type 1 diabetes. Thyrotoxicosis has a small adverse effect on glucose tolerance and causes a relatively slight upset in established diabetes. Thyrotoxicosis is sometimes detected at a very early stage in those regularly attending a diabetic clinic by the insidious and initially unexplained loss of weight. Care must be taken in treatment, as thyroid hormone enhances hepatic insulin clearance and the sudden conversion from hyper- to hypothyroidism, as may occasionally occur in the treatment of thyrotoxicosis, may be associated with sudden hypoglycaemia.

The prevalence of hypothyroidism is increased in Type 1 diabetes, and also inexplicably in Type 2 diabetes. The effects of primary hypothyroidism on diabetes are very slight, leading perhaps to a small decrease in insulin requirement. However, it is a very common disorder and frequent cause of malaise. Appropriate biochemical investigations should be undertaken if there is any doubt, because treatment with thyroxine is both straightforward and rewarding.

Addison's disease

Addison's disease, which is much more common in Type 1 diabetes than in the general population, usually presents with gradual onset of malaise, skin pigmentation, hypotension and diarrhoea, with diminishing insulin requirements and a tendency to severe hypoglycaemia.

Autoimmune polyglandular syndromes

Autoimmune polyglandular syndromes are striking but rare and include Type 1 diabetes. There are two syndromes.

1 Adrenal failure, primary gonadal failure, pernicious anaemia, hypothyroidism, alopecia and vitiligo, hepatitis, intestinal malabsorption, hypoparathyroidism and mucocutaneous candidosis.

2 Schmidt's syndrome: Graves' disease or hypothyroidism, adrenal failure, pernicious anaemia, primary hypogonadism, alopecia and vitiligo, myasthenia gravis, and probably inflammatory hypophysitis.

Coeliac disease

There is some association between Type 1 diabetes and coeliac disease. Anti-tissue transglutaminase antibodies can be detected in approximately 8% of Type 1 diabetic patients, most of whom will prove to have the clinical disease. It is always important to exclude a diagnosis of coeliac disease during the investigation of diabetic autonomic diarrhoea (page 157). If suspected on the basis of positive blood tests, a diagnostic biopsy is mandated before instituting the therapeutic gluten-free diet. Treatment is essential as there is a risk of lymphoma of the gastrointestinal tract.

Hypopituitarism and diabetes

Bernardo Houssay described in the 1930s the amelioration of diabetes following hypophysectomy. Control of diabetes after hypophysectomy may be difficult, requiring very small doses of insulin, and patients may be sensitive to small changes of insulin dose; they are at great risk of severe hypoglycaemia. A decrease in insulin requirement also occurs with the spontaneous development of hypopituitarism in cases of Sheehan's syndrome which may occur either suddenly or over several years. Indeed, a falling insulin requirement may alert the physician to the diagnosis. The authors have known two patients, in whom the diagnosis of hypopituitarism was made several years after their pregnancies, in whom insulin requirements decreased instead of increasing, indicating the onset of the disease ante-partum.

Epidemiology of Diabetes

Summary

- Diabetes is a global disease affecting people of all ages

- Diabetes has a huge impact on health and mortality especially from cardiovascular disease

- Type 2 diabetes is a disease of affluence associated with indolence and obesity

- A huge increase in Type 2 diabetes is occurring worldwide especially among malnourished people in developing countries when they become more prosperous and gain weight

- There is also a considerable increase in Type 2 diabetes in children associated with obesity

- The genetic changes in families with dominantly inherited Type 2 diabetes of youth (MODY) are increasingly identified

- The prevalence of Type 1 diabetes varies around the world tending to be lowest at the equator and highest towards the poles

- The incidence of Type 1 diabetes is increasing

Diabetes is a global disease with a huge adverse impact on health and mortality, particularly from cardiovascular disorders. It occurs at any time of life from infancy to old age. Type 2 diabetes is primarily a lifestyle disorder which accounts for around 90% of cases. It is increasing at an astonishing rate, particularly in developing countries, presenting serious logistical problems regarding the resources needed to improve the outlook for these patients. Type 1 diabetes is primarily an autoimmune disorder, and its incidence is increasing in northern European countries at an average rate of 3% per year, for very different reasons. The prevalence of both major forms of diabetes varies greatly from one part of the world to another, so that there are some areas where one or other scarcely exists while in others more than half of the adult population can be shown to have Type 2 diabetes.

Type 2 diabetes

Type 2 diabetes is a disease of relative prosperity, where the prosperity leads to overweight and physical indolence. Insulin resistance, increasing with obesity, associated with progressive failure of insulin secretion in relation to ageing underlies the development of diabetes. In 1995, it was estimated that around 135 million people had the condition and it has been calculated that this may increase to as many as 300 million by the year 2025 (Box 2.1). This increase will be particularly pronounced among poorer malnourished people living in countries such as India or China, as they move from country to town, gaining weight and becoming less active with their increased prosperity even when that is quite modest (Box 2.2). It has been suggested that evolutionary pressures may have encouraged a genotype with a survival advan-

Box 2.1 Top 10 countries for estimated number of persons with diabetes in 1995 and 2025

Rank	1995 Country	Est. no. (millions)	2025 Country	Est. no. (millions)
1	India	19.4	India	57.2
2	China	16.0	China	37.6
3	USA	13.9	USA	21.9
4	Russian Federation	8.9	Pakistan	14.5
5	Japan	6.3	Indonesia	12.4
6	Brazil	4.9	Russian Federation	12.2
7	Indonesia	4.5	Mexico	11.7
8	Pakistan	4.3	Brazil	11.6
9	Mexico	3.8	Egypt	8.8
10	Ukraine	3.6	Japan	8.5
All other countries		49.7		103.6
Total		135.3		300.0

From *International Diabetes Monitor*, April 1999, page 39, with permission.

Box 2.2 Risk factors for Type 2 diabetes

Age
Ethnic group
Family history
Western diet
Obesity
Physical inactivity
Urbanization

Box 2.3 High incidence populations for Type 2 diabetes

Extremely high incidence
Pima Indians
Nauruans

High incidence
Asian populations in UK, south India and elsewhere
Maori population in New Zealand
Polynesian populations in South Pacific
Maltese
Urbanized African and Caribbean populations
  including black American populations
Hispanic populations of Central/North America

tage in relation to food scarcity which becomes a disadvantage as the population become more prosperous and more corpulent (the thrifty genotype hypothesis).

The prevalence of Type 2 diabetes varies greatly across the world. Ethnic origin represents a very strong determinant for its development but environment is equally important. It is relatively low amongst the Mapuche Indians of Chile and the people of the Papua New Guinea Highlands, while at the other end of the scale more than half of the adult Pima Indians of Arizona are affected, and almost as many of the people in the Pacific island of Nauru (Box 2.3). In the USA, while the prevalence is approximately 7% for white Americans, as many as 15% of wealthy urban

Hispanic Americans are affected, with a somewhat lower prevalence for those on smaller incomes. Type 2 diabetes occurs equally in both sexes, any differences being largely accounted for by relative frequency of obesity in different cultures and ethnic groups.

The largest studies examining the prevalence of diabetes in the UK were conducted during the 1960s in Bedford and Birmingham. Subsequently, adult Whitehall civil servants were surveyed during the 1970s and since then smaller studies have been

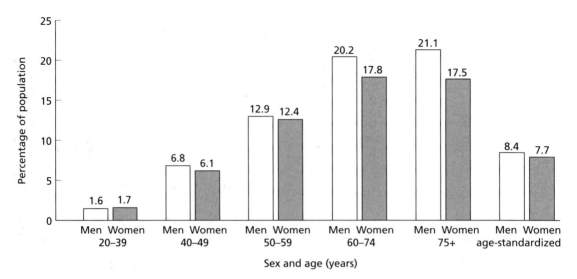

Figure 2.1 Prevalence of diabetes in men and women in the USA aged > 20 years. Included are all diagnosed and previously undiagnosed cases as defined by a fasting plasma glucose > 7.0 mmol/L. Sourced from NHANES III. ((1998) *Diabetes Care*, **21**, 518–524).

undertaken in Dorset, Oxfordshire and Ely. Every investigation has demonstrated that there are almost as many undiagnosed people with Type 2 diabetes as there are known cases. Overall, the prevalence in northern European countries is approximately 4%. In resident ethnic minorities mainly living in the inner cities of our larger conurbations, the prevalence is much higher: indeed, among UK Asians it exceeds 20%, and as many as 17% of Africans and Caribbeans are also affected.

Type 2 diabetes increases markedly with age (Fig. 2.1) which is accompanied by declining glucose tolerance and insulin secretion together with increasing insulin resistance accompanying progressive weight gain. It reaches a peak after 60 years of age and the data show that around 10% of those aged over 70 years in the UK have Type 2 diabetes.

Obesity

Obesity has a major role in the genesis of diabetes (Fig. 2.2). In non-diabetic subjects, glucose tolerance deteriorates as weight increases, with higher fasting and 2-h postprandial glucose levels. Even though obese people often have higher insulin levels than lean subjects as a result of insulin resistance, there

may still be insufficient insulin to restore blood glucose to normal, leading to diabetes as a result. The abnormalities may be reversed by weight reduction.

There is a close relationship between the prevalence of obesity and that of diabetes, and in most Western populations, 60% or more of newly presenting patients with Type 2 diabetes are obese. There is indeed a twofold increased risk of Type 2 diabetes in subjects with a body mass index between 29 and 30, increasing to sixfold when it exceeds 35.

Fat distribution, which can be roughly estimated from the waist : hip ratio (WHR) varies strikingly from those with a 'pear-shape' (gynoid, WHR < 0.7) to those who are 'apple-shaped' (android, WHR > 0.9): it is the latter who are strikingly more prone to Type 2 diabetes. This is probably because intra-abdominal, as opposed to subcutaneous, fat is more metabolically deleterious.

Type 2 diabetes in children and young people

Hitherto, childhood Type 2 diabetes was witnessed only in some ethnic minorities and in those with the rare inherited maturity onset diabetes of the young (MODY) syndromes described on pages 45 and 13. There is now growing recognition of a substantial

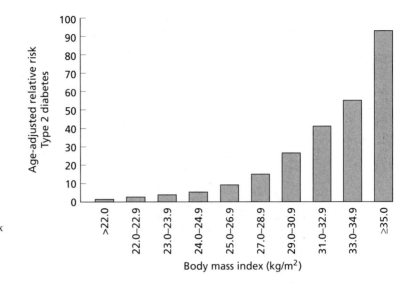

Figure 2.2 Relative risk of Type 2 diabetes according to body mass index in US women aged 30–55 years. From Colditz GA *et al.* (1995) *Annals of Internal Medicine*, **122**, 481–486.

increase of this disease in the prosperous industrialized nations. In the USA, between 8 and 45% of recently diagnosed cases of diabetes among children and adolescents are Type 2 diabetes, and the problem is increasing. It is most likely to occur at 12–14 years of age, more frequently in girls, and is strongly associated with obesity, physical inactivity and a family history of Type 2 diabetes. However, it is important to ascertain whether young people developing diabetes may have some other specific variant: thus, when young people of lean physique are discovered to have Type 2 diabetes, it is important to determine whether not they have latent autoimmune diabetes of adults (LADA). There is also evidence that in approximately one-quarter of such patients diabetes results from a specific genetic defect including those of the MODY group (pages 13 and 45) or other rare genetic syndromes.

Birth weight and Type 2 diabetes

A new concept regarding the cause of Type 2 diabetes comes from the discovery that the smaller the birth weight of an infant, the greater the likelihood that 50 years later Type 2 diabetes and coronary artery disease will develop. The chance of this occurring is greater in those who are smallest at birth and largest when 1 year old. These ideas are derived from obser-

vations of Barker and Hales who reviewed 468 men in Hertfordshire whose birth weights had been meticulously recorded by health visitors earlier in the century. Poor fetal nutrition might have an adverse effect on islet development and function, predisposing to diabetes later in life. These novel ideas are now the subject of intensive experimental and epidemiological research.

Genetic factors

The heterogeneity of Type 2 diabetes has made it impossible to identify precisely the genetic background to this disease except amongst those with some forms of dominantly inherited single gene Type 2 diabetes amongst young people (MODY, pages 13 and 45). There is nevertheless ample evidence that Type 2 diabetes has a strong genetic background. Amongst identical twins, approximately 90% are concordant for diabetes; and people with one or both parents with Type 2 diabetes have a lifetime risk of developing the condition themselves of 40 and 50%, respectively.

Microvascular complications: ethnic variations

Microvascular complications vary substantially between racial groups. This is particularly striking in the development of nephropathy which occurs much

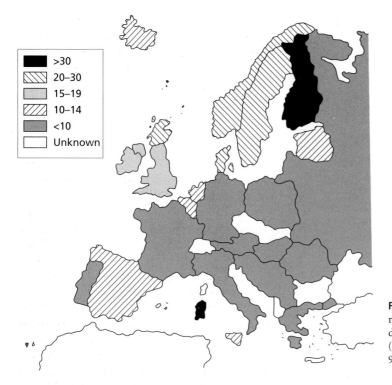

Figure 2.3 Age-standardized incidence rates per 100 000 per year of Type 1 diabetes (onset 0–14 years) in Europe. (After Green, A. *et al.* (1992) *Lancet*, **339**, 905–909.)

more frequently amongst Asians, black American and Mexican Americans than amongst white populations. The prevalence of nephropathy in Pima Indians is increased fourfold compared to that in white patients with Type 2 diabetes. In contrast, foot ulcers, which occur in more than 5% of Western white diabetic patients, are much less commonly seen in Asians (1.5%), Hispanic black people and Japanese subjects, and fewer Asians are subject to amputations. The lower incidence of foot lesions in some racial groups has been attributed to greater joint mobility associated with lower foot pressures and consequent decreased risk of ulceration. Variations in footwear are also important. Further details of ethnic variations in microvascular complications can be found in the relevant chapters of the *International Textbook of Diabetes Mellitus* (eds Alberti, Zimmet and Defronzo).

Gestational diabetes

Asians and African and Caribbean black people have a substantially increased risk of developing gestational diabetes. At King's College Hospital in London these ethnic groups accounted for 80% of gestational diabetic pregnancies. This is linked to the high risk of Type 2 diabetes in these populations.

Type 1 diabetes

The incidence of Type 1 diabetes varies some 30-fold between Scandinavia, where it is highest, and Japan, where it is lowest. Genetic susceptibility to diabetes presumably plays a large part in these differences. Apart from the very high incidence of Type 1 diabetes (30 per 100 000) on the island of Sardinia, there is a striking increase from the Equator to the North or South Poles, with the highest incidence in Finland. There are even trends within Europe (Fig. 2.3): thus, the incidence is higher in Finland than in Denmark; in Canada than southern USA; and in the southern hemisphere within New Zealand, higher in the South Island than in the North Island. Even within the British Isles there is a wide variation, ranging from

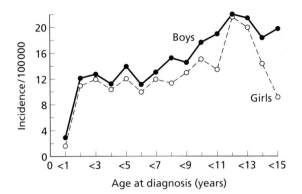

Figure 2.4 Incidence of diabetes by age at diagnosis in 1988 for 837 boys and 763 girls. (After Metcalf, M.A. & Baum, J.D. (1991) *British Medical Journal*, **302**, 443–447, with permission from the BMJ Publishing Group.)

6.8 per 100 000 in the Republic of Ireland to 19.8 per 100 000 in Scotland.

The incidence of Type 1 diabetes has been increasing rapidly over the past 20 years. Thus, in Finland, the incidence of Type 1 diabetes rose from 13 per 100 000 in the 1950s to 33 per 100 000 in the 1980s and 43 per 100 000 by 1990. Similar changes have also been noted in Scotland, Poland and North America. In the British Isles, there has been a striking increase in incidence from 7.7 to 13.5 children per 100 000 over 15 years from the early 1970s to the late 1980s. Ethnic groups immigrating into Westernized societies generally assume the prevalence of Type 1 diabetes of the indigenous population and this observation, which hints at environmental influences on a uniform genetic background risk, has not been adequately explained.

The peak incidence of Type 1 diabetes is in the early teenage years for both boys and girls, decreasing rapidly after the age of 13 years (Fig. 2.4). There is a small male excess. There is also a marked seasonal variation, most cases being diagnosed in the autumn and winter. Much research has been conducted seeking a possible environmental cause but, although much of the evidence has pointed to the implication of viral illnesses, the precipitating cause for Type 1 diabetes remains uncertain. One of the problems is that it is likely that the precipitating insult occurred many years before the clinical onset of disease. Various

environmental influences, including the early introduction of cows' milk in the baby's feed and Coxsackie viral infections have been postulated, triggering an autoimmune response that mistakenly includes islet antigens in its course. None of these hypotheses has been proven.

Genetic risks

The susceptibility to Type 1 diabetes, not the disease itself, is transmitted genetically. This is best illustrated by identical twin studies of Type 1 diabetes, where only about 30–40% of twin pairs will both develop the disease and become 'concordant'; this contrasts with more than 90% concordance for Type 2 diabetes. Approximately 1–2% of children of a Type 1 diabetic mother will become insulin dependent themselves by age 25, the risk appearing to be rather higher (about 6%) if the affected parent is a father and up to 10% if the child has a sibling with diabetes. This represents an approximately 30-fold or greater risk above the general population, but Type 1 diabetes is still an uncommon disease, with total prevalence in the UK of about one in 800 children up to age 16. The risk is higher in the rare instances where both parents have Type 1 diabetes; such couples should be advised to seek genetic counselling, although few physicians would discourage pregnancy in this situation.

Over 70% of the genetic susceptibility to Type 1 diabetes rests in the tissue type (HLA type, page 40). The onset of the diabetic process is marked by the appearance of antibodies to components of the islet cell (page 41). The development in a non-diabetic individual of three or more autoantibodies (islet cell antibodies, anti-GAD antibodies, anti-IA-2 antibodies, anti-insulin antibodies) gives an 88% chance of developing Type 1 diabetes within 10 years. The onset of diabetes is then preceded by loss of the first phase insulin response in an intravenous glucose tolerance test. Some people now request a screening test especially when there is a strong family history of Type 1 diabetes. However, there is at present no benefit to be gained from immunological screening because there is no effective action that can be taken to delay the onset of the disease. Immune suppression techniques that have been reported to delay the onset of Type 1 diabetes are both insufficiently effective and excessively hazardous to undertake as routine procedures. Attempts to induce tolerance with nasal or subcutaneous insulin, effective in some animal models, have not met with success. Attempts to alter the progress of the disease with antioxidants likewise have not been successful and further research is needed.

3

Synthesis, Secretion and Actions of Insulin

Summary

- Islets of Langerhans—their anatomy and cellular composition

- Pancreatic B cells are specialized to undertake proinsulin biosynthesis, conversion and secretion; recombinant synthesis of human insulin

- Insulin secretion is regulated by glucose and other factors

- Insulin has effects on carbohydrate lipid and protein metabolism. Its molecular actions are complex and not fully understood

- Metabolic changes in fasting and after meals aim to maintain blood glucose levels in a narrow normal range

This chapter reviews mechanisms by which insulin is produced in the body, describing both the cell biology of the insulin-producing pancreatic B cell, the biochemical steps involved in insulin synthesis and secretion, and their regulation.

A single islet of Langerhans is on average 0.2 mm in diameter and they are scattered throughout the whole human pancreas, comprising 1–2% of its total volume. Thus, an average human pancreas may contain between 250 000 and 500 000 individual islets.

The structure of the B cell is typical of a cell that is adapted to synthesize and secrete proteins (Fig. 3.1). The uniqueness of the B cell derives first from the fact that it is programmed to synthesize insulin (via its precursor proinsulin) and, secondly, in the very sophisticated mechanisms that it has developed to regulate the rate of its secretion in response to glucose.

The major function of proinsulin, the biosynthetic precursor of insulin, is to permit correct orientation of the interchain disulphide bridges in the insulin structure so that the two polypeptide (A and B) chains are completed correctly. Within 30 min of its synthesis in the B cell endoplasmic reticulum, en-

zymes in the Golgi complex have cleaved the proinsulin molecule at specific residues to form insulin (Fig. 3.2). The excised part of the proinsulin, the connecting peptide (or C-peptide for short), is stored in the B cell along with insulin and secreted at the same time. It has no clear physiological function outside the B cell but may be useful clinically. The existence of C-peptide circulating in the blood indicates the presence of residual B-cell function. This is useful in patients who are receiving insulin injections in whom blood insulin measurements would have no meaning as a measure of endogenous B-cell activity.

B cells contain substantial stores of insulin in membrane-limited granules or vesicles (Fig. 3.3). There are about 13 000 of these in the average B cell, sufficient for 24 h supply without any new synthesis. They are released by transport to the B-cell membrane along directed pathways involving microtubule and actin filaments. Once they reach the cell membrane they are then released from the cell by exocytosis (Fig. 3.1). This is the regulated pathway of secretion.

The structure of insulin (in terms of its amino acid sequence) varies little between most mammalian

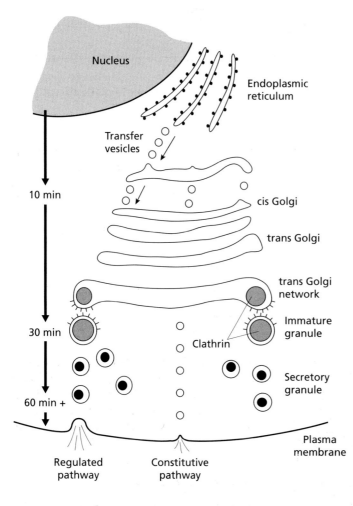

Figure 3.1 The secretory pathway in the pancreatic B cell (after Balayes *et al.* in Ashcroft & Ashcroft 1992).

species. Thus, porcine and human insulin differ by only one amino acid, and bovine insulin by three (Fig. 3.4), although rats and mice have two insulins each. The possible physiological significance of the differences in structure between bovine, porcine and human insulin is discussed later (page 87).

The B cell also synthesizes and exports a number of other proteins, although most of these are made in much smaller quantities than insulin. Perhaps the most interesting (and controversial) of these is the peptide islet amyloid polypeptide (IAPP) or 'amylin'. This is exported from B cells along with insulin in insulin granules and can, in some circumstances and in some species, be deposited outside the cells as amyloid fibrils. It is not yet clear whether these deposits, which are found surrounding the B cells in some patients with Type 2 diabetes, are a cause or, perhaps more likely, an effect of the hyperglycaemia in these patients. Similarly, it is not known whether amylin, its analogues or antagonists, may be useful in the treatment of insulin dependent (Type 1) diabetes. Further research is required to evaluate the role of IAPP in normal B-cell function and in diabetes.

Synthesis of human insulin by recombinant DNA technology

One of the first commercially important results of recombinant DNA technology in the mid-1980s was the ability to programme bacteria (usually *Escherichia coli*) or yeast to make human insulin in large

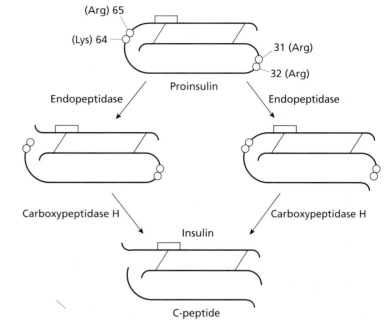

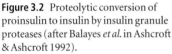

Figure 3.2 Proteolytic conversion of proinsulin to insulin by insulin granule proteases (after Balayes *et al.* in Ashcroft & Ashcroft 1992).

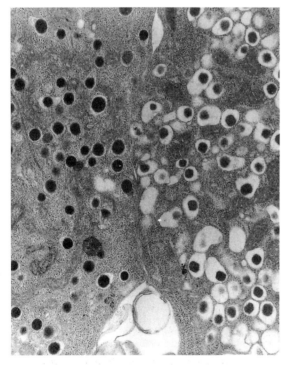

Figure 3.3 Electron micrograph of a thin section through parts of two islet cells. The cell on the right (B cell) produces insulin, the one on the left (A cell) produces glucagon. They are present in a ratio of 70 : 25 in mammalian islets.

quantities. This allowed the pharmaceutical industry to offer human insulin in unlimited quantities for the first time, in contrast to bovine or porcine insulin extracted from animal pancreas which had been the products available in the years since the discovery of insulin by F. Banting and C. Best in 1921.

Regulation of insulin secretion

The most important factor in the regulation of insulin secretion is the change in blood glucose concentrations, and B cells have a very sensitive mechanism that allows them to secrete insulin only when blood glucose levels are above fasting, but to increase rates of secretion very considerably as blood glucose concentrations increase in the range of 6–12 mmol/L (Fig. 3.5). These responses are both very sensitive and rapid, usually within 30 s of the arrival of a glucose stimulus.

This characteristic response to glucose is achieved largely by the enzyme glucokinase, which is a key regulating step in the early stages of B-cell glucose metabolism. The possibility that genetic defects in some of the enzymes of glucose metabolism might lead to the defective patterns of insulin secretion in Type 2 diabetes has excited some interest, although so

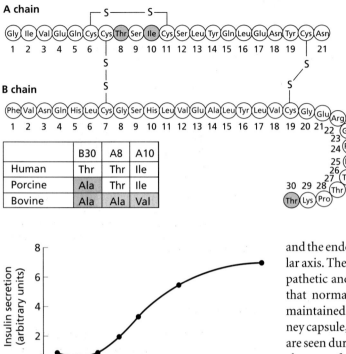

Figure 3.4 Primary structure (amino acid) sequence of human insulin. The highlighted residues are those which differ in porcine and bovine insulins, as shown in the inset (after Wood, S.P. & Gill, R. in Pickup & Williams 1991).

	B30	A8	A10
Human	Thr	Thr	Ile
Porcine	Ala	Thr	Ile
Bovine	Ala	Ala	Val

Figure 3.5 Insulin secretory responses of islets of Langerhans to increasing glucose concentrations. No stimulation is seen below a threshold value of 5 mmol/L.

far this mechanism has been identified only in the rare subset of dominantly inherited Type 2 or maturity onset diabetes in the young (MODY) (see pages 7 and 13).

Insulin secretion may be affected by a range of other hormonal and neuroendocrine factors, including gastric inhibitory peptide which may act to potentiate insulin secretory responses to glucose by raising concentrations of cyclic adenosine monophosphate (cAMP) within the B cell. This sensitizing effect on the B cell of gut hormones released during digestion may explain the greater insulin secretory response found to oral than to intravenous glucose. This relationship between gut hormones

and the endocrine pancreas is called the entero–insular axis. The islets are also served by elements of sympathetic and parasympathetic innervation. The fact that normal blood glucose concentrations can be maintained after transplantation of islets to the kidney capsule, and normal patterns of insulin secretion are seen during culture of isolated islets *in vitro* in the absence of neural influences, may suggest that this neural regulation is not critically important for the control of blood glucose in normal circumstances.

We now know that adenosine triphosphate (ATP) generated during metabolism of glucose by the B cell may, along with adenosine diphosphate (ADP), close specific potassium gates (channels) in the B-cell membrane, shutting off potassium exits down its concentration gradient. This causes the cell membrane to depolarize and calcium to enter the cell by opening voltage-sensitive gates (channels) and stimulation of secretion results (Fig. 3.6). Interestingly, the insulin-secreting sulphonylureas such as glibenclamide or glyburide (Chapter 7) may also close the same potassium channels directly through their interaction with a sulphylurea receptor. This may explain why these drugs provoke insulin secretion in Type 2 diabetic patients when B-cell glucose metabolism may be defective, resulting in insufficient ATP production. Conversely, diazoxide, a reversible inhibitor of insulin secretion used in the treatment of insulin-secreting tumours, acts by opening the same potassium channels (Fig. 3.6).

Glucose acts as the major physiological stimu-

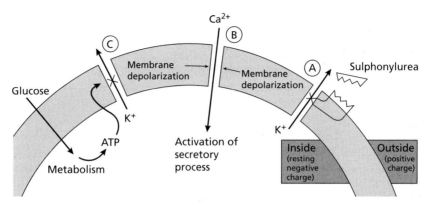

Figure 3.6 Possible mechanisms through which sulphonylureas may stimulate insulin release. (A) Sulphonylureas may bind to specific membrane receptors which act to close K^+ channels in the membrane. (B) This reduces K^+ efflux, increasing the net intracellular positive charge and tending to depolarize the membrane, which in turn promotes Ca^{2+} entry into the B cell through voltage-dependent channels in the plasma membrane. Increased intracellular Ca^{2+} levels stimulate insulin secretion. (C) Glucose may act similarly, by generating ATP within B cells which acts to close ATP-sensitive K^+ channels.

lus predominantly via activation of calcium–calmodulin-dependent protein kinase (pk-B). Agents that stimulate production of cyclic AMP (glucagon, gastric inhibitory peptide) and activate protein kinase B will modulate the insulin secretory response to glucose but not replace it. Similarly, agents that stimulate protein kinase c (carbachol; cholecystokinin) will also act as modulators, but not initiators of secretion. The complex inter-relationships between these pathways, all leading to secretion of insulin by exocytosis, is shown in Fig. 3.7.

Actions of insulin

Insulin has a bewildering array of effects on carbohydrate, lipid and protein metabolism in various tissues, as summarized in Table 3.1. All of its effects are anabolic: they encourage laying down of carbohydrate (as glycogen), lipid or protein stores. Conversely, during insulin deficiency, as in Type 1 diabetes, all of these are reversed, and the wasting of body mass characteristic of untreated Type 1 occurs. The way in which insulin can exert this variety of effects is not known. The first stage, identification of target tissues is, however, certain and involves binding of insulin circulating in the blood to specific receptors.

Insulin receptors

Not all tissues are insulin sensitive. The most important unresponsive tissue is the brain, and others are the kidney and intestine. Those tissues that are insulin dependent share a specific insulin receptor on their cell outer surfaces which causes insulin in the blood to bind to the cells and trigger its effects. The structure of the insulin receptor is known (Fig. 3.8). It is clear that insulin does not normally penetrate its target cells, and that its actions after binding are brought about inside the cell indirectly by second messengers. The nature of these is poorly understood. One of the key properties of the insulin receptor is that it can phosphorylate tyrosine residues on peptides and proteins (including itself) that contain this amino acid: it is a tyrosine kinase. Many of the effects that result from insulin receptor activation may result from this tyrosine phosphorylation. This in turn triggers changes in one or more peptides, including the insulin receptor substrates (IRS) and mitogen activated protein kinases (MAP kinase) (Fig. 3.8), which may cause activation of the enzymes that trigger the various metabolic effects of insulin. The detailed stages involved in the downstream pathways involved in insulin action appear to be very complex, but it seems likely that the detailed

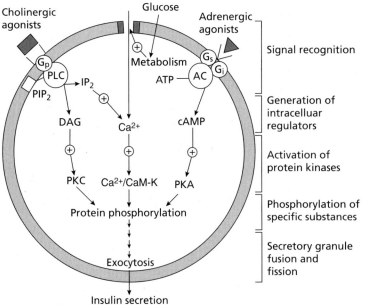

Figure 3.7 Signalling pathways which regulate the secretion of insulin. AC, adenylate cyclose; PLC, phospholipase; DAG, diacylglycerol.

Table 3.1 Physiological effects of insulin.

Process	Action	Tissue
Effects on carbohydrate metabolism		
Glucose transport	↑	Adipose, muscle
Glycolysis	↑	Adipose, muscle
Glycogen synthesis	↑	Adipose, muscle, liver
Glucose oxidation via pentose phosphate pathway	↑	Liver, adipose
Glycogen breakdown	↓	Muscle, liver
Glycogenolysis, gluconeogenesis	↓	Liver
Effects on lipid metabolism		
Lipolysis	↓	Adipose
Fatty acid synthesis	↑	Adipose, liver
Low-density lipoprotein synthesis	↑	Liver
Lipoprotein lipase	↑	Adipose
Cholesterol synthesis	↑	Liver
Effects on protein metabolism		
Amino acid transport	↑	Muscle, adipose, liver, others
Protein synthesis	↑	Muscle, adipose, liver, others
Protein degradation	↓	Muscle
Urea formation	↓	

↑, Increase; ↓, decrease.

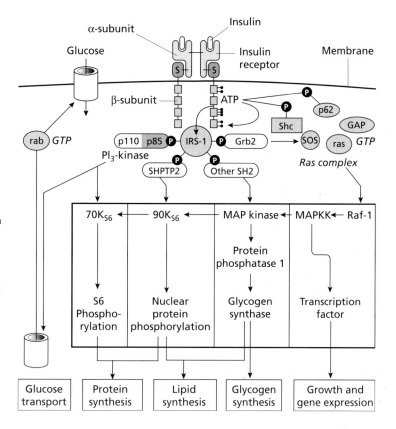

Figure 3.8 Insulin receptor substrate (IRS)-1 dependent and independent pathways in insulin signalling. The insulin receptor is capable of mediating the phosphorylation of Shc on tyrosine and the activation of Ras and mitogen activated protein (MAP) kinases in the absence of IRS-1. The interaction of IRS-1 and Grb2 can also play a part in MAP kinase signalling, but it is not required for mitogenic signalling. Shc, Ras and Grb2 are cytoplasmic proteins involved in cell signalling. (Reproduced with permission from Maratos-Flier, E., Goldstein, B.J. & Kahn, C.R. (1997) in Pickup, J.C. & Williams, G. (eds) *Textbook of Diabetes*, 2nd edn.

molecular steps that produce the metabolic effects of insulin in its target cells will be clarified in the next few years.

The major physiological aim of blood glucose regulation is to maintain a glucose supply to the brain, which is uniquely dependent on glucose as its fuel substrate. For this purpose, blood glucose is generally maintained between 4 and 7 mmol/L in the face of major fluctuations in carbohydrate intake with different feeding patterns, including starvation.

In addition to changes in insulin secretion and action, blood glucose concentrations can be affected by the following factors.

1 The rate of absorption of carbohydrate from the gastrointestinal tract. This obviously reflects the frequency and composition of food intake, but can also be modified by the addition of materials that, because of their viscosity (guar) or chemical nature (acarbose), tend to slow down rates of absorption.

2 Rates of glucose uptake and storage as glycogen, or production (from glycogen stores) or by gluconeogenesis by the liver.

3 Rates of glucose utilization in peripheral tissues — this will increase substantially in exercise.

Other hormones

Other hormones may also profoundly affect blood glucose regulation, but insulin is the *only* hormone that lowers blood glucose. In contrast, adrenaline, corticosteroids, growth hormone and glucagon can all increase the levels of circulating glucose. The metabolic balance between insulin and other hormones is therefore of great importance in maintaining blood glucose within narrow limits. Diseases of other endocrine glands apart from the islets of Langerhans may cause widespread disturbances of metabolism which include diabetes.

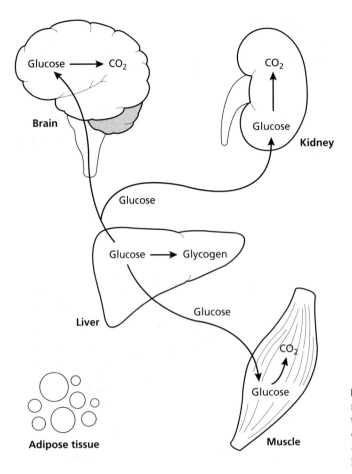

Figure 3.9 Pattern of fuel utilization following a meal containing carbohydrate or protein during the postabsorptive period (after Newsholme, E.A. & Leech, A.R. (1983) *Biochemistry for the Medical Sciences.* © John Wiley & Sons Ltd, with permission).

Growth hormone

Probably exerting its effects via production of insulin-like growth factors (IGFs), growth hormone has profound effects in stimulating growth, while insulin, perhaps by cross-reacting with IGF receptors on relevant target cells, may also have growth-provoking effects. Conversely, IGF can mimic some of the actions of insulin on carbohydrate metabolism, possibly by cross-reacting with insulin receptors. Growth hormone itself has also been shown to have anti-insulin effects, causing insulin resistance during starvation.

Catecholamines

The acute effect of catecholamines is to decrease the sensitivity of glucose utilization to insulin, by enhancing glycogen breakdown and increasing fat

mobilization. They also inhibit insulin release. These are probably the mechanisms by which intense fear can provoke hyperglycaemia.

Chronic elevation of catecholamine levels may have rather different effects, for instance, during cold exposure or during exercise training. Thus, exercise will increase the rate of utilization of all metabolic fuels, so that glycogen stores of liver and muscle are mobilized. Peripheral tissues also become more sensitive to insulin.

Adrenal steroids

Cortisol is a major counter-regulatory hormone in carbohydrate metabolism. It acts to increase gluconeogenesis, particularly in the liver, by increasing the activity of key enzymes. The absence of this powerful long-term action, for instance in Addison's disease,

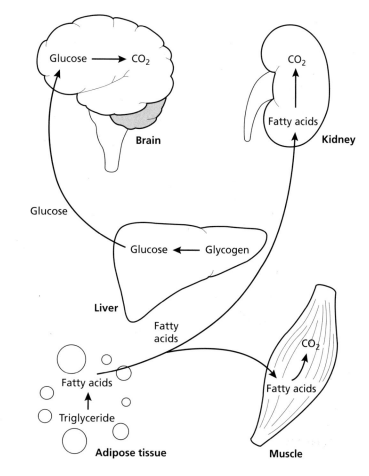

Figure 3.10 Pattern of fuel utilization during the early period of starvation. The use of fatty acid by muscle 'protects' glucose for use by the brain and other tissues (after Newsholme, E.A. & Leech, A.R. 1984. *Biochemistry for the Medical Sciences*. © John Wiley & Sons Ltd, with permission).

results in an apparent increase in insulin sensitivity (p. 15).

Glucagon

Glucagon provides the counter-regulatory hormone to insulin; it is provided from the pancreatic A cell by cellular mechanisms similar to insulin. However, the stimulus for glucagon secretion is a fall in blood glucose below 5 mmol/L, and glucagon plays an important part in preventing significant fall of blood glucose during fasting. Like the catecholamines, its primary site of action is the liver, where it binds to specific glucagon receptors which are linked to adenylate cyclase, the enzyme that causes generation of cyclic 3′,5′-AMP from ATP. Cyclic AMP, as second messenger, then induces a cascade of phosphoryla-

tion reactions which lead to mobilization of glycogen and to production of glucose from non-carbohydrate precursors by gluconeogenesis. Together these contribute glucose to the bloodstream, and will maintain blood glucose levels at 4–5 mmol/L for 12–24 h fasting. Beyond this time, longer term energy stores (adipose tissue and, ultimately, amino acids derived from protein breakdown) are required to maintain glucose concentrations during starvation.

Effects of meals and fasting

Following a meal containing carbohydrate or protein, insulin output from the B cells of the islets will be increased. This will ensure that there is a rapid transfer of glucose to tissues and the synthesis of liver and muscle glycogen as well as of triglyceride (Fig. 3.9). In normal individuals, blood glucose concentrations does not rise above 6–7 mmol/L despite very large intakes of carbohydrate or protein.

By contrast, in fasting, the lack of food, either carbohydrate or protein, results in a fall in blood insulin. The earliest consequence is a breakdown of liver glycogen, which takes place after even an overnight fast in humans. If fasting continues, both fat and protein stores are catabolized to provide energy. Fatty acids are used as a fuel and, as noted already, they will spare the utilization of glucose; gluconeogenesis is also increased (Fig. 3.10). As a result of these elaborate control mechanisms, blood glucose will rarely fall below 3 mmol/L, even in quite prolonged fasting.

Metabolic Changes in Diabetes: A Summary

Summary

- Metabolism changes in Type 1 and Type 2 diabetes, and the secondary consequences of hyperglycaemia and ketosis are profound and complex
- Consequences of chronic hyperglycaemia including effects on sorbitol metabolism, protein glycation and the development of complications

The main players in the metabolic regulatory processes that maintain blood glucose concentrations within such tight limits are clear. So what goes wrong?

Type 1 diabetes mellitus

In Type 1 diabetes the pancreatic B cells are selectively almost completely destroyed. The possible reasons for this are discussed in 'Aetiology and Genetics' (Chapter 5), but the effects of a complete lack of insulin are predictable and stem from the absence of all of the anabolic effects of insulin. Thus, the most evident metabolic changes seen in untreated Type 1 diabetes are hyperglycaemia and ketosis. In addition, wasting of body protein and fat may also be obvious, particularly if the condition has been prolonged. Hyperglycaemia is associated with intense polyuria as the renal threshold to glucose is exceeded, and the ketosis causes a serious metabolic acidosis. The hyperglycaemia may be profound and up to 100 mmol/L has been recorded in untreated cases. More usually, the figures at diagnosis range between 15 and 30 mmol/L. The blood ketones are considerably

more elevated than they are in starvation. Total ketones may be as high as 30 mmol/L in diabetic ketoacidosis, compared with about 8 mmol/L in prolonged starvation, or less than 0.1 mmol/L in healthy non-fasting adults.

These changes are the result of severe insulin deficiency and are summarized in Fig. 4.1. Insulin deficiency depresses glucose transport and glycogen synthesis in tissues such as muscle. Glucose utilization is slowed as a result of the defective activity of a number of enzymes in the glycolysis pathway. At the same time, there is a depression of protein synthesis and a corresponding increase in protein breakdown. Lack of insulin induces activation of the liver enzymes that promote gluconeogenesis. Amino acids derived from protein will therefore be converted to glucose with greater facility. Overproduction of glucose from this source complements glucose under-utilization to produce hyperglycaemia.

The increased breakdown of fat also directly follows as a consequence of insulin deficiency. A low blood insulin results in increased lipase activity in adipose tissue cells. Long-chain fatty acids so released are transported in the blood to the liver. Within the liver, they are broken down to yield large quantities of

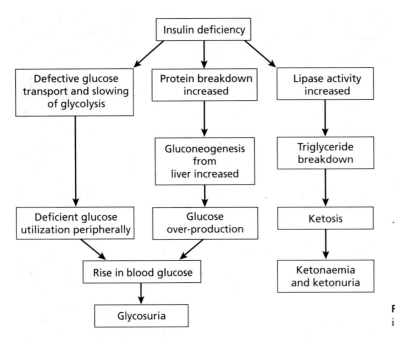

Figure 4.1 Metabolic consequences of insulin deficiency.

acetyl coenzyme A (CoA). Some of this, instead of being burnt by the tricarboxylic acid cycle, is diverted to the formation of acetoacetate. Acetoacetate is easily decarboxylated to give acetone or, alternatively, is reduced to form beta-hydroxybutyrate. Collectively, acetone, acetoacetate and beta-hydroxybutyrate are known as the 'ketone bodies'; they can be rapidly metabolized by many tissues to provide considerable amounts of energy, although when produced in large quantities they are excreted in the urine. Acetone, which is volatile, is excreted both in the breath and in the urine.

Following a meal there is failure to suppress hepatic glucose production as glucose begins to enter the circulation from the gut, and diminished peripheral uptake, both results of insulin deficiency. Lipolysis is stimulated by the combination of very low insulin levels and increased concentrations of the counter-regulating hormones glucagon and adrenaline. Consequently, plasma non-esterified fatty acid (NEFA) levels are raised. Ketone bodies are formed by partial beta-oxidation of fatty acyl CoA derivatives. Ketone bodies (acetoacetate, 3-hydroxybutyrate and acetone) therefore accumulate.

Thus, Type 1 patients show protein catabolism, negative nitrogen balance and muscle wasting.

Some secondary consequences of hyperglycaemia and ketosis in Type 1 diabetes

Hyperglycaemia results in a massive loss of glucose in the urine as the renal threshold for glucose is exceeded. This in turn induces an osmotic diuresis, and therefore dehydration. Cations such as Na^+ and Mg^{2+} are also lost in quantity in the urine. In the absence of insulin, potassium leaks from cells and plasma potassium may rise. In addition to increased blood acetoacetate and beta-hydroxybutyrate, blood lactate and long-chain fatty acids are increased.

Collectively, these contribute to produce a severe metabolic acidosis, in which the blood pH may fall to as low as 6.8. (The fluid and electrolyte changes in diabetic ketosis, and their management, are described in Chapter 10.)

Conclusions

Type 1 diabetes results from a complete absence of insulin. Not surprisingly therefore it can be treated very effectively by the replacement of that insulin. The method of delivery should ideally be as close as possible to that originally provided by the B cells, with sensitive minute by minute variations in response to changes in blood glucose. While infusion pumps that provide insulin at predetermined rates are readily available, devices that measure blood glucose and infuse insulin accordingly (artificial pancreases) are at present only satisfactory in a research situation, and not for routine clinical use. In any case the optimal route—the portal circulation—is not clinically practicable. Pancreatic and islet transplantation provide potential alternatives but shortage of diabetic pancreatic donors, and dangers of immunosuppression, make these unlikely as a realistic option for most Type 1 diabetes patients.

Transplantation of islets of Langerhans has been successful in reversing Type 1 diabetes in animal models but, until recently, not in humans. However, recent advances in techniques, and of immunosuppression, have increased the success rate to about 80%, although in only a small number of patients in specialized research centres.

Type 2 diabetes mellitus

In Type 2 diabetes there is a relative but not an absolute lack of insulin. The reserves or supply of the hormone from the B cells may decrease in middle life and become insufficient to provide adequate insulin for the high carbohydrate intake of the adult, and in some cases the increasing mass of adipose tissue, whose metabolism is controlled by insulin. Peripheral tissues may also become less sensitive to the effects of insulin (insulin resistant). It follows that the treatment of Type 2 centres not on replacement of missing insulin but rather on the lowering of insulin requirements—by reducing unrefined carbohydrate intake in the diet, together with the use of agents that can either increase B-cell production of insulin (e.g. sulphonylureas), which may also increase the sensitivity of peripheral tissues to insulin (Chapter 7), or reduce rates of glucose absorption and therefore blood glucose (guar, acarbose), or modify hepatic glucose output (biguanides).

Fasting hyperglycaemia is caused by increased hepatic glucose production, fuelled by enhanced gluconeogenesis, caused mainly by relatively low insulin levels in the blood. Basal glucose uptake is normal or increased above normal, but insulin-stimulated glucose uptake is greatly impaired. The nature of the defect is unknown, but skeletal muscle is the most severely affected. Glucose transport, glucose oxidation and glycogen formation are all decreased. Type 2 diabetes patients do not become ketoacidotic spontaneously; plasma NEFA and ketone-body levels are only slightly raised. Protein metabolism is normal and the muscle wasting typical of Type 1 diabetes does not occur. Insulin levels are sufficient to prevent excessive proteolysis.

Insulin resistance in peripheral tissues is a function of obesity, and can also occur in pregnancy (Chapter 12). The mechanism for the insulin resistance of obesity is still imperfectly understood. One reason for resistance is a reduced number of receptors in tissues because of high circulating insulin levels. High hormone concentrations suppress the number of hormone receptors present on the plasma membrane of cells ('downregulation'). In addition, there is also evidence for a defect in the mechanism for coupling the action of the receptor to subsequent biochemical events (a 'postreceptor' defect).

It has already been suggested that the B cells in Type 2 diabetes are relatively insensitive in their response to glucose. The additional stress on the islet imposed by obesity may well result in diabetes in situations in which the reserves of insulin available for secretion become inadequate.

Some consequences of chronic hyperglycaemia in diabetes

The importance of maintaining good blood glucose control in order to prevent or slow the onset of diabetic complications has been described in two landmark studies: the Diabetes Control and Complications Trial (Type 1 diabetes), and the UKPDS (Type 2 diabetes) (see page 129). It is clear that prolonged exposure to elevated glucose concentrations damages tissues initially through acute reversible metabolic changes that are mostly related to increased

Table 4.1 Acute and chronic biochemical consequences of hyperglycaemia. Reproduced with permission from Giardino, I. & Brownlee, M. (1997) In: *Textbook of Diabetes* (eds J. Pickup & G. Williams), p. 42.3. Blackwell Science, Oxford.

Acute reversible changes	Cumulative irreversible changes
Increased polyol pathway activity	Increased AGE formation on extracellular matrix
Increased NADH : NAD$^+$ ratio	Abnormal matrix binding properties
Intracellular myoinositol depletion	Disordered basement membrane structure
Increased diacylglycerol synthesis *de novo*	Increased basement membrane permeability
Increased protein kinase C activity	Increased AGE formation on nucleic acids and nucleoproteins
Increased formation of early glycation products	Increased mutation rate (in prokaryotes)
Increased free-radical formation from early glycation products	

AGE, advanced glycation end-products; NADH, nicotinamide-adenine-dinucleotide phosphate (reduced form); NAD$^+$, nicotinamide-adenine dinucleotide.

Figure 4.2 The sorbitol pathway

Figure 4.2 The sorbitol pathway. NADPH, nicotinamide-adenine-dinucleotide phosphate (reduced form); NAD$^+$, nicotinamide-adenine dinucleotide.

polyol pathway activity, decreased myoinositol and altered diacylglycerol levels, or glycation of proteins. Hyperglycaemia raises intracellular glucose levels in insulin-independent tissues such as nerve, glomerulus, lens and retina. Aldose reductase, the rate-limiting enzyme of the polyol pathway, catalyses the reduction of glucose to sorbitol, which is subsequently converted to fructose (Fig. 4.2). Sorbitol does not easily cross cell membranes and accumulates intracellularly. It may cause damage through its osmotic effects (e.g. in the lens) by altering the redox state of pyridine nucleotides (i.e. increasing the NADH : NAD$^+$ ratio); and by depleting intracellular myoinositol levels. In diabetes, myoinositol levels are decreased in some insulin-independent tissues, both as a result of sorbitol accumulation and because hyper-

glycaemia inhibits its uptake into cells. Myoinositol is a precursor of phosphatidylinositol.

Early glycation products form on proteins through the attachment of glucose to amino groups forming Schiff–base adducts. These then undergo 'Amadori' rearrangement to form stable products analogous to glycated haemoglobin. Glycation may affect the function of various proteins and could also be partly responsible for free-radical-mediated damage in diabetes. The pathways involved in these changes are summarized in Table 4.1. Chronic exposure to hyperglycaemia causes gradual, cumulative and irreversible changes in long-lived molecules such as collagen, intracellular proteins and nucleic acids. The early glycation (Amadori) products combine to form complex cross-linked structures termed advanced glycation end-products (AGE). The permanent changes induced by AGE formation may explain why restoration of normoglycaemia may not reverse tissue damage inflicted by previous exposure to hyperglycaemia. In experimental animals, treatment with aminoguanidine, an inhibitor of AGE formation, prevents diabetic damage in the retina, kidney, nerve and artery. Equally, aldose reductase inhibitors have been used to reverse changes to sorbitol production, but so far with no clinically useful effects.

The development of complications varies from individual to individual, and in some cases (e.g. nephropathy) there are likely to be strong genetic influences. In others (e.g. micro- and macrovascular

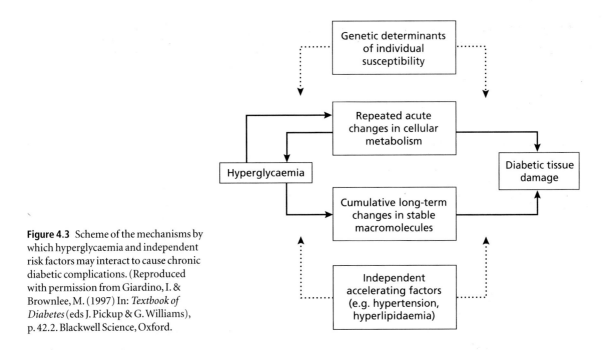

Figure 4.3 Scheme of the mechanisms by which hyperglycaemia and independent risk factors may interact to cause chronic diabetic complications. (Reproduced with permission from Giardino, I. & Brownlee, M. (1997) In: *Textbook of Diabetes* (eds J. Pickup & G. Williams), p. 42.2. Blackwell Science, Oxford.

complications), hypertension and dyslipidaemia are likely to be important factors. These relationships are summarized in Figure 4.3. Much effort is now being put into prevention of complications, both by better blood glucose control and by pharmacological interventions in key pathways.

Aetiology and Genetics

Summary

■ B cell pathology in Type 1 diabetes and its pathogenesis are reviewed, including the possible role of toxins and viruses

■ Genetics of Type 1 includes studies on twins; the dominant role of HLA haplotypes in inheritance

■ Autoimmunity—circulating antibodies, insulin autoantibodies are important markers of B cell destruction

■ Cellular immunity may be important in eliciting B cell destruction

■ Predicting diabetes—the role of genes and antibodies as predictive factors is unclear

■ Prevention of Type 1 diabetes through immunosuppression or other secondary interventions is in principle possible

■ Type 2 islet pathology

■ Type 2 genetics show complex polygenic interaction of genes and environment

■ MODY genetics show a monogenic dominant inheritance. At least five genes have been identified in different families

The application of the modern techniques of molecular genetics, and in particular the Human Genome Project, has allowed significant progress in understanding the genetics of diabetes, especially Type 1, although the precise causes of Type 1 and Type 2 diabetes are still not known. This chapter summarizes our present understanding of the genetic basis and aetiology of both common forms of the disease.

Type 1 diabetes mellitus

Islet pathology

There are striking differences in the changes occurring in Type 1 and Type 2 diabetes. The most charac-

teristic changes develop in Type 1, in which B cells of the islets are selectively destroyed and the insulin content and numbers of islets are drastically reduced; negligible amounts of insulin can be extracted from the pancreas in this type of diabetes soon after diagnosis.

This selective destruction of B cells may occur as a result of an autoimmune process, triggered by virus infection or by exposure to toxic chemicals or some other environmental cause. However, some B cells do persist, although in small numbers, in about half of people with Type 1 diabetes of less than 10 years' duration, and in 10% of those of longer duration. Evidence for B-cell regeneration is very scarce but can sometimes be found in those who have died soon after diagnosis. Infiltration of lymphocytes in

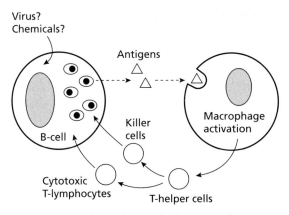

Figure 5.1 A possible mechanism for the immune destruction of pancreatic B cells in Type 1 diabetes.

or around the islets (insulitis) is the most characteristic change in Type 1 diabetes and one that is in keeping with an immune process (Fig. 5.1). It is found most frequently in children who have died suddenly soon after the onset of diabetes, but it is not common, occurring in less than 15% of pancreases examined, and up to 40% of those under 5 years of age. Insulitis affects only a few islets, and is rarely seen after diabetes duration of more than 6 months.

Pathogenesis

A combination of environmental and genetic factors which trigger an autoimmune attack on the B cells seems likely to be responsible for B-cell destruction during the onset of diabetes in genetically susceptible individuals. There may be a period of several years from the start of this process to the onset of disease symptoms, and during this period islet cell antibodies, insulin autoantibodies and antibodies to specific B-cell proteins may appear in the circulation (see below). They probably represent markers of B-cell destruction rather than a primary cause. In the UK, approximately 15% of all people with Type 1 diabetes have a positive family history, with at least one first-degree relative affected by the disease. The corollary to this is that the majority of people with diabetes do not have a first-degree relative with diabetes and approximately 90% of cases are 'sporadic'. The chances of the child of a Type 1 patient developing the disease at some time are increased compared with the chil-

dren of unaffected individuals (page 40). With increased knowledge of diabetes susceptibility genes, along with use of antibodies to islet cells (ICA), insulin autoantibodies (IAA) and glutamic acid decarboxylase antibodies (GAD), it may be possible to provide an accurate prediction in populations as well as in families in the near future (page 43).

Evidence of the operation of environmental factors on the aetiology of Type 1 diabetes comes from many virus studies, from observation of the effects of some toxic chemicals and from the changing geographical incidence of Type 1 disease.

Toxic chemicals

Ever since the discovery of the highly diabetogenic chemicals alloxan and streptozotocin there has been continuing interest in chemicals which destroy B cells. For instance, alloxan has been extensively used to produce an insulin-deficient diabetes in animals, although there is no evidence to incriminate it as a cause of diabetes in humans. Streptozotocin, which is a nitroso derivative, behaves similarly to alloxan although it is more selective in its effects on the B cells; both these substances may give rise to islet cell antibodies. There has also been a suggestion from Iceland that smoked mutton (which contains toxic *N*-nitroso compounds) may cause diabetes. Several drugs used in the treatment of other conditions may induce diabetes. Among them is the thiazide diuretic diazoxide, used in the treatment of hypertension. The effects of this drug are rapidly reversible and are probably elicited via the adenosine triphosphate (ATP) dependent potassium channel in the B-cell membrane (see pages 26–27); it has been used in the treatment of insulin-secreting tumours.

Coxsackie and related picorna viruses

The sera of people newly diagnosed with Type 1 diabetes may contain higher titres of antibody to Coxsackie B4 than those of controls. Further evidence for Coxsackie involvement has come from a few cases of overwhelming Coxsackie infection. In two cases, viruses isolated from the patients induced diabetes in mice. Research in animals has indicated that only certain strains of Coxsackie are diabetogenic and such strains may be relatively uncommon in humans, where they arise by virus mutation.

The case for a viral factor in the aetiology of human diabetes is also supported by a large number of experimental models in which diabetes has been produced by viruses in animals. At least 20 viruses are at present known that attack the islets of Langerhans in animals. Prominent among these viruses are the small RNA viruses known as the picorna group. Diabetes definitely attributable to this virus was first noted in cattle during an outbreak of foot-and-mouth disease in southern Italy. Another picorna virus, encephalomyocarditis (EMC) virus, may produce severe diabetes in mice.

Type 1 diabetes in the UK shows a marked seasonal incidence, with a peak incidence in the autumn and winter months; similar relationships have been shown in several other parts of the world. The reason for this observation is still unclear; it might represent the unmasking of a latent diabetes by non-specific virus infection.

Changing pattern of Type 1 diabetes in other countries

Further evidence for a role for environmental factors in the aetiology of diabetes is seen in the changing incidence of diabetes with time in some European countries (page 21), and in the north–south gradient seen in Europe, with a higher incidence in northern European countries such as Finland than in countries bordering the Mediterranean.

Genetics of Type 1 diabetes

The fact that patients tend to have a family history of diabetes has been known for many centuries. However, the exact mode of inheritance is complex and not completely understood, not least because of the heterogeneity of diabetes itself. It is now clear that it is factors that predispose to Type 1 diabetes that are inherited, rather than Type 1 diabetes itself. Recent studies of the genome of families in which two or more children have Type 1 diabetes, as well as of the twins of people with diabetes, have done much to clarify the situation. There are at least two genetic loci that may predispose to Type 1 diabetes, which have been confirmed in several studies. The human leucocyte antigen (HLA) status of the individual is the single major determinant, accounting for about 50% of genetic risk (see below).

The structure of the insulin gene which is located on the short arm of chromosome 11 is now known in detail. Mutations in the structure of the gene itself may lead to the production of abnormal insulins by the B cell, similarly to the production of abnormal haemoglobins. There are only very few families in which insulins with an abnormal structure have been identified, and when diabetes develops it has been very mild and never Type 1. More abnormal insulins are likely to be described in the future. Changes in the sequence of nucleotides flanking the insulin gene, on the other hand, have been recorded more commonly than in control subjects. These changes could determine the rate at which insulin is produced; while such changes may be important as markers for diabetes, their functional significance is not clear at present.

Studies on twins

Studies on identical twins provide particularly valuable information on the relative roles of genetics and the environment in the pathogenesis of diabetes. The largest of such studies was conducted by Pyke *et al.* and now includes over 300 pairs of identical twins, one or both of whom have diabetes. The most important findings in this group relate to concordance rates among the major classes of people with diabetes: almost two-thirds of the Type 1 twins were discordant (i.e. only one had diabetes), showing that genetic factors cannot be the sole cause of diabetes. By comparison, there is almost complete concordance in the Type 2 identical twins (i.e. both have diabetes) which implies that genetic factors are the chief determinants of this condition.

The unaffected twin of a Type 1 patient may, however, display lymphocyte abnormalities which disappear with time. These abnormalities include an increase in the number of activated T lymphocytes. Mild but persistent metabolic abnormalities have also been recorded in this unaffected group. These observations are consistent with the possibility that some common environmental factor may have initially affected both twins, although only one subsequently shows changes progressing to total B-cell destruction.

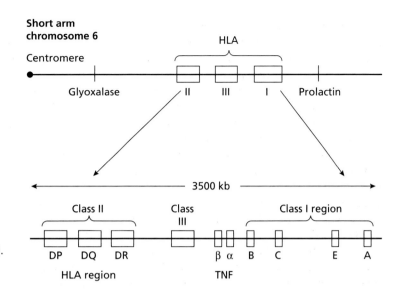

Figure 5.2 Gene map: short arm of chromosome 6 (after Hitman, G.A. & Marshall, B. in Pickup & Williams 1991). HLA, human leucocyte antigen; TNF, tumour necrosis factor.

Role of the HLA system

The major histocompatibility complex antigens (MHCs) are adjuncts to several types of immunological activity. They are glycoproteins present on the surface of cells, and they are coded by genes on the short arm of chromosome 6 (Fig. 5.2). In humans, the major histocompatibility antigens are termed HLA antigens (or human leucocyte-associated antigens), because they were originally found on human leucocytes. They are subdivided into three main groups. Class I MHC molecules are needed for the lysis of cells infected with viruses, and they are present on all cells. Class II molecules (e.g. HLA-DR) have a more limited distribution and are necessary for the activity of T-helper cells. Class III molecules are associated with the action of complement. An association of Class I antigens (HLA-B8 and B15) with Type 1 diabetes has been known for some time, but more recently Class II antigens (HLA-DR3 and DR4) have been found to be much more closely associated. More than 90% of Type 1 patients show either DR3, DR4, or both together; the relative risks are shown in Table 5.1. In contrast DR2 appears to be protective against diabetes.

These haplotypes are also common in the general population, 60% possessing either DR3 or DR4, and cannot provide specific prediction markers of Type 1 susceptibility. Attempts have therefore been made to

Table 5.1 Approximate relative risk for Type 1 associated with HLA-DR haplotypes.

HLA-DR haplotype	Relative risk
DR3 alone	5
DR4 alone	7
DR3 and DR4	14
DR2	0.1

examine the association with several subsets of either DR3 or DR4; the discovery of a very close association with the *DQ* gene may also be relevant. There is also some association of Type 1 diabetes with the complement (Class III) genes which play an important part in clearance of immune complexes and viral neutralization.

These HLA associations with Type 1 diabetes apply to populations of northern European origin; other associations may be relevant in different racial groups.

Autoimmunity

Circulating antibodies to islets

The possibility that an autoimmune response could be associated with the onset of diabetes was suggested by the lymphocytic infiltration sometimes seen at postmortem around the islets in Type 1 diabetics. In

Table 5.2 Classes of inflammatory cells involved in cellular immunity (see Fig. 5.1).

Type	Subgroup	Functions
Lymphocytes		
T lymphocytes	T-helper lymphocytes	Activate B lymphocytes, cytotoxic T cells and T-suppressor cells
	Cytotoxic T lymphocytes	Lysis of target cell
	T-suppressor lymphocytes	Inhibit cell-mediated and humoral immune responses
B lymphocytes		Differentiate into plasma cells; synthesize immunoglobulins
Killer cells		Lysis of target cells
Antigen-presenting cells		
Macrophages		Ingestion and processing of antigens
Dendritic cells		Presentation of antigen and class II antigens to activate T-helper cells. Release of interleukin 1 and tumour necrosis factor-alpha

the 1970s, antibodies against islets were detected in the serum of people with diabetes who had other autoimmune endocrine disorders. Most patients with Type 1 diabetes are now known to have circulating islet cell antibodies (ILA's) although the titre of these decline during the first 12 months after presentation. These are specific for the B cell, while islet cell surface antibodies (ICSA) react with the A, D or B cells in the islets. Antibodies to specific proteins that are present within B cells have also been identified. The most important of these are antibodies to GAD (probably the 64-kDa antigen identified some years earlier) and its associated proteins of a lower molecular weight. Antibodies to a 37-kDa protein (probably tyrosine phosphatase IA-2) have also been identified in Type 1 diabetes. These antibodies may appear in the sera years before the onset of the disease; they are identified most readily in genetically predisposed relatives of people with Type 1 diabetes. Not all people who possess any of these islet cell antibodies develop diabetes, although those with two or three antibodies appear to be at higher risk of diabetes. There is still no certain method of predicting development of Type 1 diabetes in any individual, even within families. Complement-fixing antibodies are also found in diabetes associated with other autoimmune endocrine disorders. Islet cell antibodies may be directly cytotoxic to islets in culture. However, because islet function is normal in some patients with islet cell antibodies, they might only represent markers of damage from some other cause.

Insulin autoantibodies

The appearance of autoantibodies to the insulin molecule itself has been described in newly diagnosed Type 1 patients. These antibodies have to be distinguished from those insulin antibodies induced by the injection of insulin from different species into patients in the course of treatment. They may appear before the onset of clinical diabetes. They too may indicate previous islet cell damage.

Cellular immunity

Apart from possible damage by circulating antibodies, the effects of different classes of inflammatory cells (summarized in Table 5.2) may also be important. These include cytotoxic T cells, and macrophages (which can produce lymphokines) as well as natural killer cells. The mechanisms of the action of monokines and lymphokines are summarized in Table 5.3. The mode of action of these cells is complex and often involves the participation of cell surface glycoproteins, namely the MHCs already described. A speculative model of the role of cellular immunity in the destruction of B cells is shown in Fig. 5.1. These cellular events at the onset of diabetes are difficult to study, except in the rare instance of the death of a Type 1 patient during development

Table 5.3 Mechanism of action of monokines and lymphokines.

	Actions
Monokines (produced by monocytes and macrophages):	
Interleukin-1	Induces interleukin-2 release from T-helper cells
Tumour necrosis factor-alpha	Cytotoxic to tumour cells *in vitro*
Lymphokines (produced by lymphocytes and T-helper cells):	
Interleukin-2	Stimulates division of activated T and B cells
Interferon-gamma	Activates macrophages Increases HLA Class I and II antigen expression on cell surfaces

of the disease. Indirect methods of study, for example by examining peripheral lymphocytes, are therefore undertaken and have shown a marked increase in the number of activated lymphocytes in the blood of patients with newly diagnosed Type 1 diabetes.

An alternative approach is to use animal models. The best known of these is the BB (or Biobreeding) rat. This mutant animal develops diabetes after 60–120 days associated with marked insulitis. There is marked hyperglycaemia, and ketosis. Transfer of lymphocytes from afflicted rats to normal rats results in transfer of the diabetes. Clearly, in these animals, the cell-mediated destruction of B cells results in diabetes.

Predicting diabetes

It is now possible to assess the risk of Type 1 diabetes developing in first-degree relatives of those who already have the disease. The Barts–Oxford (BOX) family study found that relatives with ICAs only had a risk of progression to diabetes of 8% at 10 years. In those who also had IAAs the risk was about 84%, compared to 61% when combined with GAD antibodies. ICAs occurring together with the 37-kDa (IA2) antibody gave a risk of 76% and was associated with rapid progression to the disease. In the presence of three or more antibodies the risk was 88%. It is therefore possible to predict the chances of developing diabetes from the range and titre of these antibodies.

In the future, prediction may become important not only to advise the individual, but also because methods of preventing diabetes in those at risk could become a reality.

Prevention of Type 1 diabetes

Because of the immunological changes associated with the onset of Type 1 diabetes, attempts have been made to prevent it by immunosuppression. While immunosuppression can successfully reverse the diabetes of the BB rat, results have been less encouraging in humans so far. Initial attempts with steroids with or without azathioprine were unsuccessful, but there is now evidence that ciclosporin A can produce a remission (avoiding insulin use) in a small proportion of patients if started within 6 weeks of diagnosis. Unfortunately, the benefit is only present as long as ciclosporin is continued, indeed it may be lost despite continued therapy. There are unacceptable side-effects, notably renal impairment. Clinical use is therefore unjustifiable and attempts are continuing to develop an alternative effective agent with less toxicity.

The value of any such agent, however, requires the very early diagnosis of diabetes, and would necessitate identification of those about to develop the disease if it is to be widely effective in preventing Type 1 diabetes. None the less, the observation that an immune attack on islet cells can be reduced by immunosuppression is clearly of great importance in understanding the cause of diabetes, and opens the possibility of prevention of Type 1 by suitable intervention in susceptible individuals in the future.

Other approaches to the prevention of Type 1 diabetes are undergoing extensive multicentre trials at the time of writing this book. The use of large doses of nicotinamide, which may alter the immune response, has been investigated by the European Nicotinamide Intervention Trial (ENDIT) which involved screening 22 000 relatives and randomizing 422 of them to treatment or placebo. Unfortunately it was shown to have no detectable effect. The use of parenteral insulin in the prediabetic period has been reported to preserve B-cell function, but a major trial has failed to confirm this effect.

Table 5.4 Causes of Type 2 diabetes. There are likely to be relationships between reduced insulin secretion and increased insulin resistance.

Reduced insulin secretion (B-cell defects)
Fetal malnutrition (page 19)
IAPP accumulation (page 24)
Faulty glucose sensing
   GLUT 2 (glucose transporter) abnormality
   Glucokinase defect (page 44)
Faulty insulin processing
   Pro-insulin cleavage defect

Increased insulin resistance (increased peripheral glucose
   uptake/decreased hepatic glucose output)
Android obesity (page 18)
Insulin receptor defect
Insulin gene defect (very rare)
Post-receptor defect
   Insulin receptor substrate abnormality
Circulatory antagonists (pages 29–30)
   Glucagon, cortisol, growth hormone, catecholamine
   Fatty acids/ketone bodies
   Anti-insulin antibodies
   Anti-insulin receptor antibodies
Glucose toxicity
   Hyperglycaemia itself causes reduced insulin secretion and
    glucose transport

Associations of Type 2 diabetes with many other genetic abnormalities are now described—these include polymorphism of the glucokinase gene; mitochondrial DNA mutation (page 13) and many rare genetic syndromes (page 7). IAPP, islet amyloid polypeptide.

Type 2 diabetes mellitus

Some potential causes of Type 2 are discussed in Table 5.4. To date no single major causative factor has been identified despite massive efforts in this direction.

Islet pathology

In Type 2 diabetes, the pancreas may contain normal numbers of islets, and extractable insulin may differ little from normal. There is therefore no absolute insulin deficiency but rather a relative deficiency in comparison of the body's needs. Islet amyloid polypeptide (IAPP) (see page 24) produced in the B cells may be deposited around them as amyloid deposits.

In Type 2 diabetes, subtle biochemical changes are present that prevent the normal insulin response to a glucose stimulus and may also prevent the effectiveness of insulin at its target sites (insulin resistance) (page 35).

Genetics of Type 2 diabetes

Type 2 diabetes has a strong genetic component, including high concordance in monozygotic twins, familial clustering and differences in prevalence between different ethnic groups. Analysis of the genetic components is much more difficult than for Type 1 diabetes because of considerable heterogeneity within the disease state, with variable contributions of obesity, defective insulin secretion and insulin resistance. The most commonly used approach to identification of Type 2 associated genes has been to identify and evaluate the role of candidate genes that, in physiological terms, seem likely to be involved. Despite analysis of large numbers of candidate genes, only two relatively rare forms of diabetes have been definitively linked to individual genes, and a mitochondrial point mutation has been identified that leads to diabetes, myopathy and deafness. It may account for less than 1% of Type 2 diabetes.

Maturity onset diabetes in the young

In dominantly inherited maturity onset diabetes of the young (MODY), a relatively rare single-gene defect in the production of glucokinase, a key enzyme in the early stages of metabolism of glucose, may account for about 15% of the cases (Table 5.5). Failure of metabolism of glucose results in a reduced insulin secretory response to glucose. This finding has stimulated a search for other candidate genes (and proteins) among the enzymes involved in glucose metabolism.

MODY is a rare (3% of all cases) form of diabetes which shows a monosomal dominant (single gene) form of inheritance. It has therefore been much studied by geneticists in the hope that it might give clues to the genetics of mainstream Type 2 diabetes. The results are interesting in that while each family with MODY has only a single gene

Table 5.5 Comparison of the different subgroups of maturity onset diabetes of the young.

Gene: Nomenclature:	Glucokinase MODY 2	HNF-1alpha MODY 3	HNF-4 alpha MODY 1	HNF-1 beta MODY 5	IFP-1 MODY 4
Chromosomal location	7p	12q	20q	17q	13q
Frequency in a large UK series	15%	65%	5%	1%	<1%
Penetrance of mutations at age 40 years	45% diabetes 95% impaired fasting glycaemia	>90%	>80%	>90%	Limited data
Onset of hyperglycaemia	Early childhood (from birth)	Adolescence Early adulthood	Similar to HNF-1 alpha	Similar to HNF-1 alpha	Early adulthood
Severity of hyperglycaemia	Mild with minor deterioration with age	Progressive. May be severe	Progressive. May be severe	Progressive. May be severe	Limited data
Microvascular complications	Rare	Frequent	Frequent	Retinopathy observed	Unknown
Pathophysiology	Beta cell dysfunction	Beta cell dysfunction	Beta cell dysfunction	Beta cell dysfunction	Beta cell dysfunction
Abnormality of glucose sensing	Yes	No	No	No	No
Other phenotypical features	Reduced birth weight	Low renal threshold and sensitivity to sulphonylureas	Low plasma triglyceride levels	Predominant renal phenotype; cysts; renal failure; genital malformations	Pancreatic agenesis in homozygotes

mutation, there are in fact several forms of MODY and several quite different genes involved, as shown in Table 5.5.

The effect of glucokinase mutations on insulin secretion could have been predicted but the role of the transcription factors (HNF's) could not have been anticipated, and provide a new area for research in B-cell biology. Meanwhile, MODY has brought diabetes into the arena of 'genetic medicine' because patients can be advised with certainty about the exact genetic basis of their condition.

Clinical Presentation and Treatment

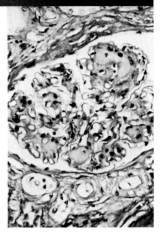

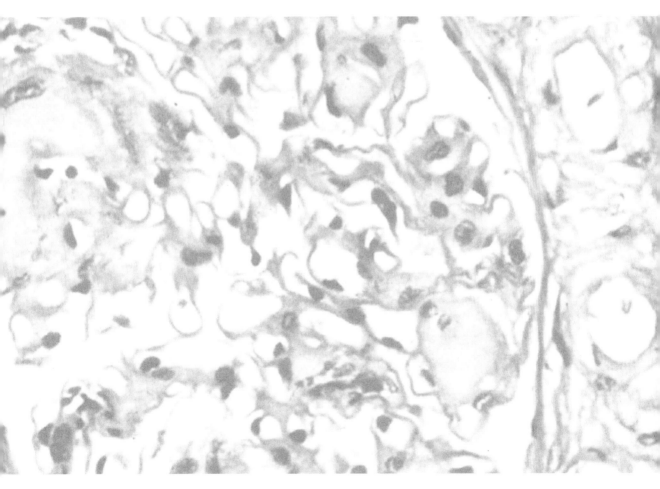

Clinical Features of Diabetes

Summary

- A careful clinical history of the severity of symptoms is the best guide for assessing appropriate treatment

- Thirst, polyuria, weight loss, fatigue and/or pruritus vulvae are the most frequently reported symptoms; Type 2 diabetes can however often present apparently in the absence of any symptoms

- Some patients with Type 1 diabetes present in diabetic ketoacidosis; and some with Type 2 diabetes in hyperosmolar nonketotic diabetic 'coma' (HONK)

- Complications of diabetes are sometimes present at the time of diagnosis of Type 2 diabetes: these include retinopathy, neuropathy (sometimes symptomatic painful neuropathy), and proteinuria. Major arterial disease is often detected at diagnosis in these patients

- Full physical examination is required at presentation, paying special attention to the presence or absence of complications associated with diabetes

- Skin changes include necrobiosis lipoidica diabeticorum or granuloma annulare. Vitiligo may be associated with Type 1 diabetes. Acanthosis nigricans is seen in cases of insulin resistance in some patients with Type 2 diabetes

Clinical presentation

'The history of diabetic symptoms is of the greatest importance and an accurate appreciation of their severity far exceeds an estimation of the blood sugar as a means of assessing the need for treatment.' [From John Malins, *Clinical Diabetes Mellitus*, Eyre & Spottiswoode, 1968]

The diversity of the clinical presentation of diabetes together with varying perceptions of the patients themselves often combine to conceal the diagnosis of diabetes which should, in theory at least, be very straightforward (Box 6.1). Thirst is the most prominent symptom of diabetes. Patients may drink huge volumes of fluid. However, the common use of fizzy drinks with a high glucose content by thirsty people with a vague malaise, may cause extreme hyperglycaemia, polyuria and dehydration. Some patients observe that they have a 'dry mouth' but deny thirst and occasionally, when dehydration develops, they may describe difficulty with speech or swallowing. Even this obvious symptom is sometimes overlooked and we have known of patients where investigations for speech defects or dysphagia have been undertaken before the correct diagnosis has been established. A dry mouth is ascribed by some patients to various drugs (antidepressants or diuretics in particular) without any thought of the possibility of diabetes. Rather curiously, a few patients never seem to develop thirst even in the presence of severe hyperglycaemia.

Polyuria, especially nocturia, is a major symptom

Box 6.1 **Classical symptoms of diabetes**

Thirst	Dry mouth
Polyuria	Nocturia
Weight loss	Wasting
Balanitis	Pruritus vulvae
Fatigue/tiredness	
Myopia	

---

and not to be confused with the frequency and urgency of micturition associated with urinary tract infections. Nevertheless, many patients are given antibiotics without considering the diagnosis of diabetes which is overlooked. The volumes of urine are sometimes huge, causing thirst and eventually dehydration. In the young, enuresis, and in the elderly, urinary incontinence, may develop as a result of polyuria. Some patients are extensively investigated for urological or gynaecological causes of frequency, nocturia, pruritus vulvae or balanitis before the diagnosis is made.

Many patients, both those with Type 1 and Type 2 diabetes, describe weight loss at the onset of diabetes, which often causes concern regarding the possibility of some grave disorder. In Type 1 diabetes the weight loss is sometimes both acute and profound, causing a cadaveric appearance. We have seen patients whose weight loss has been overlooked or even diagnosed as anorexia nervosa. Weight loss occasionally develops despite a substantial increase in appetite and food intake, especially in the young. Some obsessional patients who keep daily records of their weight throughout life notice weight loss as a very early symptom occurring before the development of other symptoms leading to the diagnosis of Type 2 diabetes. Diabetes should always be considered as a potential diagnosis in any patient describing weight loss when no other cause has been discovered.

Fatigue and tiredness are common symptoms of untreated diabetes. They are often attributed by patients to ageing or overwork and may be accompanied by excessive somnolence and a tendency to fall asleep. Alleviation of these symptoms by treatment is exceptionally rewarding, many patients describing a new sense of energy and well-being, even by those who had previously denied any symptoms at all. Tiredness is not a feature of adequately treated diabetes although many patients, usually those with a mild depressive tendency, continue over many years to believe so.

Pruritus vulvae is a presenting symptom in about two-fifths of Type 2 diabetic women and is associated by women with Type 1 disease as indicative of lost glycaemic control; this, and balanitis in men, is a result of monilial infection which occurs more readily in the presence of glycosuria. Doctors often fail to recognize the potential relevance of this symptom and patients are frequently treated for symptomatic relief without any thought of the possibility of diabetes. The rash in some patients with pruritus vulvae involves the entire perineum and upper parts of the thighs and may be extremely disagreeable. Balanitis in men is much less common. Inflammation and pruritus of the prepuce and glans penis develops and causes some men to go to clinics for sexually transmitted disease before diabetes is diagnosed. Phimosis needing circumcision occasionally develops. Treatment of diabetes and reduction of glycosuria leads to complete resolution of both pruritus vulvae and balanitis.

The development of myopia at the onset of diabetes is not uncommon; occasionally it is the presenting symptom and astute opticians will send such patients straight to a diabetic clinic (page 150). The most common explanation is osmotic change in the lens of the eye and the vitreous, leading to changes in refraction, rather than diabetic retinopathy or maculopathy or early development of cataract, all of which may also occur in newly diagnosed Type 2 diabetes (rarely at diagnosis in Type 1 diabetes as the prodromal illness is usually much shorter). Patients should be warned not to return to the optician for refraction until the diabetes is controlled.

The intensity of symptoms varies greatly: in general, they are more severe and more acute in Type 1 than in Type 2 diabetic patients. The duration of symptoms amongst Type 1 diabetic patients is usually recorded as a few weeks, but it may be as little as a few days or be found to extend over several months or longer if a very careful history is taken. At times, transient yet characteristic symptoms are noted with hindsight to have occurred 1 or 2 years previously. Sometimes, symptoms appear to begin during intercurrent illness. Transient hyperglycaemia is known to occur occasionally during illnesses in the prediabetic phase, especially in small children and in maturity onset diabetes of the young (MODY). A few patients present in ketoacidosis; this occurs either when the diabetes is very acute in its onset, or on occasions after two or three visits to a doctor who has failed to recognize the diagnosis of diabetes. These patients usually come to Accident and Emerency departments weak, thin and dehydrated and with all the features of ketoacidosis described on page 89. Type 2 diabetes can occasionally present with ketoacidosis and this is believed to be a result of very high levels of anti-insulin stress hormones resulting from some other severe illness. Diabetic ketoacidosis in young or middle-aged black and Asian adults (not always with an obvious precipitating illness) may also represent transient insulin dependence but, in all other cases, diabetic ketoacidosis is diagnostic of Type 1 disease and means a lifelong requirement for exogenous insulin therapy.

Identification of Type 1 diabetes depends in practice on specific clinical features. Rapid development of thirst, polyuria and substantial weight loss over days, weeks or sometimes months, all point to Type 1 diabetes. They lead to wasting and physical weakness, and ultimately vomiting and dehydration. Insulin is always needed immediately and should never be delayed. If it is not given, ketoacidosis is inevitable. About one-fifth of cases of ketoacidosis develop in previously undiagnosed cases, sometimes when their symptoms have been overlooked during preceding weeks. Drowsiness, dehydration and overbreathing (together with acetone in the breath) are the chief features of ketoacidosis, always indicating the need for urgent admission to hospital with administration of intravenous fluids and insulin.

The presentation of Type 2 diabetes is, in general, less acute. Patients may complain of only one or other of the characteristic symptoms and even then only on careful questioning. Malaise and fatigue are common. Symptoms develop over very variable periods, most frequently over several weeks or months, and may even have been treated for long periods, sometimes for years. Even such characteristic and disagreeable symptoms as pruritus vulvae can be present for a long time if the diagnosis of diabetes has been overlooked. A white crystalline deposit on trousers and shoes from splashes of urine loaded with sugar is sometimes noticed by men.

A few patients present with hyperosmolar nonketotic (HONK) coma, or when patients with intense thirst drink huge volumes of fizzy, sugary fluids such as Coca-Cola, lemonade and Lucozade.

Increasing numbers of Type 2 diabetic patients are found to have diabetes at routine screening examinations when either urine or blood tests are performed. Although some of these patients admit that with hindsight they were aware of characteristic symptoms, many deny them altogether, becoming aware of their previous malaise and loss of energy only after starting treatment.

Sometimes diabetes is diagnosed because of acute complications such as infections of skin and genitourinary tract. Older Type 2 diabetic patients may present for the first time as a result of chronic diabetic complications; their presence indicates the existence of long-standing unrecognized diabetes which is sometimes confirmed by examination of old medical records and discovery of unnoticed glycosuria or hyperglycaemia years before. In the UK Prospective Diabetes Survey (UKPDS), 50% of patients (all newly diagnosed with Type 2) had complications at diagnosis and it is estimated that on average people have had diabetes for 11 years before diagnosis. Many of these complications are not severe and are found during assessment for diabetes but foot sepsis or ulceration presenting in an Accident and Emergency department frequently indicates a diagnosis of diabetes, and investigation of failing vision from cataracts, or less commonly from retinopathy, sometimes leads to the discovery of diabetes. Painful neuropathy rarely occurs as a presenting symptom although sensory neuropathy is more common. Although proteinuria (nephropathy) is not uncommonly present at diagnosis in older patients, diabetes does not normally present with renal failure.

Another situation in which diabetes may be diagnosed is in patients presenting with evidence of macrovascular disease including angina, myocardial infarction, stroke, transient ischaemic attacks and peripheral vascular disease.

The symptoms of diabetes are so well known that it is surprising that the diagnosis is so often overlooked. Measurement of plasma glucose should be routine in any medical consultation where suspicion of diabetes exists or when symptoms have not been accounted for.

Other important questions at first assessment

Because of vascular risk, it is important to quantify exercise, diet and smoking habits. Alcohol intake must also be assessed. Family history may give clues about specific forms of diabetes and social history should include patients' experience of diabetes in their community, work habits and make special reference to driving.

Clinical features identifying Type 1 diabetes

Physical examination of the diabetic patient

• A full general examination should be performed in all patients, whether they are presenting with newly diagnosed diabetes or with long-standing diabetes presenting to a physician for the first time. Newly presenting Type 1 diabetic patients are often wasted from loss of fat and muscle bulk; they may be dehydrated, the tongue furred, and there is sometimes the scent of acetone on the breath. (Note that only half of the populatoin can smell acetone—it is important for a diabetes health care professional to know into which half of the population they fall!)

• Height and weight are documented and body mass index determined.

• A urine test is required to establish the presence of proteinuria or acetone. The standard bedside tests measure acetone and acetoacetate. Occasionally the predominant ketone is 3-OH butyrate: such patients may show small amounts or, very rarely, no ketones in the urine.

• Insulin injection sites should always be examined to discover evidence of fat hypertrophy, or other problems resulting from faulty technique.

• If pruritus vulvae or balanitis are mentioned by the patient, the genitalia should be examined to discover the extent of the monilial rash which may be very extensive. Balanitis causes an inflamed, cracked and sometimes swollen foreskin which is very unpleasant.

• Blood pressure must always be recorded, using a large cuff for the obese.

• Visual acuity must be measured, both uncorrected and corrected if necessary by having the patient look through a pin hole. This focuses light on the macula and corrects refractive errors. Corrected acuity that is worse than uncorrected may indicate maculopathy.

• The fundi are always examined at diagnosis and this must be performed through dilated pupils in a darkened room; although retinopathy is rarely present at diagnosis in the young, it becomes increasingly common amongst older patients (page 146).

• Examination of the feet is essential, first to discover any deformities, which may need active measures to prevent ulceration; or indeed to discover unreported blisters, ulcers, sepsis or ischaemic lesions of which the patient is unaware. The condition of the skin should be noted, looking particularly for athlete's foot, cracked skin and evidence of callus, all of which increase the risk of infection and ulceration.

• Neurological testing of the feet is performed in order to detect the presence of neuropathy. Details of this neurological examination are described on page 173.

• The presence of peripheral vascular disease should be assessed by examination of foot pulses; if both dorsalis pedis and posterior tibial pulses are absent, popliteal and femoral pulses together with evidence of femoral bruits should be sought.

• The hands are usually normal, but in those with long-standing diabetes, 'cheiroarthropathy' is sometimes seen (Fig. 6.1); this results in a mild, fixed curvature of the fingers which makes it impossible to place the hand and fingers flat on a smooth surface. This defect is accompanied by some tightening of the skin over the fingers and is thought to be brought about by a collagen defect. It causes no disability. Other changes in the hands are caused either by me-

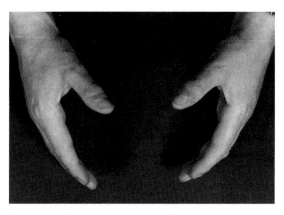

Figure 6.1 'Cheiroarthropathy': a mild fixed flexion deformity of the fingers is common in patients with long-standing diabetes.

dian nerve compression (carpal tunnel), or by ulnar nerve compression causing interosseous muscle wasting. Very rarely, burns on the fingers occur in the presence of severe sensory loss caused by peripheral neuropathy.

The liver

Liver enlargement occasionally occurs in uncontrolled diabetes as a result of fatty (rarely glycogen) infiltration. Liver function tests often produce abnormal results , although jaundice is not a feature. Hepatomegaly resolves completely as diabetes is controlled, and liver function test results return to normal. Hepatomegaly associated with a slate-grey skin pigmentation is a result of haemochromatosis (page 11). It also occurs in patients with the rare conditions of lipoatrophic diabetes and eruptive xanthomas. Hepatic cirrhosis is not a feature of clinical diabetes, although a small percentage of patients with idiopathic cirrhosis are diabetic. Insulin resistance, hyperinsulinaemia and glucose intolerance are characteristic of cirrhosis.

Skin manifestations

Necrobiosis lipoidica diabeticorum (Fig. 6.2) is an uncommon and unsightly blemish of the skin which affects a few people with diabetes, 75% of them

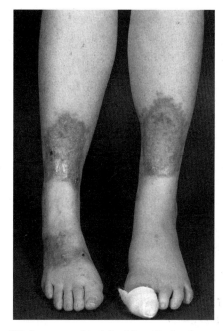

Figure 6.2 Severe necrobiosis lipoidica affecting the anterior aspects of the legs and right foot.

women. It is unrelated to other diabetic complications, or to duration of diabetes. The shin is the most common site of involvement, although lesions can appear almost anywhere. The base of the lesion is characterized by atrophic skin with obviously dilated capillaries (telangiectasis) and a slightly raised pinkish rim; ulceration sometimes occurs. The lesions are indolent, very slowly increase in size and rarely resolve. There is no effective treatment and most women apply cosmetic preparations to ameliorate the appearance of the blemish. Application of topical steroids can be tried although with little effect.

Granuloma annulare is related histologically to necrobiosis; it consists of a raised pinkish lesion, sometimes in a circular configuration, occurring on the hands or feet. Its relationship to diabetes is dubious.

Vitiligo, a common autoimmune disorder causing patchy skin depigmentation, may have an association with Type 1 diabetes.

Eruptive xanthomas (Fig. 6.3) are occasionally seen in uncontrolled diabetes, especially Type 2 patients. Crops of multiple 2–5 mm yellowish papules

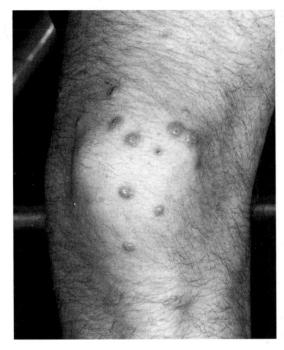

Figure 6.3 Xanthomatous rash occasionally seen in uncontrolled diabetes.

with surrounding pink haloes develop rapidly especially on the elbows, knees and buttocks. These changes are associated with exceptionally severe hyperlipidaemia involving all lipid fractions; the serum has a milky appearance, and the retina has an unusual hue sometimes described as 'peaches and cream' associated with very pale arteries and known as lipaemia retinalis. The severe hyperlipidaemia causes spurious lowering of serum sodium which is artefactual. The lesions disappear over a few weeks once the diabetes has been controlled.

Xanthelasmas affecting the eyelids are not a feature

of diabetes *per se*, although in some instances are related to the presence of hypercholesterolaemia.

Carotenaemia occurs if large quantities of carrots (or pumpkin, sweet potato or tomatoes) are eaten and leads to deposition of carotene in the stratum corneum causing yellow discoloration of soles and palms. Its only association with diabetes is because of the alteration of dietary habit and the excessive consumption of the relevant vegetables.

Other rare skin conditions associated with diabetes are acanthosis nigricans and lipoatrophy, described on page 12.

Generalized pruritus is not a feature of diabetes. It remains uncertain whether or not skin sepsis is related to diabetes.

The laboratory examination of the patient with diabetes is detailed in Box 6.2.

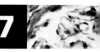

Management of Type 2 Diabetes

Summary

- Type 2 diabetes mellitus is a progressive disease of insulin resistance with increasing loss of insulin secretory capacity throughout life

- The intensification of therapy with time is to be expected and patient and professional should be aware of this from the beginning

- As Type 2 diabetes mellitus is a lifestyle disease, management must always include practical advice about lifestyle factors

- While adequate insulin secretory reserve remains, it is appropriate to start by treating the insulin resistance and there is evidence to support the use of metformin as first-line therapy therapy in overweight patients

- Insulin secretagogues and/or insulin replacement therapy will be needed over time and should be introduced as soon as the patient's individualized targets for glucose control are no longer being met by other means

- Weight reduction is very beneficial in the overweight and obese but must be considered in its own right. Glycaemic control can be improved separately from weight reduction, although in the obese patient, weight reduction may be essential to achieve good results

- Patient education is essential and home monitoring is an important element of self-management

- The published evidence does not support the use of home blood glucose monitoring in diet- and exercise- (and many tablet) treated Type 2 diabetic patients and urine monitoring should be considered

- Home blood glucose monitoring is necessary in the patient at risk for hypoglycaemia and once insulin therapy is introduced, in order to allow the patient to make dose adjustments

- Good glycaemic control substantially diminishes risk of microvascular disease in Type 2 diabetes but may need to be advanced beyond current treatment guidelines to make a major impact upon macrovascular disease

- Active management of other cardiovascular risk factors is crucial

- Regular review for the development of complications and their active management form an essential part of therapy

Three important principles underlie the proper management of Type 2 diabetes:

1 *Type 2 diabetes* is a lifestyle disease
2 *Type 2 diabetes* is a progressive disease
3 *Type 2 diabetes* is a major risk factor for premature cardiovascular disease.

Other important points to remember are that each patient will have a variable degree of insulin resistance and insulin secretory failure, both of which can be treated; comorbidities such as hypertension, hyperlipidaemia and obesity require active management; engaging the patient in his/her management is crucial.

Principles of dietary management

All patients with Type 2 diabetes require active dietary management throughout their disease. Weight loss in the obese is extremely valuable but is separate from dietary manipulations to control blood glucose. It is important to separate the two in both the patient's and the professional's mind. Obese patients will have often tried dieting for weight reduction in the past with variable lack of success and a patient's failure to lose weight, while regrettable, is not an excuse for failure to intensify other therapy where needed to achieve glycaemic targets.

Where appropriate, dietary advice should also encompass minimizing salt intake to help blood pressure control and the diabetic diet needs also to target circulating lipid levels.

Timing of meals

For glycaemic control, the aim is to provide a diet that results in gradual changes in blood glucose over time, so that the failing pancreas can cope with demand. Meal timing is important: patients should be advised to take regular moderate-sized meals, spread evenly throughout the day, rather than small snacks and one large meal when they are hungry once a day.

Carbohydrates

Ideally, 60% of the total caloric intake is provided from carbohydrate, although this is not easy to achieve. The eating of complex carbohydrates ('starchy' foods) such as bread, potatoes, pasta and rice in moderate amounts with each meal should be encouraged. In theory, the less refined the better (wholemeal bread, brown rice and pasta, etc.), but the benefit is quite small. Complex carbohydrates cause a slower rise in blood glucose concentration than simple sugars which are very rapidly absorbed, such as sugar itself, non-diet soft drinks, jams, honey, fruit tinned in fruit juice, cakes and sweet biscuits. Such high-sugar items should be replaced where possible with low-sugar alternatives such as diet versions of soft drinks and possibly jams, or eaten in small quantities in mixed meals. Some authorities classify foods by 'glycaemic index' — the size and shape of the blood glucose curve compared to that of glucose itself. Although this can give helpful information, it is not widely useful as eating mixed meals alters the absorption profile of glucose from each component. Soluble fibre, such as found in pulses and broad beans, is particularly effective at this.

Foods made specifically for diabetic patients are generally unhelpful — the sorbitol in them causes diarrhoea (and is high in calories, as is fructose), they have a short shelf life and they are expensive. The patient would do better to eat moderate amounts of regular foods in mixed meals, where other foods taken at the same time will slow the absorption of the glucose. The exception is the use of diet soft drinks and sugar substitutes, such as aspartame, which can be helpful.

Patients need to be warned against fresh fruit juice carrying the label 'no added sugar'; one does not add sugar to something that already contains a large amount and a glass of fruit juice may contain several fruits with no structure to retard the absorption of the sugar. In contrast, items of fresh fruit are to be encouraged with a caution against grapes and dried fruit where the tendency is to eat too many at once.

Vegetables contain virtually no sugar or fat and can be eaten freely.

Fat

No more than 30% of the caloric intake should be from fat and at least half of this should be polyunsaturated or monounsaturated (olive oil). Patients should be encouraged to replace animal fats and oils with their vegetable equivalents and to move from full cream to semiskimmed, or from semiskimmed to skimmed milk. Patients should be advised to avoid fried foods, to trim visible fat off meat and to replace red meats such as pork and beef with low-fat animal protein alternatives such as chicken and fish or vegetable proteins. Patient should be encouraged to find low-fat alternatives for favourite foods: thick oven chips are better than conventional french fries and turkey bacon can be usefully substituted for the real thing!

Protein

Apart from the advice in connection with reducing higher fat animal proteins, it is not usual to restrict protein in the diabetic diet. There is evidence that removing animal protein from the diet may provide benefit in reducing the progression of renal disease, but it is not usual significantly to restrict protein intake except in cases of frank renal failure. Outside this setting, it is rare to advise any reduction in patients' protein intake, unless it is unusually large.

Alcohol

Current evidence suggests that alcohol has potentially beneficial antioxidant properties. However, the rule of moderation is very important in diabetes! Patients should be advised that alcohol is a potent source of calories, and beer and cider of rapidly available carbohydrate. Low-alcohol beers are high in sugar and vice versa and it is preferable to use conventional alcohol in moderate quantities. Alcohol intake becomes a problem for patients on insulin or insulin secretagogues; after an initial hyperglycaemia (less marked with wines and some spirits than with beers and lagers), there is a drive towards hypoglycaemia as gluconeogenesis is suppressed. Delayed hypoglycaemia, occurring the following morning before or even after breakfast can be a major problem, particularly for insulin users.

Dietetic advice needs to be culturally sensitive and is best given by a qualified dietitian with knowledge of his/her local population. It is important to try to provide positive dietary advice—*do* this, *replace* that with the other—rather than delivering a list of prohibitions. Attempts should be made to accommodate patients' favourite foods, if only on an infrequent 'treat' basis.

Exercise

There are several studies showing that quite modest amounts of exercise can prevent diabetes in susceptible populations and the consensus is that about 30 min of reasonably brisk exercise no less than four times a week might well prevent the doubling in diabetes prevalence we are expecting. Indeed, lack of exercise is probably a bigger problem than overeating and there is some evidence that a fit overweight person is healthier than a thin sedentary one. It follows that such exercise is also useful in treating hyperglycaemia once diagnosed.

Advice must be practical; younger patients may be keen to take up a new sport but older patients particularly may find difficulty fitting exercise into daily life. If exercise is not enjoyable or easily accommodated into lifestyle it will not be continued.

Patients who do not exercise at all should be encouraged to take up brisk walking, gradually building up to half an hour at least every other day. Practical advice such as telling patients to walk additional bus stops on journeys into work and to use stairs rather than lifts and escalators at work are all helpful. There are some diabetic complications that require particular care. Patients who are planning to take up walking or jogging need to be checked for peripheral neuropathy and in any event should be given advice about wearing natural wool or cotton socks and well-fitting sports shoes. They should inspect their feet after exercise, and jogging or running on concrete pavements should be discouraged where possible.

Patients wanting to take up more vigorous sport should be tested for asymptomatic ischaemic heart disease by exercise ECG testing.

Isometric exercises, where the patient is exercising against resistance, such as weight training, should be discouraged for patients with hypertension or significant retinopathy: walking, bicycling and team sports are to be preferred. Swimming is an ideal exercise but does take some effort to fit into a busy lifestyle and very obese patients may be uncomfortable about appearing in a swimsuit in public.

Professional diabetes services are not currently particularly good in helping patients adopt healthier lifestyles and much could be learnt from the exercise programmes of, for example, cardiac rehabilitation.

Oral hypoglycaemic agents (Table 7.1)

When diet and exercise fail to achieve glycaemic control, medication is needed but it must be understood by both patient and professional that this is in addition to, not instead of, persistent lifestyle management. Oral agents to reduce blood glucose fall into one of three categories:

1 *insulin sensitizers*;
2 *insulin secretagogues*; or
3 *retardants of glucose absorption* from the gastrointestinal lumen.

All require residual insulin secretory capacity in the patient to be effective. Drugs from the three groups can be used in combination as the glucose secretory defect progresses with time. One of the failings of the profession is not to increase medication rapidly enough to achieve optimal glycaemic control over time. It is also important to know when to move from tablet therapy to insulin. Because of progressive insulin secretory deficiency, all patients with Type 2 diabetes are likely eventually to require insulin for glycaemic control, if they live long enough.

Insulin sensitizers

Metformin

Metformin is the one clinically useful example of the drug class of biguanides. Biguanides were described in 1957 but the precise mechanism of their action is unknown. They reduce hepatic gluconeogenesis, increase peripheral glucose uptake and also reduce the absorption of carbohydrate from the gut lumen. Because metformin works on insulin sensitivity, and with only endogenous glucose stimulated insulin secretion, it virtually never causes hypoglycaemia on its own and patients using it with diet and exercise do not need routinely to self-monitor blood glucose.

The major side-effects of metformin are gastrointestinal, particularly diarrhoea. However, the drug is usually well tolerated if started gradually (e.g. 500 mg after breakfast for 2 weeks, 500 mg b.d. for 2 weeks, and then 500 mg t.d.s., returning to the lower dosage if side-effects are encountered) and is taken after meals. Minor malabsorption, particularly of vitamin B_{12}, is reported but is rare.

Biguanides have been associated with lactic acidosis but with metformin this is almost exclusively in patients with renal failure. Metformin should be discontinued when creatinine, measured 6 monthly, begins to rise, as creatinine elevation is indicative of a marked decline in glomerular filtration rate (GFR). Some authorities continue to use metformin until creatinine is over 200 μmol/L but as metabolic problems tend to occur unpredictably in acute decompensation of mild chronic renal failure, it is our policy to stop metformin as soon as the creatinine starts to rise, even within the normal range and certainly once it is over it.

Because lactate is cleared through the liver, metformin should not be used in patients with significant hepatic abnormality, although it will produce benefit in the poorly treated obese patient with abnormal liver function associated with hepatic steatosis. It can be used in patients with cardiovascular disease, although better avoided if the patient is on major treatment for cardiac failure, with the risk of dehydration and impairment of renal blood flow.

Metformin has long been recognized as a suitable first-line agent for obese Type 2 diabetes as it is the only oral hypoglycaemic agent associated with no weight gain or even weight reduction. Cynics suggest it is because of the associated mild gastrointestinal discomfort but this is unjustified. The UK Prospective Diabetes Study (UKPDS) demonstrated a significant survival advantage for Type 2 patients started on metformin as first-line therapy, with less cardiovascular mortality, although it should be noted that they only used the drug in obese patients.

Addition of metformin to diet and exercise regimens can be expected to reduce HbA_{1c} by up to 2%.

Thiazolidinediones

These relative newcomers bind to a nuclear receptor (the PPARγ receptor) and upregulate the transcrip-

Table 7.1 Commonly used oral hypoglycaemic agents.

Drug	Dosage	Metabolism/ excretion	Side-effects	Comments
Insulin sensitizers				
Metformin	500 mg t.d.s. to 1 g b.d.	Renal excretion	Gastrointestinal Lactic acidosis B_{12} malabsorption	Avoid in renal impairment, hepatic, cardiac failure. Start slowly and monitor renal function
Thiazolidinediones				
Pioglitazone	15–30 mg/day		Weight gain Fluid retention	Useful alternative to metformin
Rosiglitazone	4–8 mg (limit to 4 mg if using with sulphonylurea)		Anaemia Gastrointestinal Fatigue Other	
Insulin secretagogues				
Sulphonlyureas				
Chlorpropamide	250–500 mg mane	Renal	Hypoglycaemia Weight gain Allergy	Avoid in renal impairment or elderly
Glibenclamide	2.5–10 mg mane		Abnormal LFT Rare: Photosensitivity Blood dyscrasias	
Tolbutamide	500 mg t.d.s.	Hepatic metabolism	Chlorpropamide enhances ADH 1	Slightly weaker than others.
Gliclazide	40 mg mane– 160 mg b.d.			Useful in renal impairment and elderly
Glipizide	5–15 mg mane, 20 mg in divided doses	Renal and hepatic		Useful in younger, fit Type 2 where good control needed
Glimepiride	1–4 mg/day	Renal		
Gliquidone	15 mg mane– 60 mg t.d.s.	Hepatic		
Metiglinides				
Repaglinide	0.5–4 mg pre meal	Hepatic	Hypoglycaemia Gastrointestinal allergy	Take before meals and skip dose if not eating
Nateglinide	60–180 mg pre meals			
Inhibitors of glucose absorption				
Guar gum	5 g pre meals		Flatulence Diarrhoea Other	
Alpha-glucosidase inhibitors	50–100 mg t.d.s.	Only 2% absorbed	Gastrointestinal Abnormal LFTs	Start gradually. Take with food

tion of insulin responsive genes, resulting in increased expression of glucose transporters and insulin receptors at cell surfaces. The two currently available examples are rosiglitazone and pioglitazone, with similar actions, although a reportedly better effect on circulating lipid profiles with the latter. These agents are lipotrophic, enhancing maturation of adipocytes, and their use is commonly associated with weight gain. It is suggested that most of this is in subcutaneous rather than intra-abdominal fat and therefore not metabolically damaging but the cosmetic results can be a problem. Other side-effects include fluid retention and an anaemia thought to be dilutional, which makes these drugs ineligible for patients with cardiac failure. Peripheral oedema may be problematic for patients with incipient diabetic foot disease and care should be taken not to encourage oedema in patients with neuropathy or peripheral vascular disease. Because of rare but severe hepatotoxicity with an early example of this drug class, 2-monthly monitoring of liver function is recommended but there is no evidence that either pioglitazone or rosiglitazone are hepatotoxic.

Thiazolidinediones have been demonstrated to be more efficacious than placebo if added to either metformin or a sulphonylurea. Because of the problems with fluid retention, they are not indicated in conjunction with insulin and at the time of writing there was no good evidence to show their efficacy as a third-line agent, although it is likely there will be benefit there. They can be expected to reduce HbA_{1c} levels by 1–1.5% and one of their major uses is as an effective insulin sensitizer for people who cannot tolerate metformin.

Insulin secretagogues

Sulphonylureas

The hypoglycaemic action of sulphonamides was recognized during a typhoid epidemic in Vichy France, where antibiotics were used in malnourished people. From this observation, sulphonulyreas were developed, the first two being the short-acting tolbutamide and the long-acting chlorpropamide. Tolbutamide (and, by association, sulphonylureas in

general) suffered a reverse when the University Group Diabetes Program (UGDP) study found a higher rate of cardiovascular events in patients on the drug in the 1960s. Considerable doubt has since been cast on that result and these agents have become a mainstay of Type 2 diabetes treatment. They act by stimulating insulin release from beta cells through a pathway independent of glucose metabolism, using their own cell membrane receptors. The natural ligand for the sulphonylurea receptor is not known but the receptors comprise a binding region (SUR) and incorporate a potassium channel (Kir), the closing of which causes cell membrane depolarization, calcium influx and insulin secretion. Because they cause artificial insulin secretion, independent of glucose metabolism, they can cause hypoglycaemia which is commonly both neuroglycopenic and prolonged. Patients rescued from severe hypoglycaemia on sulphonylureas need admission to hospital for observation and glucose support over 48 h, until the drug has cleared. Sulphonylurea therapy is associated with weight gain, although much of this may relate to the cessation of glycosuria, in which the patient can be losing up to 500 kcal/day. Allergic reactions are also possible in patients sensitive to sulphonomides.

Alcohol, aspirin, sulphonamides and monoamine oxidase inhibitors may enhance the hypoglycaemic effect of sulphonylureas but, apart from alcohol, the hazard is probably small. Warfarin and sulphonylureas interact, to enhance the action of each.

The use of long-acting agents such as chlorpropamide and glibenclamide is discouraged, particularly in the elderly or those with renal impairment where they must be avoided because of the risk of prolonged hypoglycaemia. Shorter-acting tolbutamide, gliclazide or glipizide are to be preferred, although this advice may be reconsidered in the light of evidence suggesting improved compliance with once daily medications. Glipizide can effectively be given once a day until the dose exceeds 15 mg and is probably more effective than gliclazide. It is 50% metabolized by the liver, 50% excreted through the kidneys. Gliclazide is to be preferred in patients with renal impairment or in the very elderly, as it is fully metabolized to inactive compounds. Tolbutamide shares this benefit and is much cheaper but is a much larger tablet to swallow.

Other sulphonylureas include glimepiride and gliquidone.

Metiglinides

These are recently developed shorter-acting insulin secretagogues which act through a receptor different from the sulphonylurea receptor. They are probably more dependent on glucose for their effect than sulphonylureas and, because of this and their relatively short action, might have some clinical advantages, although a reduced rate of hypoglycaemia has yet to be demonstrated. Metiglinides can be taken immediately before food and omitted if a meal is omitted, which may give the patient some dietary freedom. Because of their fast action they are thought to target postprandial hyperglycaemia, although the survival benefits of controlling postprandial rather than basal blood glucose for any given HbA_{1c} is currently unproven. On the basis of the present evidence, these drugs are probably best reserved for patients with very erratic eating patterns and for patients who experience unacceptable hypoglycaemia with conventional sulphonylureas but inadequately controlled HbA_{1c} when they are stopped. The two agents on the market at the time of writing are repaglinide and nateglinide. They have not been compared with each other. Nateglinide is currently being tested as an agent to slow the development of Type 2 diabetes, based on the hypothesis that its fast action may counteract the loss of first phase insulin response to intravenous insulin which is an early sign of pancreatic failure.

Agents that retard glucose absorption from the gut

Guar gum

This acts as an additional source of soluble fibre and reduces absorption of carbohydrate from a meal. The doses are large and their use is associated with flatulence. They are not in common use.

Alpha-glucosidase inhibitors

These agents competitively inhibit the brush border enzyme that breaks down complex carbohydrates to monosaccharides for absorption. Taken at *exactly* the same time as the meal (tell the patient take the tablet after the first mouthful of food to be sure), they slow glucose absorption and spread it out both geographically along the gut and also in time. This produces a slow sustained rise in blood glucose from a meal, which a failing pancreas finds easier to handle. The subsequent presence of undigested carbohydrate in the lower bowel produces severe flatulence, which has limited their popularity. These agents absolutely require adequate insulin secretory reserve and are therefore best used early in the progression of Type 2 diabetes at the initial failure of diet and exercise alone. There is some evidence that their effect (essentially that of good dieting!) may help match glucose absorption to absorption of exogenous soluble insulin for Type 1 patients and, anecdotally, they have been used to offset the symptoms of 'reactive' (non-diabetic) hypoglycaemia.

Acarbose is the most commonly used of these agents in the UK. Only 2% of the drug is absorbed, making it very safe, although reversible abnormalities of liver function have been reported.

Combination therapy (Figure 7.1)

The preferred first-line agent for overweight and obese Type 2 diabetic patients is metformin and it is common practice and efficacious to add a sulphonylurea in increasing doses when metformin can no longer achieve adequate glycaemic control. Sulphonylureas (or insulin) are recommended in thin patients, particularly if there is on-going weight loss secondary to hyperglycaemia. UKPDS suggested a possible increase in mortality in patients on the metformin–sulphonylurea combination but this has widely been considered a statistical quirk. The combinations are still commonly used. An alternative is to add a thiazolidinedione to either metformin or a sulphonylurea, anticipating a further lowering of HbA_{1c} of around 1–1.5% and this is certainly a practical alternative if the patient cannot tolerate metformin. At the time of writing, the evidence of benefit for adding a thiazolidinedione to metformin *and* a sulphonylurea in triple therapy is lacking, so the combination is not recognized by the   National

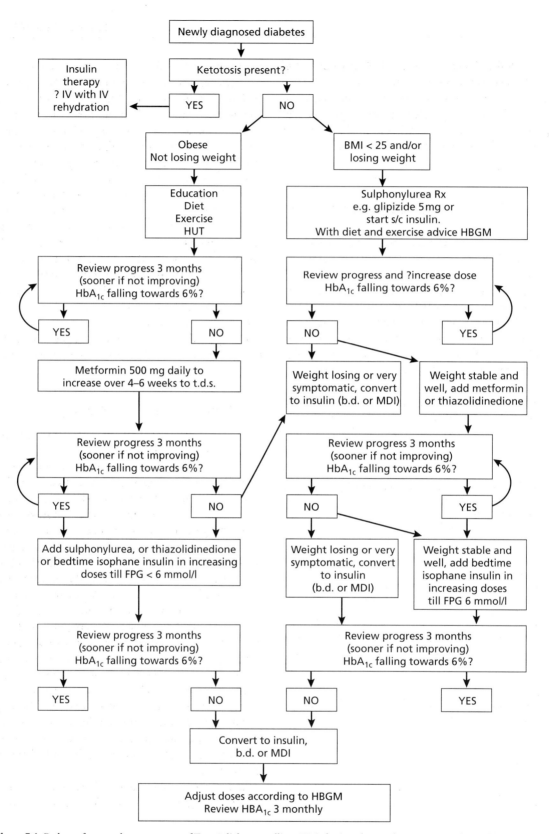

Figure 7.1 Pathway for staged management of Type 2 diabetes mellitus. FPG, fasting plasma glucose; HBGM, home blood glucose monitors; HUT, home urine testing; MDI, multiple daily injection therapy.

Institute for Clinical Excellence (NICE) in the UK but it is likely to work in some patients. Both metformin and sulphonylureas can be used with insulin as the insulin secretory defects of the Type 2 patient progress over time but thiazolidinedione–insulin therapy is not recommended because of fears of fluid retention.

Insulin therapy in Type 2 diabetes (Table 7.2)

Insulin usage in Type 2 diabetes is rising, as an appreciation of the need for strict glycaemic control to prevent microvascular (and possibly macrovascular) complications gains ground. Exogenous insulin becomes necessary as the patient's insulin secretory reserve deteriorates over time but it remains underused in these patients because of fears of insulin therapy both from the patient and the professional. Professional fears include the awareness of insulin resistance and the suspicion that very large doses will be needed in a Type 2 patient; fear of causing weight gain (usually a result of reduced glycosuria) and dislike of inconveniencing the patient with injections. This is

interesting in that this last fear does not extend to excessive use of glucose monitoring. Patient fears include fear of injections (previous experience of which will have been painful intramuscular inoculations and not always competent phlebotomy, using a needle which is orders of magnitude larger than the insulin syringe needle); fear of weight gain; fear of hypoglycaemia (less of a problem in early Type 2 diabetes); in some cases fear of loss of employment; an association of insulin therapy with terminal complications of diabetes (because of health professional reticence with insulin in older friends and relatives); and cultural issues related to injected drugs which vary from population to population. These fears need to be overcome if we are to achieve normoglycaemia in Type 2 diabetic patients and diminish their premature mortality and morbidity.

In Type 2 diabetic patients, there is good evidence that insulin can be effectively combined with oral agents.

Overnight insulin with oral agent therapy

For a description of the different types of insulin therapy available see pages 67 and 70.

The use of bedtime intermediate-acting insulin with oral agents during the day is based on the concept of Type 2 diabetes as a disease of fasting hyperglycaemia, following which the blood glucose remains high all day. There is some evidence for this concept, as the lowest plasma glucose in Type 2 patients treated with diet tends to be not fasting but before the evening meal. Research studies have shown the successful reduction of HbA_{1c} of the order of 1.5–2% with minimal weight gain (compared to other methods of intensifying therapy) in Type 2 patients treated with intermediate acting isophane or ultralong-acting analogue insulin given at bedtime in association with metformin during the day. The patient is instructed to increase his/her insulin dose by 2–4 units every time he/she measures a fasting plasma glucose more than 6 mmol/L on four successive mornings. This can leave patients on very large doses of insulin but does produce substantial benefit and control.

Recent data suggest the new long-acting insulin analogue glargine may work well used in combina-

Table 7.2 Indications for insulin therapy in Type 2 diabetes.

Absolute indications
1 Diabetic ketoacidosis or hyperosmolar coma
2 Pregnancy or the desire for pregnancy (in women)

Relative indications
1 *Inadequate control by other means*
  • Symptomatic hyperglycaemia especially if including weight loss (this is irrespective of the age or comorbidity of the patient)
  • HbA_{1c} too high for optimal achievable prevention of chronic complications (this could be as low as 7% in a young healthy patient and infinite in an elderly patient with terminal other disease)

2 *Intercurrent events*
  • Severe infection with loss of glycaemic control
  • Surgery or other procedure requiring prolonged fasting in any patient on more than diet and exercise
  • Myocardial infarction
  • Probably stroke

3 *Diabetic complications*
  • Renal failure
  • Possibly painful neuropathy

tion with oral agents as a once a day insulin regimen but its benefits over conventional intermediate-acting insulins in Type 2 diabetes remain to be confirmed.

Use of pre meal fast-acting insulin as first-line insulin therapy

There has been much recent discussion about the importance of postprandial glucose of a patient with diabetes and its complications. This stems from the observation that impaired glucose tolerance is a risk factor for cardiovascular disease but there is no evidence that treating post meal hyperglycaemia other than as a way of generally reducing the HbA_{1c} has any survival advantage. Nevertheless, some authorities do recommend the use of short-acting soluble insulins or fast-acting insulin analogues before meals as a way of first insulinizing patients with Type 2 diabetes inadequately controlled by other means. There have been no direct comparisons of this method with overnight insulin, full intensified insulin therapy with basal as well as meal insulin or twice daily mixed insulin.

Twice daily mixed insulin

This is still a widely used method of applying insulin therapy in Type 2 diabetes. The principle is that fast-acting insulin taken before breakfast and the evening meal will cover the subsequent meal and the delayed or intermediate-acting insulin will cover a meal eaten about 6 h later or the night. It is more efficacious in Type 2 than in Type 1 patients, because the residual insulin secretory reserve in the former smooths out the mismatch between insulin requirement and insulin replacement. Weight gain can be substantial.

Basal bolus therapy in Type 2 diabetes

Insulin-requiring Type 2 diabetes can reasonably be treated as Type 1 (see Chapter 8) although this is not as yet a universally accepted policy. However, the introduction of pre meal insulin is a reasonable next step for a patient who is failing to maintain good control on overnight insulin and daytime oral hypoglycaemic agents, leaving the patient on three pre-meal

and one bedtime injection each day. Residual insulin secretion means most Type 2 patients will not need more than one basal intermediate-acting insulin each day.

Aims of therapy in Type 2 diabetes

UKPDS showed a significant reduction in development and progression of microvascular disease in Type 2 diabetes with improved glycaemic control. Reduction in macrovascular disease between intensive and conventional glycaemic control did not reach statistical significance but the fact that these patients were newly diagnosed; the evidence that impaired glucose tolerance is a risk factor and the fact that intensified therapy in UKPDS did not normalize blood glucose control, have all supported suggestions that glycaemic control in Type 2 diabetes needs to be very tight indeed to make a significant impact on cardiovascular mortality. It is currently recommended that attempts are made to get the HbA_{1c} down to the upper end of the non-diabetic range (in DCCT aligned assays this means under 6.5 or even 6%) if feasible. While it is no longer acceptable for a patient with a reasonable life expectancy to leave glycated haemoglobin at 8% or more, control of blood glucose must be incorporated into the management of other risk factors, some of which may take precedence for a time.

Management of blood pressure in Type 2 diabetes

The proper management of blood pressure to appropriate targets is critical in Type 2 diabetes and is discussed in Chapter 20.

Lipid lowering

This is obviously an important part of cardiovascular prevention and is dealt with in Chapter 19.

Obesity

The obese patient is insulin resistant, often with poor glycaemic and blood pressure control. Comorbidities such as osteoarthritis interfere with the patient's ability to exercise. Tackling the obesity alone is difficult. Intensive dietary input may be useful and exercise should be encouraged. In the severely obese, consideration may be given to the use of food absorption inhibitors such as orlistat (Xenical) or centrally acting appetite suppressants such as sibutramine, although uncontrolled hypertension and psychiatric illness are contraindications to the latter. In extreme cases, weight reduction surgery may be undertaken. Certainly, in the short term this produces weight loss and substantial metabolic improvement. However, it should only be performed in centres with considerable expertise as these patients have a high intraoperative risk. Keyhole techniques may help make these procedures safer.

Monitoring of therapy

All patients with Type 2 diabetes should have an HbA_{1c} check every 3 months or so to ensure that their treatment is still adequate and to institute intensification of therapy early as control deteriorates. They also need a check of renal function if on metformin. There is no good evidence to suggest that teaching patients with Type 2 diabetes to measure blood glucose regularly at home provides biomedical benefit. Indeed, it seems to increase stress levels without delivering improved glycaemic control. On this basis, patients with no risk of hypoglycaemia (those on diet and exercise and insulin sensitizers) should be adequately managed on urine testing — they should aim for urines that are usually free of glucose and use the appearance of glycosuria as an indication of deteriorating control and the need to seek advice. The 3-monthly HbA_{1c} will then provide further evidence about the adequacy of their glucose control.

Home blood glucose monitoring becomes important when insulin therapy is started so that patients can self-adjust doses. It may also be of importance in tightly controlled patients on insulin secretagogues where hypoglycaemia is a risk of intensification of therapy and is a useful skill for the management of intercurrent illness.

Management of Type 2 diabetes during illness

For minor illnesses, hyperglycaemia is likely but probably does not require treatment, apart from encouragement of intake of sugar-free fluids. The hyperglycaemia of stress may be partially offset by any associated anorexia. At these times it is useful if the patient can test their blood glucose levels, as this will support any decisions they make about self-management if not eating. Four-hourly testing is recommended. It is usual to suggest continuing oral agents if blood glucose is over 9 mmol/L and/or urine remains negative for glucose (and ketones). A glass of fresh fruit juice, milk, soup, ice cream, yoghurt and cereal can be tried in place of usual meals. Tablets can be withheld if blood glucose is low or urine tests negative, and restarted as glucose levels rise or glycosuria occurs. Medical intervention will be required if the illness persists for more than 48 h. If the stress of the illness is severe enough to precipitate symptomatic hyperglycaemia, patients may need to intensify treatment and may require hospitalization for insulin therapy.

Type 2 diabetic patients on anything other than diet and exercise are likely to require hospitalization and intravenous insulin for more serious illness and for surgical procedures requiring them to be nil by mouth. This is certainly true for patients on more than tiny doses of insulin secretagogues, where stopping eating exposes them to risk of hypoglycaemia and stopping their tablets to uncontrolled hyperglycaemia. There are good data from the insulin and glucose infusion in acute myocardial infarction (DIGAMI) study to show the benefits of insulin therapy in patients with and after myocardial infarction and on surgical intensive care units. It is likely that similar data will shortly be available to confirm or refute the benefits of insulin therapy in acute stroke. Because of concerns that some ionic contrast media used in radiology may precipitate renal impairment, it is usual to stop metformin 48 h before and restart 48 h after procedures such as angiography, intravenous pyelography, etc. These issues are dealt with more fully in Chapter 11.

8

Management of Type 1 Diabetes Mellitus

Summary

- Type 1 diabetes mellitus is an insulin deficiency disease appropriately treated with insulin replacement

- Insulin treatment regimens need to replace both basal insulin, to control endogenous glucose production, and meal-related requirements

- Dietary restrictions have traditionally been used for improved glucose control because of the imperfections of exogenous insulins

- People with diabetes can be taught to use insulin flexibly to minimize lifestyle restrictions, using multiple daily insulin injections

- New insulin analogues and insulin delivery systems do offer the potential for more physiological insulin replacement but conventional insulins can be used very successfully in flexible regimens too

- Regular home blood glucose monitoring is essential for good control

- The target for insulin replacement should be the re-establishment of normal metabolism, however:

  - Targets may need to be modified in line with clinical states; and

  - Optimal regimens need to be modified in line with patient choice

- Non-glucose risk factors for microvascular and macrovascular disease need active management, separate from the insulin replacement therapy

- Regular review for the development of complications and their active management form an essential part of therapy

Type 1 diabetes is a disease of insulin deficiency. Logically therefore the treatment should be by replacement of insulin alone. Because of the inadequacies of currently available insulin therapies, it is traditional also to prescribe dietary restrictions and modifications designed to allow the achievement of good glycaemic control with minimal risk of hypoglycaemia. Dietary advice is needed to deal with the pharmaco-dynamics of exogenous insulins, which differ significantly from those of endogenous insulin. However, times are changing. There is now good evidence to show that many patients can be taught enough about food values and insulin requirements to manage their own insulin flexibly and virtually without dietary restriction. This is changing the way we think about insulin usage. Furthermore, new insulins are being developed that have more physiological action profiles which may help patients achieve normoglycaemia more readily than previously.

History

Insulin was discovered in 1921 and rapidly became available as a therapy for people with Type 1 diabetes. Early insulins were extracted from animal (cow and pig) pancreas, differing from human insulin in three and one amino acids, respectively. These early insulins were soluble and fairly short acting. However, these insulin preparations contained significant amounts of other pancreatic polypeptides which encouraged the formation of binding antibodies that complicated their action. From the mid-1930s, inclusion of retardants of insulin absorption from their site of injection under the skin, such as zinc and protamine, created intermediate- and long-acting insulins, designed for delayed or prolonged action. In 1972, chromatography was used to separate out insulin from other pancreatic peptides and to produce highly purified or monocomponent insulins, each of which had a faster onset and shorter duration of action than their less pure peer. At the beginning of the 1980s, with the coming of age of molecular biology, the human insulin gene was introduced into microorganisms such as bacteria or yeast in order to produce large amounts of insulin with the molecular structure of human insulin. This was expected to be less immunogenic than even the monocomponent insulins and have potential advantages for human patients, although the antibody formation with human insulin is similar to that seen with highly purified pork insulin. The human insulins, because they are synthetic, can theoretically be produced in unlimited quantities, supplying the world's insulin needs at less cost. However, they were not introduced as cheaper versions of the older forms. Further developments of molecular biology have allowed the synthesis of new insulin analogues with small changes in the amino acid sequence of the human insulin molecule which confer specific pharmacokinetic properties deemed to be desirable.

Exogenous insulin has to be injected subcutaneously as it would be digested if taken by mouth.

Short-acting insulins (soluble) can also be given intravenously, or even intramuscularly, if necessary in emergency situations. Insulin can also be delivered into the peritoneal cavity, from whence about 50% is absorbed directly into the portal vein of the liver. This may have some advantages, including possibly less risk of hypoglycaemia, but is an expensive and complex procedure only currently available as a research tool. Other research efforts are examining the possibility of delivering insulin through the pulmonary alveoli so that it could be inhaled rather than injected. Long-term safety data are awaited and this is not yet available in routine clinical practice.

Currently available insulin preparations
(Table 8.1)

A scheme of the time course of action of the various insulins currently available is shown in Fig. 8.1. These profiles are dictated by the rate at which the insulin is absorbed from the subcutaneous injection into the circulation from where it is active. The index profile considered is that of conventional soluble insulin but this forms hexamers in solution which have to be broken down into dimers and monomers for absorption. This delays and prolongs the action of the insulin, relative to the pharmacokinetics of endogenous insulin. In intermediate- or delayed-acting insulins, the absorption of insulin is retarded by excess amounts of protamine or zinc in the insulin preparation. It should be noted that the absorption of conventional insulins shows marked intrapatient variability, so that the time course of action is never wholly predictable. Insulins are available as highly purified extracts from animal pancreas or biosynthetically by insertion of the insulin gene (human or modified) into bacteria (*crb*, *prb*) or yeast (*pyr*). Human insulin made by enzymatic modification of animal insulin is no longer listed in the *British National Formulary*.

Ready-mixed insulins

Of limited use in Type 1 diabetes, there do exist a number of insulin preparations which contain both a

Table 8.1 Commonly used types of insulin for subcutaneous injection.

Generic name	Onset	Peak	Duration	Examples
Fast-acting insulins				
Soluble (regular)	30 min	2–4 h	6–8 h	Human Actrapid
Human				Humulin S
Pork				HumanVelosulin
Beef				Pork Actrapid
				Hypurin Porcine Neutral
				Hypurin Bovine Neutral
Monomeric insulins	15 min	50 min	3–5 h	NovoRapid
				Humalog
Intermediate-acting insulins				
Isophane insulin	2 h	4–8 h	12–18 h	Human Insulatard
				Humulin I
				Pork Insulatard
				Hypurin Porcine Isophane
				Hypurin Bovine Isophane
Insulin zinc suspension insulins crystalline	2 h	4–8 h	12–24 h	Human Monotard
				Humulin Lente
				Hypurin Bovine Lente
				Human Ultratard
				Humulin Zn
Long-acting insulin analogues				
Insulin glargine	2 h	none	18–36 h	Lantus
Biphasic insulins				
	One peak as soluble			Human Mixtard 10, 20,
	One peak as intermediate			30, 40 and 50
				Pork Mixtard 30
				Hypurin Porcine 30/70 mix
				Humalog Mix25 and Mix50
				Novomix 30

fast- and a delayed-acting insulin. Such 'premixed' insulins can be useful in patients with very regular lifestyles (see below) and may also be useful in Type 2 diabetes (see page 64).

Novel insulin analogues

The fast-acting analogues (Humalog and Novo-Rapid) have small changes in their molecular structure which make the molecules less likely to stick together than conventional human or animal insulins, which tend to form hexamers in solution. The two analogues remain largely monomeric in solution and are absorbed more quickly from the subcutaneous depot. This accounts for their faster onset, sharper peak and shorter duration of action. They give better control of the immediate post meal blood glucose but may not last until the next insulin injection becomes active. Their use is associated with reduced risk of nocturnal hypoglycaemia (see Chapter 9). The monomeric insulins are designed as meal-related injections. Synthetic insulins with flatter and more prolonged absorption profiles relative to isophane and lente insulins are beginning to be available. These include insulins that are insoluble at physiological pH (e.g. Lantus) or which have an attached fatty acid chain binding them to albumin for slow release. These insulins have theoretical benefit as

(a) Multiple daily injection therapy 1

(b) Multiple daily injection therapy 2

(c) Twice daily mixed insulins

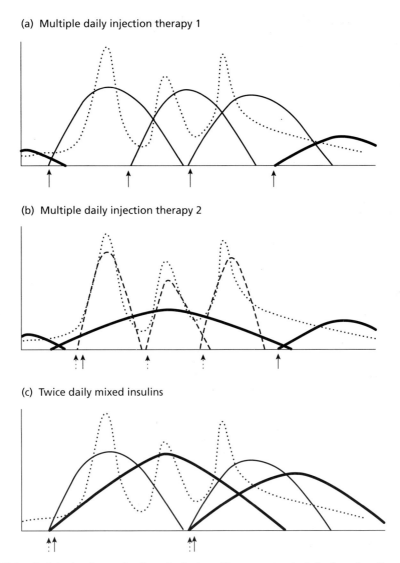

Fig. 8.1 Multiple daily insulin injection therapy. In all panels, the dotted line represents the daily plasma insulin profile of the healthy person eating three meals a day. The up arrows represent the timing of the insulin injections, the down arrows food. (a) Pre meal soluble insulin (solid line) with bedtime isophane (heavy solid line). Note that the rise in insulin after soluble injections before meals is quite slow, which may result in postprandial hyperglycaemia, followed by relative hyperinsulinaemia in the late postprandial period, risking hypoglycaemia before the next meal. The latter is dealt with by ingesting snacks between meals. (b) Pre meal insulin analogues (hatched line) with twice daily isophane (heavy solid line). The faster absorption of the analogue allows better control of the postprandial glucose and the shorter duration of action reduces the drive to hypoglycaemia in the night. The independent replacement of all basal insulin (daytime as well as night-time) prevents running out of insulin between meals. Sometimes, extra isophane is also needed at the evening meal time to avoid running out of insulin before the onset of action of the bedtime isophane. (c) Twice daily mixed insulins (heavy solid lines). There is significant hyperinsulinaemia between meals and often in the middle of the night, with risk of hypoglycaemia. Paradoxically, the overnight isophane, given in the mixture before the evening meal, may not last until the following morning, especially when the evening meal is taken early. Moving this dose alone to bedtime (often with a dose reduction) may be very effective, still allowing a mixed dose to be used in the morning to avoid the patient needing to inject at lunchtime.

background replacement but their clinical advantages remain to be proven.

Inhaled insulin

As a response to people's natural reluctance to self-inject, many attempts have been made to provide an insulin that can be taken by other routes. The oral route has proven impossible to date (although research continues) but nasal insulin has been studied and there are currently major attempts to develop and market insulins to be taken by inhalation. The insulin is absorbed across the alveolar membranes of the lungs, which are about the area of tennis court. Initial studies show favourable absorption profiles for a fast-acting insulin, akin to those of monomeric analogue insulin, but the bioavailability is poor compared to subcutaneous insulin, making this an expensive option. There is an urgent need to demonstrate that there will be no long-term detrimental effects on the lungs before these insulins can be generally accepted. It is the opinion of the author that the major role for inhaled insulin will be if its availability makes insulin therapy more acceptable to people who need it but not to survive—Type 2 diabetic patients in suboptimal control on other therapies. For all but a few Type 1 patients with needle phobia, the injections themselves are not the worst part of their treatment regimen.

Physiological insulin secretion

The healthy human pancreas secretes a background of insulin, delivered directly to the liver, throughout the 24-h period. The principal action of this, with balanced secretion of its antagonist glucagon, is to control endogenous glucose production so that it precisely matches glucose uptake by brain and peripheral insulin-sensitive tissues and blood glucose concentration is maintained within a narrow normal range. Because of diurnal variation in insulin sensitivity, insulin secretion is minimal around 2–3 a.m., rising slowly thereafter to the fasting value. In addition to this background of insulin, the healthy pancreas produces a short-lived insulin secretory burst in response to meals. Exogenous insulin re-

placement therapy aims to reproduce as closely as possible this physiological profile, using mixtures of the insulins described above (Fig. 8.1).

Multiple daily injection therapy (intensified insulin therapy)

Using currently available insulins, the closest approximation to normality is to try to replace background insulin with one or more daily injections of an intermediate- or long-acting insulin in modest doses and use a soluble insulin or a fast-acting analogue before meals. With soluble insulins, the injection is best taken approximately 30 min before a meal is eaten. Because of the long duration of soluble insulin action (relative to the normal prandial insulin peak from a healthy pancreas), these preprandial injections are often also expected to provide the background insulin between meals. An intermediate- or long-acting insulin is then taken at bedtime, intended to remain active through to the following morning to control the fasting blood glucose. Problems with this regimen include the relatively long action of the soluble insulin, which usually means that if enough is taken to cover the immediate postprandial need, hypoglycaemia will supervene before the next meal. The patient is committed to taking snacks between meals to offset this. Replacing the background insulin with twice daily intermediate-acting insulin (before breakfast and before bed) and using smaller doses of soluble insulin before meals, intended just for the meal, may give more stable control. Smaller doses of any insulin are absorbed more quickly than larger doses, because they have a larger surface area : volume ratio, so there may be slightly less tendency to hypoglycaemia between meals.

Using monomeric analogues instead of soluble insulin before meals, the injection must be taken immediately before eating a carbohydrate-containing meal, or hypoglycaemia may ensue. These insulins provide better control of the postprandial blood glucose. However, the patient may run out of insulin before the next meal-related dose. This can be dealt with by incorporating one or two additional injections of intermediate-acting insulin at breakfast and/or at another meal time to provide a stable background. There may be less need to snack between meals with analogues, especially if the meal-related dose is minimized by the provision of adequate background insulin replacement.

Approximately 40–60% of a patient's total daily insulin requirement should be in the background insulin, with the remaining 60–40% divided between meals. In general, patients require most insulin for breakfast, least for lunch and an intermediate amount for the evening meal, almost irrespective of the sizes of these meals, because of diurnal variations in insulin sensitivity and in activity level. Doses should be adjusted on the basis of home glucose monitoring records. Patients should be encouraged to test before meals and at bedtime and adjust their doses every few days to achieve target preprandial glucose levels of around 4–7 mmol/L and, if testing after meals, 6–9 mmol/L 90 min to 2 h after meals. These adjustments are best made prospectively, on the basis of the readings made over the previous few days, trying to correct patterns where readings are consistently outside the target range at particular times of day. It is also appropriate to adjust single doses in anticipation of increased food intake or exercise, and to take small corrective doses for unexpectedly high readings, provided in the latter case that recurrent need for correction is followed by an appropriate prospective adjustment in routine dose to obviate the problem. Self-adjustment on this scale requires the patient to be well educated and confident in the workings of insulin, food and exercise on his/her body.

The quoted target ranges are the ideal, and patients may need higher goals if they have difficulty in testing frequently or making appropriate adjustments to their insulin.

When converting from a simple regimen to a more intensive flexible regimen of twice daily basal injections and soluble or analogue injections before meals, the total daily dosage should be reduced by about 20%. Thereafter, 50% of the residual total insulin dosage is put into the background insulin (equally divided between the morning and evening injections) and 50% is used for meal control—divided between the three main meals, again with most for breakfast and least for lunch. If patients can be taught to estimate the carbohydrate content of their meals correctly, they may choose to vary the dose of the meal insulins accordingly, with the greatest ratio of insulin : carbohydrate for breakfast and least for lunch.

Modified multiple daily injection regimens

Some patients find injecting in the middle of the day inconvenient or embarrassing. This particularly applies to schoolchildren. In this circumstance, the lunchtime insulin injection can be replaced by intermediate-acting insulin administered at breakfast, in the expectation that it will reach its peak action 6 h later. Intermediate-acting insulin can be combined with fast-acting insulin for breakfast in the same syringe, provided the injection is given rapidly after mixing to prevent loss of the fast-acting insulin effect. Such a regimen may work very well for a patient whose meal times are predictable and conventional, with approximately 6 h between breakfast and lunch, although a snack is required mid morning and mid afternoon if good control is to be maintained and hypoglycaemia avoided. Readymixed insulins, in various ratios, are available and can be used to simplify the injection before breakfast but allow much less flexibility and no independent adjustment of the breakfast and lunchtime insulins.

Twice daily mixed insulins

Use of twice daily mixed insulin should not be encouraged in Type 1 diabetes. They have been popular for many years because in theory the mixture of a short- and an intermediate-acting insulin before breakfast provides insulin for breakfast and lunch while a similar mix before the evening meal provides insulin for the evening meal and overnight. The problems include inflexibility, postprandial hyperinsulinaemia, as the action of the soluble insulin wanes and the intermediate-acting insulin begins, and the failure of the pre evening meal intermediate-acting insulin to provide adequate cover for the night. Its peak action will occur in the middle of the night when it is least needed thereby causing nocturnal hypoglycaemia, and there is a likelihood, particularly if the evening meal is taken early, of the insulin not lasting through to the following morning. Where the soluble insulin in these regimens is replaced by fast-acting analogue, slightly better post breakfast and post evening meal control may be achieved and nocturnal hypoglycaemia may be less of a problem.

Twice daily mixed insulin regimens are acceptable in patients where tight control is not desirable for other reasons, or for patients who are unable to deal with a more flexible and physiological regimen. They may provide respectable control in Type 2 diabetes where there is residual endogenous insulin secretion. While we do not recommend using these regimens in Type 1 patients, if a particular patient is achieving good control, satisfactory lifestyle and no problematic hypoglycaemia by using one, the regimen should not be changed just for the sake of it!

Diet in Type 1 diabetes

It is important to encourage patterns of healthy eating in Type 1 diabetes because of the increased risk of vascular disease. Therefore, the dietary principles outlined in Chapter 2 are appropriate. Patients should know the advantages of consuming a diet that obtains no more than 30% of the total energy content from fat, with at least half that fat being unsaturated or polyunsaturated. They should also know that eating and drinking simple sugars, such as non-diet fizzy drinks, fresh fruit juice, jams, cakes and other similar foods will produce a rapid rise in blood glucose concentrations, which cannot easily be handled by exogenous insulins. Likewise, the fairly even spread of caloric intake in regular meals taken throughout the day is important to help achieve good glycaemic control and control fat metabolism and avoid hypoglycaemia. However, it should be recognized that the real exigencies of the Type 1 diabetic diet are dictated by the inadequacy of exogenous insulin regimens, rather than the nature of the disease itself. This does not make them less important clinically but it is important to recognize why the patient's food intake is so rigidly controlled in Type 1 diabetes, so that research can be appropriately devoted towards improv-

ing the treatment regimens to enable Type 1 diabetic patients to enjoy the same dietary freedoms and make the same choices as the non-diabetic. This is in sharp contrast to the Type 2 diabetic patient where poor diet and lifestyle are major contributors to the disease process and are therefore a legitimate target for therapy.

In order to deal with the relative hyperinsulinaemia post-meal created by exogenously injected insulins, it is usual to instruct Type 1 diabetic patients to consume three meals a day at roughly 6-h intervals, interspersed with carbohydrate-containing snacks. One of the biggest problems for the patient is the insistence upon eating at times when they would not normally choose to do so but, if aiming for tight control with good postprandial glucose readings and an absence of hypoglycaemia before the next meal and in the night, snacking between meals and at bedtime is almost unavoidable.

Historically, patients were taught to 'carbohydrate count' or estimate the grams of carbohydrates contained in different foods so that the carbohydrate content in each meal and snack could be prescribed to match the prescribed insulin dose. This rigidity became deeply unpopular and for many years UK dietitians have advocated the principles of healthy eating only, in the expectation that insulin would be prescribed to match the food taken. This is still widespread practice, and has obvious potential health benefits, but it does mean that the diabetic patient in tight control is often on a very rigid lifestyle pattern and cannot easily accommodate deviations from routine. There is now evidence that it is possible to use carbohydrate counting very differently and teach patients how to adjust meal-related injections of soluble or monomeric insulin flexibly at the time of eating, judging the dose according to estimated carbohydrate content, general principles and personal experience. Such patients will describe their doses in ratios (units of insulin to grams or portions of carbohydrate) rather than as fixed doses. One of the limitations of such flexible regimens is the absence of an ideal background insulin and two or more injections of isophane insulin are usually used. These types of regimens have been in use in Europe for many years and have recently been introduced into the UK as the

Dose Adjustment for Normal Eating (DAFNE) project. Patients require full skills training in replacing insulin matched to desired food intake and exercise and this has been delivered to date in five day teaching packages, using principles of adult education and a set curriculum, by specially trained diabetes educators. The aim of the programme is to allow patients to achieve good glycaemic control while eating flexibly and to render them more independent of professional advice.

Continuous subcutaneous insulin therapy (pump therapy)

The most flexible insulin replacement regimen currently available to patients is insulin pump therapy. A monomeric insulin (such as NovoRapid) is placed in a syringe-like reservoir and is inserted into a small pump that will deliver the insulin through a cannula attaching the reservoir to a subcutaneous needle worn by the patient, at rates that are programmed into the pump. The pump can be activated to deliver measured bolus doses of insulin, which are effectively the same as pre-meal injections on intermittent insulin regimens.

The advantage of pump therapy is that background insulin is delivered at a steady rate, without the peak and trough effect of intermediate- or long-acting insulins. This basal rate can be varied according to the time of day to accommodate patients who, for example, have a significant rise in insulin requirements towards the morning (the 'dawn phenomenon'). A patient can also afford to miss meals as his/her background insulin replacement is independent of meal-related boluses.

One of the problems of insulin pump therapy is that its benefits have not been unequivocally demonstrated in many randomized controlled trials. There have been many demonstrations of improved control with the institution of pump therapy, but invariably the starting of pump therapy includes a major educational input in which patients are taught to estimate the carbohydrate content of their meals and learn the ratio of insulin analogue required for each unit of carbohydrate to be consumed. Intensive education is

very important with pump therapy as, in the absence of any subcutaneous depot of insulin, any interruption to insulin flow will rapidly result in hyperglycaemia and ketosis. Patients undertaking pump therapy, to be safe, need to commit themselves to at least four times daily blood glucose monitoring and, if they are to achieve good blood glucose control, also need to understand how to use the information from their home glucose monitoring to adjust their doses both at the time of doing the blood test and prospectively. Failure to do this makes pump therapy dangerous because of the increased risk of hyperglycaemia and ketosis, and also less effective.

In the randomized controlled trials that do exist, there is a consistent suggestion of small but significant improvement in glycated haemoglobin (of the order of about 0.5%) and there is good evidence of reduction in severe hypoglycaemia. The main evidence-based indication for insulin pump therapy can therefore currently be considered to be problematic hypoglycaemia not amenable to optimization of conventional therapy. It is also logical to assume that pump therapy may also be appropriate for patients with a marked dawn phenomenon. If fasting hyperglycaemia is a result of inadequate duration of action of intermediate- or long-acting insulins, pump therapy is a good current solution, although an effective long-acting analogue may be another option. These indications apart, there are patients who prefer the lifestyle achieved using an insulin pump, an option that is now available if they are prepared to pay for it.

Pump therapy, while not expensive compared to many treatments for other chronic diseases, is expensive compared to conventional insulin therapy administered by needle or pen devices. At the time of writing, the pump itself costs slightly over £2000 and the additional running costs in terms of reservoirs and plastic cannulae (which can be quite sophisticated and include devices to allow them to be disconnected and reconnected without introducing air and often using flexible non-metal 'needles') costs £1000 to £3000 each year. There is also the additional health professional input required for educating the patient in pump usage, although this is a short-term cost for each individual. Ultimately, well-educated pump users should become more independent of their professional teams, being able to adjust their insulin appropriately themselves.

Developing therapies

No current therapy for Type 1 diabetes is ideal. What is needed is a method of restoring glucose-sensitive insulin delivery. 'Closing the loop' by linking an insulin delivery device such as a pump to an on-line glucose monitor is considered an important target, the achievement of which is mostly limited by the absence of a glucose monitor that will work consistently and reliably *in vivo*. Glucose measurement *in vivo* is plagued by difficulties, including the need for consistent calibration and the tendency of the body to isolate foreign bodies with an inflammatory or scarring response. Methods examined include enzyme-based methods similar to those used in current home blood glucose meters but made suitable for wearing, and the use of infrared spectroscopy. A device that measures interstitial glucose every 5 min over a period of up to 3 days using a probe inserted into the subcutaneous tissue (the Continuous Glucose Monitoring System of Minimed/Medtronic) shows most promise and is already in clinical use as a monitoring device. One study using an intravascular device to measure blood glucose suggested that closing the loop was possible over 48 h but there was still a rise in postprandial glucose as the system has to measure a rising glucose before increasing insulin delivery. Another consideration is the need for the patient to be wearing two devices—a colleague has likened this to John Wayne wearing a holster on each hip!

It follows that replacing the original islets may be the most desirable way of restoring glucose-responsive insulin secretion. Whole organ pancreas transplantation can restore normoglycaemia reasonably reliably now but remains a major operation still generally reserved for people undergoing renal transplantation for diabetes-induced end-stage renal failure. Infusing only the isolated islets (into the portal vein of the liver) is a much less traumatic procedure but only recently successful in achieving insulin independence. Success depends on acquiring skill in the difficult techniques of separating the islets from the rest of the pancreas, good coordination between transplant teams and expert interventional radiology and the improvement of immunosuppressive regimens. Eliminating the need for steroids seems to have been a very important step but immunosuppression remains complex and needs to be more focused and safer before islet transplantation becomes acceptable as a routine therapy. Meanwhile, the apparent need for more than one donor per patient to achieve insulin independence also limits the extension of the technique. Even with two donors, only about 20% of the normal insulin secretory capacity is restored with current techniques and as yet the long-term function of the grafts has to be demonstrated. Research into growing islets in culture or developing new sources of glucose-responsive insulin secreting cells remains a high priority. Until these problems and those of immunosuppression are solved, islet transplantation is reserved for those in whom insulin therapy is failing in a very major way. Suitable patients for what is still a research procedure are those with recurrent severe hypoglycaemia despite optimization of conventional therapy, where there is evidence of benefit. Another possible indication may be rapidly advancing early complications (renal impairment makes the immunosuppressive regimens in current use too toxic), again despite optimized medical therapy.

Techniques of insulin injection

Insulin is injected into subcutaneous fat. The favoured sites are shown in Fig. 8.2. Specifically designed disposable syringes with attached needles are available in three syringe sizes for use with U100 insulins—0.3, 0.5 and 1.0 mL, taking a maximum of 30, 50 and 100 units, respectively. Needle sizes also differ—6, 8 or 12 mm, with the shortest being most suitable for slim people and children. Two techniques for injection are recommended—either vertically down through the skin, or at a 45° angle into a fold of skin pinched up between the fingers. The skin should be clean but it is not necessary routinely to use an alcohol wipe. If insulins are to be mixed in one syringe before administration, it is important not to contaminate the soluble insulin (clear) vial with

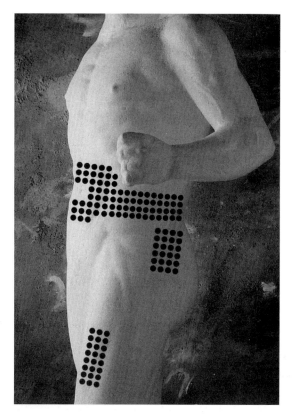

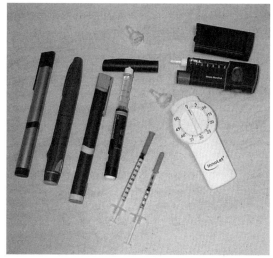

Fig. 8.3 Examples of insulin injection devices. Photograph courtesy of Dr Stephen Thomas.

Fig. 8.2 Appropriate sites of injection for insulin. Photograph reproduced from the UK DAFNE teaching materials by permission of the DAFNE Steering Committee.

intermediate-acting insulin (cloudy), as surplus retardant in the latter may compromise the fast action of the soluble insulin. The soluble insulin should therefore be drawn up first and the intermediate-acting insulin then added into the syringe. If air is injected into the vials before insulin extraction, the sequence should be 'air into the cloudy, air into the clear; draw up clear, draw up cloudy'. For economic reasons, patients should be asked to reuse disposable syringes for up to 3 days.

The use of pen devices with a reservoir of 3 mL insulin which can be injected through a detachable needle without need to draw up the insulin from a separate vial has greatly facilitated multiple daily injection therapy (Fig. 8.3). The pens are designed so that the dose can be entered by dialling a number.

When the device is activated, the dialled dose is delivered. Care must be taken that all air is removed from the reservoirs or 'cartridges' by injecting a couple of units into the air with the pen held pointing upwards prior to injection. The needle should be replaced for each injection with pen devices, although some patients reuse each needle several times, leaving it *in situ* in between. This is not advisable because it increases the risk of air entering the cartridge (so the air-clearing step is important) and because modern needles are very fine and breakages have been reported. Also important is adequate mixing of non-soluble insulins. They do not mix well in the narrow pen cartridges and repeated inversion about 20 times is necessary to ensure mixing. Failure to do this may mean that insulin given towards the end of the life of a cartridge has a very different concentration from at the beginning, an additional cause of glycaemic instability.

After injection, the patient should leave the needle in the skin for a few seconds (e.g. while counting slowly to 10). Failure to do this may allow insulin to leak back along the needle track, and the patient receiving less (and variable) amounts with each dose. This problem is noted as a droplet of insulin on the skin after injection.

Side-effects of insulin therapy

Oedema and weight gain

When insulin therapy is instituted rapidly in a very underinsulinized patient, the insulin may cause salt and water retention and clinically obvious although temporary oedema. Reducing glycosuria (which can account for up to 500 kcal/day) also promotes weight gain. Insulin also inhibits lipolysis and protein breakdown. Patients report that insulin stimulates appetite, although it is not known whether this is a response to a general improvement in well-being. It is important to guard against regimens where patients feels the need to eat extra food to avoid hypoglycaemia—in such circumstances the insulin dose should be reduced.

Lipohypertrophy

Fatty lumps at injection sites are common and occasionally so large as to be unsightly. They tend to develop if injections are repeatedly given over a very limited area of skin. For this reason it is best to vary the site of injection from day to day. Lipohypertrophy is rarely troublesome but once present tends to persist: the occasional very large fatty tumour may even require surgical removal. Furthermore, if insulin is repeatedly injected into a fatty lump the rate of absorption may be delayed.

Insulin allergy

This is very rare and in most cases presents as urticaria at the site of injection. It is usually caused by the preservatives in the insulin solution rather than the insulin itself and can sometimes be treated by changing the insulin preparation or manufacturer. In refractory cases insulin allergy can be treated by desensitization.

Hypoglycaemia (see also Chapter 9)

The major acute side-affect of insulin therapy is hypoglycaemia. This is a risk whenever the exogenous insulin levels are higher than the endogenous insulin level would be at that time in a healthy person. Times of particular risk are between meals and in the middle of the night, although hypoglycaemia can occur at any time. The insulin user must be instructed in physiological processes that increase the risk of hypoglycaemia. The two major offenders are intermittent exercise and intermittent alcohol consumption. Both cause delayed hypoglycaemia and patients need to reduce the overnight insulin and sometimes also the fast-acting insulin the next morning after unusual exertion or alcohol consumption—and especially after both. Omission of a meal is another common cause of hypoglycaemia. Hypoglycaemia is discussed in more detail in Chapter 9.

Glucose monitoring

The insulin-treated Type 1 diabetic patient should undertake regular home blood glucose monitoring. Good glycaemic control, of the degree indicated by research trials as conferring protection from the development of microvascular complications, can only be achieved by a well-motivated patient with a good understanding of the workings of their insulin and food interaction. For convenience, it is usual for the patient to test before meals and before bed and if the glucose targets are achieved at this time and the HbA_{1c} is within the target range for the patient, postprandial glucose monitoring on the basis of present evidence is probably not essential. However, postprandial monitoring becomes very important if the patient is experiencing problems with glycaemic control or if the HbA_{1c} is significantly higher than suggested by preprandial glucose levels. In this circumstance, it is common to find that the patient is underinsulinized for meals and skipping snacks between meals, resulting in high postprandial glucose levels with no hypoglycaemia by the next meal respectively. Postprandial monitoring should be undertaken 90 min after completion of meals, with the possible exception of in pregnancy (see Chapter 12). This is because of the near impossibility of matching the absorption of insulin and food, with high risk of a transient post meal glucose peak, which conventional soluble insulins cannot manage without increased risk of hypoglycaemia. Postprandial glucose monitoring may become more important if the present hypothesis that postprandial hyperglycaemia causes increased risk of macrovascular disease for any given HbA_{1c} is proved correct.

Ideal glucose targets are around 4–7 mmol/L pre meal, 6–9 mmol/L post meal. It is usual to suggest to patients on soluble insulins that the pre-bedtime snack glucose should be between 7 and 9 mmol/L to diminish the risk of nocturnal hypoglycaemia. This last is probably not necessary in patients using monomeric analogues. Some patients who cannot achieve such tight goals fear for their future, and it is important neither to frighten nor discourage them in their efforts. HbA_{1c} should be the best possible without creating problematic hypoglycaemia. HbA_{1c} values of 6.5–7% are usually considered a good compromise in DCCT aligned assays. Such tight targets should only be recommended to patients who are motivated to achieve them and who develop a good understanding of their insulin regimen. It is important to stress the risks of low (as well as the upper) limits of the normal range in order to avoid hypoglycaemia, which is potentially very dangerous. All patients should have access to a glycated haemoglobin measurement approximately every 3–4 months so that they can establish for themselves that they are remaining within target.

Typically, home blood glucose monitoring is performed by the patient on a droplet of capillary blood expressed from a tiny stab wound in the fingertip. The skin is punctured by a small lancet and it is important to recognize that modern spring-loaded devices, used with monitors that require only a tiny blood drop, are essential — old fashioned hand-held lancets and devices needing large blood drops are unacceptably painful and difficult to use. The finger should be clean, as glucose on the finger will result in falsely high readings and newsprint and other chemicals may make the reading artificially low, but dry, as damp will cause the blood to spread over the finger rather than drop onto the device. Alcohol wipes should not be used. A warm finger bleeds more efficiently than a cold one. The side of the finger is marginally less painful than the very tip. The blood is dropped onto a reagent pad on a test strip specifically designed for the particular meter and calibrated to it. The chemical reaction triggers a signal, in the old days colorimetric but now electronic, and the meter gives a reading, usually calibrated to compare to plasma glucose. Common failings include insufficient blood on the reagent pad (less common with modern devices), contaminated skin and omitting to calibrate meters to the specific batch of strips in use. More commonly, the blood tests simply are not performed! Making a hole large enough to bleed in a very sensitive body region is uncomfortable as well as inconvenient. Devices that take blood from less sensitive areas, such as the forearm, are beginning to appear but there are concerns that at least some of these give readings that lag behind fingertip capillary blood glucose measurements to a potentially dangerous degree.

Meters often store several glucose readings but beware of encouraging the patient to depend on the meter memory for observing his/her control. The best use of the memory is to avoid the need to write down the result every time a test is made but the patient should be encouraged to download these memories into a glucose diary every few days, so he/she can look for patterns in their glucose control and make adjustments to their therapy. For this, the meter's clock needs to be working! Professionals should also be sensitive to the extreme difficulty people have in admitting to 'failing' and the great psychological pressure not to record results that are way out of range.

The availability of continuous glucose monitoring emphasizes the imperfections of currently available insulin regimens, with a high detection of hypoglycaemia and wide swings in plasma glucose levels.

Urine monitoring

It follows that urine monitoring for glucose is only recommended when the patient cannot use home blood glucose monitoring. Properly used, urine monitoring can give useful information about periods of hyperglycaemia but it must be realized that glycosuria reflects a blood glucose exceeding the renal threshold for glucose (usually 10 mmol/L although it may be higher in the elderly and is lower in pregnancy) during the period of urine production. Because the aim is to achieve urine tests negative for glucose, they cannot establish the presence of hypoglycaemia. Urine monitoring for ketones is a useful skill so that patients can assess their insulin lack when ill.

Management of non-glucose factors in Type 1 diabetes

Patients with Type 1 diabetes require regular monitoring for the risk factors for complications and for early complications themselves. If found, these need active management. The management of hypertension, hyperlipidaemia and specific complications is dealt with in the relevant chapters.

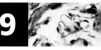

Hypoglycaemia

Summary

- Hypoglycaemia is defined in diabetes as a plasma glucose concentration of less than 3.5 mmol/L

- Hypoglycaemia is an inevitable event in patients using exogenous insulin but therapy must be managed to minimize risk of severe hypoglycaemia. It is also a risk in Type 2 patients treated with insulin secretagogues but is minimal in Type 2 patients on diet, exercise and/or insulin sensitizers alone

- Severe hypoglycaemia is defined as an episode in which the patient was unable to treat him/herself because of cognitive incapacity induced by the low blood glucose

- Problematic hypoglycaemia includes the occurrence of severe episodes and of episodes which are asymptomatic as the latter may predispose to severe episodes

- The risk of problematic hypoglycaemia is minimized by seeking out and then avoiding exposure to plasma glucose levels of less than 3 mmol/L

- Nocturnal hypoglycaemia is common, especially in patients using twice daily mixed insulin regimens, and is often asymptomatic

- Patients with problematic hypoglycaemia during waking hours must avoid dangerous situations (such as driving) until their awareness of minor hypoglycaemia is restored

- Patients and their families need education to help them understand why hypoglycaemia occurs and how to manage acute episodes

- The hypoglycaemia of sulphonylurea therapy is commonly neuroglycopenic and may be very prolonged

- Patients on insulin and insulin secretagogues should always be asked about hypoglycaemia experience

Hypoglycaemia (literally 'low glucose in the blood') is the main and most feared acute effect of insulin therapy and can also complicate therapy with insulin secretagogues. It occurs because pharmacologically raised insulin levels are not responsive to falling insulin requirements and may remain elevated at inappropriate times. The body has a good system of neuroendocrine defences against hypoglycaemia, so severe episodes in general only occur where two abnormalities are present:

1 *pharmacological elevation* of circulating insulin; and

2 *defects* in the normal counterregulatory response.

Both occur together in diabetic patients treated with exogenous insulin or insulin secretagogues.

Definitions

The British surgeon, Whipple, decreed that for an episode to be diagnosed as hypoglycaemia, three features were required:

1 *symptoms* compatible with a low blood glucose concentration;

2 *measurement* of a blood glucose concentration below the normal range; and

3 *resolution* of the symptoms by elevation of the plasma glucose (Box 9.1).

Medical textbooks commonly state that the biochemical definition of hypoglycaemia is a plasma glucose of less than 2.8 mmol/L, or even 2.6 mmol/L for women. These definitions were coined to define spontaneous pathological hypoglycaemia such as may be induced by insulin-secreting tumours but they are not appropriate for routine management of diabetes. The normal postabsorptive venous plasma glucose range in humans is 3.5–5.5 mmol/L and there is danger to the diabetic person in accepting plasma glucose levels that are much below that range. These dangers include loss of cognitive ability and the development of asymptomatic hypoglycaemia, both of which occur during exposure to plasma glucose levels of around 3 mmol/L. Less than 3.5 mmol/L is therefore probably the best definition of biochemical hypoglycaemia in diabetes. Whipple's triad, adapted to incorporate this biochemical definition and adapted also to include episodes for which the patient him/herself is unaware, becomes appropriate for diabetes (Box 9.1).

Clinically, hypoglycaemia is traditionally divided into mild (symptomatic, self-treated) and severe (where cognitive function is impaired to an extent that the patient requires treatment by another person). Within each category, there are degrees; thus, some authorities introduce a further category of 'moderate hypoglycaemia' where self-treatment is possible but with significant disruption to daily life, and severe hypoglycaemia is sometimes taken to mean only those episodes where parenteral therapy (intramuscular glucagons or intravenous glucose) has been administered and/or consciousness has been lost with or without seizure. In assessing a patient's hypoglycaemia experience, however, one should document frequency (and, if possible, typical timing) of mild self-treated episodes and severe episodes and one should also inspect the home glucose records (or ask the patient so to do) for episodes of biochemical hypoglycaemia — levels of less than 3 mmol/L for which they had no awareness. One should also ask if family and friends notice the hypoglycaemia before the patient does — or, more particularly, if family and friends can correctly identify hypoglycaemia of which the patient is not aware. Such asymptomatic hypoglycaemia, of both types, predisposes in most patients to more severe episodes.

Symptoms of hypoglycaemia

The symptoms of hypoglycaemia (Box 9.2) are conventionally described as 'autonomic' (sweating, shaking, palpitations, anxiety, feeling hot); neuroglycopenic (confusion, inability to concentrate, slurred speech, drowsiness) and miscellaneous (blurred vision, hunger). Patients describe other symptoms such as tingling in the lips or face. As long as the patient can recognize the symptoms for what they are at a time when blood glucose is high enough to support brain function to the extent that the patient can make a sensible response to the hypoglycaemia, the episode is mild and self-treated. It should be noted that in young children, less able to express themselves, neurological signs such as irritability and drowsiness become more prominent. Neurological symptoms such

---

Box 9.1 **Whipple's triad**

Diagnosis of hypoglycaemia
1 Symptoms compatible with low blood glucose
2 Low glucose concentration measured in blood or plasma
3 Relief of symptoms on restoration of circulating blood/plasma glucose concentrations

Whipple's triad adapted for diabetes
1 Symptoms *or signs* compatible with low blood glucose
2 Plasma glucose <3.5 mmol/L
3 Relief of symptoms and signs by restoration of circulating blood/plasma glucose concentrations

---

Box 9.2 **Presentation of acute hypoglycaemia**

Symptoms

Autonomic	Neuroglycopenic	Other
Sweating	Difficulty in speaking	Hunger
Shakiness	Loss of concentration	Blurred vision
Feeling hot	Drowsiness	Weakness
Feeling anxious	Dizziness	
Nausea		
Pounding heart		

Signs

Pallor	Confusion
Tremor	Irritability
Perspiration	Slurred speech
Tachycardia or bradycardia	Lethargy
Widening of pulse pressure	Coma
	Seizure
	Hemiparesis

Additional manifestations in children
Headache
Aggression
Argumentativeness
Foolishness
Naughtiness
Irritability
Sadness
Sleepiness
Nausea
Nightmares
Convulsions

Asymptomatic hypoglycaemia
Home blood glucose test of < 3 mmol/L with no symptoms
Family and friends recognizing hypoglycaemia when patient does not

From:
Amiel SA. Hypoglycaemia associated syndrome. The Ernst Freeidrich Pfeiffer Memorial Lecture. *Acta Diabetol* 1998; 35: 226–231.
Ross LA, McCrimmon RJ, Frier BM, Kelnar CJ, Deary IJ. Hypoglycaemic symptoms reported by children with Type 1 diabetes melllitus and by their parents. *Diabetic Medicine* 1998; 15: 836–843.

as unsteadiness and loss of coordination and difficulties with speech and vision feature in hypoglycaemia in the elderly.

Defences against severe hypoglycaemia

The dangers of hypoglycaemia lie primarily in the loss of cognitive ability. The brain is normally dependent on glucose as its main fuel source and, as it stores very little, requires a constant supply from the circulation. The body is designed to maintain that supply in the face of very large variations in glucose intake (fasted vs. fed state) and tissue consumption of glucose (rest vs. exercise). Small falls in glucose availability trigger a counterregulatory response: cessation of pancreatic insulin secretion and release of glucagon disinhibit endogenous glucose production from the liver and restore circulating glucose levels. Greater falls in glucose availability trigger adrenaline release from the adrenals and stimulate the sympathetic nervous system, inhibiting peripheral glucose uptake and further enhancing endogenous glucose production by providing more substrates for gluconeogenesis via lipolysis and proteolysis.

In diabetes, these counterregulatory responses are impaired. Insulin levels are artificially maintained in the face of a falling blood glucose concentration by the persistence of injected exogenous insulin or the continued action of sulphonylureas on the beta cells. In Type 1 diabetes and late Type 2 diabetes, where insulin secretion (assessed by C-peptide levels) is lost, glucagon responses to hypoglycaemia are also defective. The patient is then dependent upon the adrenergic and autonomic responses and, most importantly, the associated symptoms (especially the symptom of hunger) to alert them to the falling blood glucose so that they can stop the episode by eating carbohydrate. In general, these symptomatic responses occur at a higher glucose level than that associated with significant confusion—if the symptoms do not occur in timely fashion, the patient is unlikely to be able to coordinate a sensible eating response in time to avert significant loss of cortical function.

The main determinant of the glucose level triggering symptomatic and autonomic responses to hypoglycaemia seems to be the glucose level to which the patient is accustomed. Thus, poorly controlled patients may feel symptoms of hypoglycaemia at normal glucose levels, while patients who have experienced much hypoglycaemia (< 3 mmol/L) in the recent past may not mount an autonomic response until plasma glucose has fallen below 2.5 mmol/L, at which time cognitive dysfunction can already be detected.

Severe hypoglycaemia

Severe hypoglycaemia is most common in Type 1 diabetic patients with long disease duration; patients who have been severely hypoglycaemic in the past and those on many forms of intensified insulin therapy. Severe hypoglycaemia rates were three times higher during intensified insulin therapy than in conventional therapy in the Diabetes Control and Complications Trial (DCCT), but it is noteworthy that overall hypoglycaemia rates fell in both groups as the trial progressed, suggesting that the services became more experienced at supporting intensified therapy regimens. The relationship between severe hypoglycaemia risk and HbA_{1c} was near linear—more hypoglycaemia the lower the HbA_{1c}—but it is of interest that, at any one HbA_{1c}, the rate appeared to be higher in the intensively treated patient group. The reason for this is not clear.

Severe hypoglycaemia is less of a problem in Type 2 patients but not insignificant. One-tenth of the problem in a disease that is about 10 times more common gives very similar incidences! In Type 2 diabetes, severe hypoglycaemia is a particular problem with insulin secretagogues such as sulphonylureas, especially the longer acting ones. The presentation is commonly neuroglycopenic (confusion and loss of cognitive ability). In one study of severe hypoglycaemia in elderly Americans, 48% of patients presenting to Accident and Emergency departments had loss of consciousness or lethargy, 7% syncope and 6% seizure. Small numbers of patients had had a stroke, myocardial infarction or injury associated with the hypoglycaemia. In the UK, the rates of severe hypoglycaemia recorded by an ambulance service were not that much lower in insulin-treated Type 2 diabetic patients than in Type 1 patients. This may reflect the current UK practice of starting insulin when oral hypoglycaemic agents can no longer maintain control, probably reflecting exhaustion of insulin secretory capacity. Insulin deficiency is associated with increased risk of severe hypoglycaemia.

Asymptomatic hypoglycaemia and failure of the neuroendocrine responses to hypoglycaemia are strongly associated with increased risk of severe hypoglycaemia. Similar counterregulatory failure can be induced experimentally by prior exposure to hypoglycaemia, suggesting that it is an adaptation to recurrent hypoglycaemia that causes hypoglycaemia unawareness and increased risk of severe hypoglycaemic events. Certainly, strict avoidance of exposure to blood glucose levels of < 3 mmol/L in daily life restores subjective awareness, and to a large extent the normal counterregulatory hormone responses to those that have lost them, but is not always easy to achieve.

Clinical management of acute hypoglyaemia (Box 9.3)

Mild episodes are self-treated. Ideally, a home blood glucose test is carried out before treating to confirm the diagnosis, as this may help decide dose adjustments to avoid hypoglycaemia later, but in practice this is often not performed. A plasma glucose reading of less than 3.5 mmol/L confirms that hypoglycaemia was the cause of the symptoms, although many patients can reach lower glucose levels without symptoms. A reading of less than 3 mmol/L, with or without symptoms, is always considered to be hypoglycaemia, as cognitive dysfunction is detectable at this level.

Oral treatment of a hypoglycaemic episode should include some readily available carbohydrate such as glucose in tablet form, ideally 15–20 g (e.g. Dextrosol, 5–6 tablets); fresh orange juice (200 mL); Lucozade (100–150 mL) or other non-diet drink. If a meal is not imminent, some complex carbohydrate should then be taken to maintain the glucose until the next meal, such as two semisweet biscuits or a slice of bread. Chocolates such as Mars Bars are popular with patients but not ideal as the fat in the chocolate retards the absorption of the glucose, delaying recov-

---

Box 9.3 Treatment of acute hypoglycaemia

Mild
15–20 g rapidly absorbed carbohydrate orally, e.g.

Lucozade	100–150 mL	approx. half tea-cup
Fruit juice	150–200 mL	approx. tea-cup full
Lemonade	150–200 mL	approx. tea-cup full

or non-diet cola
Repeat after 5 min if no improvement
Then:
Either
Take meal within 60 min with usual dose of insulin, if appropriate
or
10 g starchy carbohydrate (e.g. slice of bread) if meal within next 1–2 h
or
20 g starchy carbohydrate (e.g. 2 slices of bread) if meal not for 2 h or at night

Check blood glucose at 30 min to ensure has recovered to > 4 mmol/L

Severe
Intramuscular glucagon 1 mg
Should be effective within 10 min
Then
20 g rapidly absorbed carbohydrate and, when recovered
40 g starchy carbohydrate (e.g. 2 slices of bread)

or

Intravenous glucose 75 mL 20% glucose
Repeat in 5 min if no effect
Then:
20 g rapidly absorbed carbohydrate and, when recovered
40 g starchy carbohydrate (e.g. 2 slices of bread)

Do not use 50% glucose unless through a central venous line

---

ery. One problem with hypoglycaemia is the tendency to overtreat, leading to posthypoglycaemic hyperglycaemia. This is compounded by the release of counterregulatory hormones which can induce an insulin-resistant state lasting several hours.

In severe hypoglycaemia, if the patient is still conscious, another person may administer glucose in one of the forms above. However, giving oral glucose is dangerous if the conscious level is suppressed, as inhalation may occur. Glucagon 1 mg can be given intramuscularly and produces recovery within 10 min. Family members can be taught to give this. If medical personnel are in attendence, e.g. in the Accident and Emergency department, intravenous glucose is appropriate, using 75–125 mL of 20% glucose or 150–250 mL of 10% glucose. Fifty per cent glucose is too strong and very toxic to veins and should not be used. Once conscious, the patient can be fed a carbohydrate-containing snack to maintain glucose levels until the next meal.

Some attempt should be made to ascertain the cause of a hypoglycaemic episode in order to prevent recurrence (see below). However, it is important to recognize that in Type 1 diabetic patients, although a dose reduction may be advised, the next meal will require an insulin injection, and injections should not be omitted because of current hypoglycaemia. Patients on sulphonylureas who present with severe hypoglycaemia need admission for observation as the effect of the drug is likely to be prolonged.

Clinical management of the patient with hypoglycaemia unawareness and severe hypoglycaemia

Assessment of hypoglycaemia risk is an important part of the diabetic review, particularly in Type 1 patients (Box 9.4). They should be asked about episodes of severe hypoglycaemia and also about frequency of episodes of mild symptomatic hypoglycaemia and frequency of biochemical hypoglycaemia (levels of 3 mmol/L or less on home testing when they feel fine) and episodes when hypoglycaemia is diagnosed by others around them. Nocturnal hypoglycaemia is often asymptomatic and patients should be questioned about night sweating, which may be evidence of nocturnal hypoglycaemia. Be aware that Type 1 patients often do not recognize hypoglycaemia as a problem unless it is severe and so do not mention it.

In Type 2 patients, especially if elderly, ask about episodes of feeling hungry, sweaty and shaky, resolved by eating quickly and also about episodes of feeling odd or being confused relieved by eating.

Box 9.4 Assessment of hypoglycaemia experience

Mild episodes (self-treated)?
How often? Any typical time?

Nocturnal episodes?
Symptomatic?
Night sweating?

Asymptomatic episodes?
Detected by family or friends?
Home blood glucose monitoring < 3 mol/L with no symptoms?

Severe episodes?
Episodes needing assistance?
Episodes needing emergency services?
Episodes with loss of consciousness or seizure?
Episodes affecting work?

Does patient
Drive?
Operate machinery?
Drink alcohol or exercise intermittently?

Ask patient's relative or close friend!

Asking relatives is often very illuminating!

If a patient is suspected of problematic hypoglycaemia (severe episodes or clear evidence of hypoglycaemia unawareness) the following steps must be taken.

Instruct for risk avoidance

First, ascertain that the patient is not putting him/herself or others at risk—people who are really hypoglycaemia unaware must not drive, for example, until the problem is resolved. In cases of uncertainty, explain that the patient must *always* test his/her blood glucose before driving—and at 90-min intervals on long drives—and document the result. In a person with normal awareness, driving with a blood glucose of 5 mmol/L or higher is safe, but in unawareness 7 mmol/L is a safer cut-off. This advice is pragmatic rather than evidence-based but deaths of patients and other road users have occurred and in the eyes of the law the hypoglycaemic diabetic person is driving under the influence of drugs. Judges are more understanding if it is clear that the person has been behaving responsibly. Glucose tablets or sugary drinks should always be available in the car but prevention is better than cure. If a hypoglycaemic attack occurs while driving, the patient must stop at once, remove him/herself from the driving seat and treat the episode. He/she should not resume driving until the blood glucose has recovered and then with extra care—reaction times are slower to recover from hypoglycaemia than symptoms.

Patients who have had a severe hypoglycaemic episode other than while asleep at night must inform the DVLA and must not drive until they have been clear of such episodes for 3 months—and regained any lost awareness. The legal and practical aspects of hypoglycaemia are considered further in Chapter 21.

Examine insulin regimen and home blood glucose records for evidence of a pattern of recurrent hypoglycaemia

Times of high risk are at night (when counter-regulatory responses are less vigorous and symptoms do not occur) and pre-meal—especially in patients who do not snack before meals. Taking a diary of the patient's typical day, in terms of times of rising, eating and exercising is often helpful as quite commonly a correctable problem is identified, particularly in patients not using flexible insulin regimens, such as omitted snacks, or failure to appreciate the effects of intermittent exercise or alcohol consumption. Twenty-four hour monitoring of the interstitial glucose by a system such as Minimed's continuous glucose monitoring system (CGMS) may help identify patterns of hypoglycaemia. The system records over 3 days and may reveal patterns that can suggest appropriate places to modify the treatment regimen.

Exercise
Look particularly for hypoglycaemia in the night and morning after vigorous exercise, especially if the exercise is unusual for the patient. Vigorous exercise such as running, tennis, squash, swimming, athletics or sustained exercise such as taking long walks or cycling, not only cause hypoglycaemia at the time (most patients are aware of this and either eat to cover the exercise or reduce the insulin active at the time) but

may also exhaust muscle and liver glycogen stores, which then spend the next 18–24 h vigorously taking up glucose to replenish themselves. This is a time of high risk of hypoglycaemia unless background insulin (usually the overnight insulin) is reduced by between 10 and 40% depending on the degree of exercise, relative to the patient's usual lifestyle. Bear in mind that, for the couch potato, doing a monthly shop to replenish the contents of the freezer may be the equivalent to the fitter man's skiing holiday!

Alcohol
Alcohol, which in the acute phase increases blood glucose, suppresses gluconeogenesis, which the patient needs to maintain blood glucose levels after 6–8 h fasting, e.g. overnight. Alcohol therefore is also associated with hypoglycaemia in the night or next morning. In young people, taking some alcohol with exercise at night, as in dancing in clubs, can have profound effects on glucose control and reductions of around 20% (more if no food is taken) in overnight insulin is a good place to start.

Consider possible external contributors to hypoglycaemia risk (Boxes 9.5 and 9.6)

Acute elevations of growth hormone and cortisol are probably not critical in recovery from acute hypoglycaemia but both hormones need to be present in at least basal amounts and deficiencies of either can cause frank hypoglycaemia. Addison's disease is rare but autoimmune disease is more common in Type 1 diabetes and it needs to be considered. Likewise, coincidental growth hormone deficiency as can occur with Sheehan's syndrome after pregnancy or after hypophysitis. Hypothyroidism is associated with delayed insulin clearance by the liver and care needs to be taken when treating hyperthyroidism, because of the risk of overshooting into hypothyroidism with high risk of hypoglycaemia in a treated diabetic patient. Renal impairment affects insulin clearance and increases the risk of hypoglycaemia in insulin-treated patients and in Type 2 patients using insulin secretagogues such as glibenclamide and chlorpropamide, which are normally renally excreted and should not be used in these patients. Liver failure, where glycogenolysis and gluconeogenesis may be im-

---

Box 9.5 **Contributors to hypoglycaemia risk**

Insulin therapy
Insulin secretagogue therapy

Plus
Previous exposure to hypoglycaemia
Long duration diabetes
C-peptide negativity
Hypoglycaemia unawareness

Exercise
Alcohol

Hypothyroidism
Hypoadrenalism
Hypopituitarism
Growth hormone deficiency
Renal impairment
Liver failrue

Drugs (Box 9.6)

Box 9.6 **Drug interactions with insulin secretagogues as a possible contributor to hypoglycaemia risk**

Inhibition of gluconeogenesis
Alcohol

Displacement from albumin binding of insulin secretagogues
Aspirin
Warfarin
Sulphonamides
Trimethoprim
Fibrates

Decreased renal excretion of insulin secretagogues
Aspirin
Probenecid
Allopurinol

Decreased metabolism of insulin secretagogues
Warfarin
Monoamine oxidase inhibitors

Intrinsic insulin secretagogue activity
Aspirin
Non-steroidal anti-inflammatory drugs

Increased peripheral glucose uptake
Aspirin

From McAuley, & Frier, B.M. (2001) In: *Diabetes in Old Age* (eds Sinclair, & Finucane). © John Wiley & Sons Ltd, with permission.

---

paired, can also be associated with hypoglycaemia but is likely to be clinically manifest in other ways first.

Few other drugs cause hypoglycaemia *per se* but some interact with oral hypoglycaemic agents (Box 9.6). Some may displace sulphonylureas from their albumin-binding site. Salicylates can cause hypoglycaemia in a variety of ways. It is reported that beta-blockade interferes with subjective awareness of hypoglycaemia and it is true that some beta-blockers diminish some of the autonomic symptoms. In general, sweating is increased. Certainly, beta-blockers should not be withheld from diabetic patients with a good cardiovascular indication but cardioselective agents should be chosen.

A link has also been reported between angiotensin-converting enzyme (ACE) inhibition and increased risk of severe hypoglycaemia but this remains unproven and ACE inhibitors should not be withheld from diabetic patients in whom they are indicated.

It is always sensible to advise intensification of home blood glucose monitoring and, in a well-controlled patient, temporary reduction in insulin

dosage, when starting any new drug that might conceivably have impact on glucose control.

Adjust therapy to avoid hypoglycaemia without encouraging overall loss of control

If a pattern or cause for recurrent hypoglycaemia is found, the insulin or drug regimen should be adjusted to avoid hypoglycaemia in future. There is nothing wrong in patients using different doses of bedtime insulin at weekends for example, if their weekly work is sedentary but they have an active sporting life at weekends. For nocturnal hypoglycaemia, the evidence suggests that moving the overnight intermediate-acting insulin from before the evening meal to bedtime is beneficial, and use of shorter acting analogue insulins before the evening meal may help, although care must be taken to avoid loss of control with hyperglycaemia between the evening meal and the onset of the action of the bedtime insulin. We have found that redistributing the total insulin dose, reduced by 20%, divided equally between meal doses of soluble insulin and two equal doses of intermediate-acting insulin as background can be helpful when there is problematic nocturnal hypoglycaemia. The new long-acting insulin analogue, Lantus, may also be associated with less risk of hypoglycaemia in the night.

Perhaps the most important aspect of treating high risk of severe hypoglycaemia is to provide clear guidance as to the importance of a lower limit to the glucose values considered appropriate. 'Make 4 the floor', a slogan of Diabetes UK, suggests that as a target, no pre-meal plasma glucose should be less than 4. In other words, dose adjustment is needed if pre-meal plasma glucoses are often less than 4 to prevent this recurring. When using conventional soluble insulins, the pre-bed plasma glucose range is often recommended to be higher, e.g. 7–9 mmol/L, and a bedtime snack is encouraged to diminish risk of nocturnal hypoglycaemia. Some authorities suggest an even higher lower limit to the glucose target range for first thing in the morning (5.5–7.5 mmol/L) as this is after the longest break in eating in the day. Focus on the institution of a lower limit to the desirable glucose range is preferable to simple 'relaxation of control' which may stop the hypoglycaemia but at the risk of a raised HbA_{1c} and increased risk of long-term complications. In many cases, stopping problematic hypoglycaemia may be associated with a fall in HbA_{1c} as the rebound hyperglycaemia is lost too.

A few patients seem to tolerate recurrent hypoglycaemia better than the generality, recording plasma glucoses of just under 3 mmol/L with no loss of awareness of slightly lower levels, no confusional hypoglycaemia and no severe hypoglycaemia. However, it is not safe to assume that the patient with multiple low readings in your clinic is one such!

Insulin species and hypoglycaemia

Hyperinsulinaemia is the cause of hypoglycaemic episodes in the treatment of diabetes — either caused by insulin secretagogues or exogenous insulin. As described in Chapter 7, some drugs are associated with more hypoglycaemia than others, particularly the longer acting or more powerful sulphonylureas. With exogenous insulin, the problem is compounded by the unphysiological nature of the insulin replacement (peripheral vs. portal, non-physiological action profiles, not responsive to glucose). There is growing evidence that some insulin replacement regimens may be associated with less hypoglycaemia at particular times of day—the new insulin analogues, Humalog, NovoRapid and Lantus are all reported to cause less nocturnal hypoglycaemia than conventional insulins, as described above and in Chapter 8. Among the conventional insulins, concerns that the use of human as opposed to animal insulins cause greater problems with hypoglycaemia have not been substantiated by research. Mechanistic studies comparing responses to hypoglycaemia induced by the different species have found no major or consistent differences and a recent meta-analysis and a systematic review of the published literature confirms this. There are differences in the pharmacokinetics of the various insulins but these have not resulted in detectable differences in hypoglycaemia. Reversal of problematic hypoglycaemia has been achieved by regimen alterations, while not changing the insulin species used and it is essential to seek other causes of problematic hypoglycaemia. However, some patients remain uncomfortable using human insulin and many with problematic hypoglycaemia are convinced that the use of human insulin is to blame. It is appropriate to support such patients by prescribing the insulin species with which they feel most comfortable. However, this should not be at the expense of leaving patients on inappropriate regimens and doses. A potential problem is the fear that the bad press human insulin has received may block people's willingness to try new insulins when the evidence suggests they might achieve benefit. However, it is important to respect the individual patient's experience of their insulin and to work with it to achieve the best results possible.

Diabetic Hyperglycaemic Emergencies

Summary

- Diabetic ketoacidosis (DKA) is the hallmark of the insulin deficiency of Type 1 diabetes mellitus

- Hyperglycaemia (which may not be extreme); ketosis and acidosis are all required for diagnosis

- 25% of cases are newly presenting Type 1 diabetes, the rest are associated with stress, illness or insulin withdrawal in established disease

- A common cause is incorrect professional advice to Type 1 patients who are anorexic to stop their insulin

- Vomiting in a Type 1 patient should be considered DKA until proven otherwise and is an absolute indication for hospitalization

- Type 2 patients may present with DKA in association with severe intercurrent illness, and sometimes in African and Caribbean patients, DKA may be the presenting feature of a diabetes which later does not require insulin therapy

- The treatment of DKA is always an emergency and includes rehydration, intravenous insulin therapy and potassium replacement, as well as treatment of any underlying pathology

- The mortality of DKA remains 2–10% and should be reduced by close monitoring of fluids, electrolyte and glucose status during treatment

- The initiation of therapy should be driven by protocols but these need adjusting in light of individual progress once treatment has started

- Confusion most closely relates to osmolality and is an indication for admission to intensive care

- Hyperosmolar non-ketotic states (HONK) occur in Type 2 patients, typically undiagnosed people who have been consuming high energy drinks to compensate for thirst and lethargy

- HONK has a high mortality

- Treatment is as for DKA, but the patients are more insulin sensitive (so 50% DKA insulin recommendations are appropriate) and more likely to experience clotting problems, so anticoagulation is advisable

- Lactic acidosis is very rare but may occur if metformin is inappropriately prescribed to a Type 2 patient with renal impairment

Diabetic ketoacidosis

Diabetic ketoacidosis (DKA) occurs in severe insulin deficiency and also in cases of insulin lack with marked elevation of stress hormones. It is the hallmark of Type 1 diabetes and 25% of cases represent newly diagnosed diabetes, the rest being DKA complicating other illness or insulin withdrawal in established diabetes. It can also occur as the presenting feature of Type 2 diabetes either in adults, typically of African or Caribbean ethnicity who present with the features of DKA but after treatment are later found not to require insulin therapy, or in Type 2 patients exposed to severe stress such as a myocardial infarction or severe sepsis.

To diagnose DKA, three features are required:
1 *hyperglycaemia*, although in well-hydrated patients this may not be severe;
2 *ketosis*; and
3 *acidosis*.

The main features at presentation are as follows.
1 *Dehydration*.
2 *Whole body potassium depletion*, although the initial plasma potassium may be high secondary to the dehydration and acidosis—low plasma potassium at presentation indicates a sicker patient who has been sliding into DKA for longer or who has had a prolonged antecedent period of very poor diabetic control.
3 *Respiratory compensation for the metabolic acidosis.* Hyperventilation is common and sometimes progresses to the sighing, deep respirations of Kussmaul's respiration.
4 *Impaired consciousness level.* Patients are usually drowsy but if there is significant confusion, should be managed on an intensive therapy unit as these patients are very severely ill. The degree of confusion correlates best to the degree of hyperosmolality.

Secondary features are:
1 *vomiting and gastroparesis* and risk of inhalation pneumonia;
2 *leucocytosis* in the presence or absence of infection;
3 *elevated serum amylase* in the presence or absence of pancreatitis; and
4 *hypothermia* even in the presence of infection.

The initial assessment should include estimation of the severity of all of the above, plus a check for an underlying precipitating cause, usually infection or, in older patients, myocardial infarction.

Initial management

If the patient is significantly confused or is comatose, the respiratory tract must be protected, if necessary by intubation and a nasogastric tube placed. Intravenous access must be established and in an older patient or where there is supine hypotension, a central line is recommended. A quick assessment for complicating factors such as physical injury, including head injury, and any history of recent illness or drug ingestion should be sought.

Blood should be tested at the bedside for glucose concentration and sent for urgent laboratory assessment of potassium, urea and creatinine, venous bicarbonate and arterial blood gases for pH or hydrogen ion concentration. The osmolality can be calculated from the formula

$$2 \times (Na^+ + K^+) + glucose + urea$$

and should be no more than 296. The sodium result needs to be corrected for the hyperglycaemia:

$$measured\ Na^+ + glucose - 5/3.$$

The major priority is rehydration. The patient in DKA may be many litres in deficit and although the total deficit should be corrected over 48 h, initial rehydration needs to be fast—for an adult, 0.5 L normal saline should be given rapidly, with the next 0.5 L over 30 min (Box 10.1).

Insulin is the next priority and is given intravenously. The subcutaneous route is too risky in a dehydrated but soon to be rehydrated patient. Insulin infusion can be started after the first 0.5 L of fluid has been given—6 units/h of soluble insulin is usual, or for a child 0.1 units/kg body weight/h.

Potassium needs to be considered next (Box 10.2). Adding potassium to the infusion fluids is performed when the measured potassium begins to fall or is less than 4.5 mmol/L. It is useful also to monitor the ECG, on a lead that shows the t waves clearly, as the flattening of peaked t waves indicates declining plasma potassium.

Box 10.1 **Suggested initial fluid replacement in DKA in adults**

0.9% sodium chloride	0.5 L	over 30 minutes
0.9% sodium chloride	0.5 L	next hour
0.9% sodium chloride	1.0 L	next 2 hours
0.9% sodium chloride	1.0 L	next 4 hours
0.9% sodium chloride	1.0 L	next 4 hours
0.9% sodium chloride	1.0 L	next 8 hours

• Rate may need to be increased in cardiovascular shock, or reduced in co-existing disease or renal disease or in the elderly (use a central line)
• Replace with 5% glucose once plasma glucose <15 mmol/l
• Convert to 0.45% saline if **measured** (uncorrected) sodium rises above 150 mmol/l

---

Box 10.2 **Potassium replacement in DKA in adults**

• Monitor every 2 hours initially and then every 4 hours until stable.
• Give when plasma level known to be normal or low

Plasma potassium	Amount of KCL*
Less than 3	40 mmol/hour
3–4	30 mmol/hour
4–5	20 mmol/hour
5–6	10 mmol/hour
Greater than 6	stop potassium

* some authorities recommend half KCl and half KPO$_4$

Box 10.3 **Use of bicarbonate in DKA**

• Consider only if pH ≤ 6.9
• Use 200 ml of 2.74% HCO⁻ over 30–60 min
• **NEVER USE 8.4% SOLUTIONS**
• Only repeat if pH remains ≤ 6.9
• Bicarbonate reduces plasma potassium. This may be useful in severely hyperkalaemic patients but if potassium is low, 15 mmol KCl may be given with the bicarbonate above

---

It is not usual to give bicarbonate unless the measured pH is less than 7, as the dissolution of the bicarbonate can exacerbate intracellular acidosis (Box 10.3). However, with very acidotic patients, the acidosis can impair myocardial contractility so it is usual to infuse bicarbonate very cautiously.

Fluid balance is crucial in the management of these patients and output as well as input needs to be recorded. In an unconscious patient a urinary catheter is necessary for this, although scrupulous care must be taken to minimize risk of infection. For hypotensive or elderly patients, a central line to monitor fluid replacement is needed and if the patient complains of abdominal pain, or is unconscious with no audible bowel sounds, a gastric tube should be placed to keep the stomach empty.

'Make haste slowly' might be considered the watchword of management of the DKA patient — fluids and insulin need to be started very rapidly but once established gradual restoration of normality is preferable. Blood glucose should be measured at the bedside hourly — after the initial fall in response to rehydration, the rate of fall of blood glucose that is desirable is no more than 5 mmol/L/h. Once the blood glucose reaches 15 mmol/L or less, it is advisable to reduce the insulin infusion rate to 3 units/h (0.05 units/kg body weight/h in children or those weighing less than 50 kg) and replace the saline infusion with 5% glucose, to keep plasma glucose around 10–11 mmol/L. Very rapid fall in blood glucose concentration is believed to increase the risk of complications such as cerebral or pulmonary oedema. Nevertheless, it is important to maintain the insulin infusion rate at this level until the ketones have cleared, if necessary by maintaining the glucose level with more concentrated glucose solutions (e.g. 10%). Potassium levels must be monitored particularly carefully in this situation but too early a reduction in insulin infusion rate (for example by reversion to a standard glucose, potassium and insulin (GKI) or sliding scale insulin regimen) will leave the patient normoglycaemic and still ketotic.

Any associated pathology such as infection or myocardial infarction should be managed actively.

The UK inpatient mortality for DKA is quoted as

being between 2 and 10%. Some of this will relate to any underlying pathology—the elderly patient developing DKA secondary to a myocardial infarction or pneumonia will do less well than the young person who has stopped his/her insulin for 2 days. Many complications of therapy should be preventable by careful monitoring of fluid replacement, blood glucose and potassium in particular. Almost all hospitals and all diabetes textbooks have protocols for the management of DKA (Fig. 10.1) but it is important to realize that while these work very well for the initial management, they may need modifying for the particular patient's needs and progress thereafter.

Complications of DKA include:
· Death from hyperosmolaltiy and acidosis.
· Cerebral oedema.
· Cardiac or respiratory arrest from hypokalaemia.
· Renal failure from dehydration, especially in the presence of intercurrent renal disease.
· Pulmonary oedema.
· Disseminated intravascular coagulation.
· Thrombocytopenia from phosphate depletion.
Except with very late presentations, most deaths from the above should be preventable. The degree of coma is one of the most important prognostic signs at presentation.

Concluding treatment after diabetic ketoacidosis

Once the ketones have cleared substantially from the urine (usually 24 h after the ketonuria resolved to 0 or +) the patient may be moved onto a standard intravenous sliding scale for insulin with continued intravenous fluid and glucose replacement, or if eating, can be placed on a regimen of pre-meal fast-acting insulin and bedtime delayed-acting insulin. If the former, 24 h of standard sliding scale insulin gives a useful guide to the patient's 24 h insulin requirements for the next day—25% of the total dose given as soluble insulin before meals and 25% as an intermediate isophane insulin at bedtime is a good guide. Requirements may fall over the next few days as the patient recovers and as the insulin resistance of hyperglycaemia begins to resolve.

For patients with established Type 1 diabetes, insulin requirements should return to premorbid levels once the acute illness has settled. For newly diagnosed Type 1 diabetic patients, immediate access to diabetes education services should be made available so that the patient and his/her family can be reassured about their condition and the future, learn about taking insulin in the way that suits them and their diabetes best and also be taught how to monitor blood glucose at home. Most patients newly presenting with DKA will have true Type 1 diabetes. However, some, particularly those of African or Caribbean ethnicity, may not need insulin after the first few weeks. This can only be established over time and it is perfectly appropriate to discharge these patients too on appropriate doses of insulin, which can be adjusted or withdrawn under careful supervision later in the diabetes clinic.

Pitfalls in diabetic ketoacidosis

Other metabolic acidoses can mimic DKA in some of its features and a differential diagnosis is given in Box 10.4.

Abdominal pain and vomiting are common features of DKA and patients may present as an apparent acute abdominal emergency. Surgery needs to be deferred until metabolic stability has been established by which time the presence or, more commonly, absence of an underlying acute abdominal complication can be more reliably established. While it is true that acute appendicitis could trigger DKA in a Type 1 diabetic person, it is more usual that the appearances of an acute abdominal emergency settle as the metabolic emergency resolves.

The unreliability of serum amylase for diagnosing acute pancreatitis; a leucocytosis for diagnosing underlying infection and a normal body temperature for excluding infection have already been mentioned. Antibiotics should be started based on clinical suspicion, rather than relying on the above.

The ketones measured by most strip tests are acetone and acetoacetate. Occasionally, 3-hydroxybutyrate is the predominant ketone body, and strip tests may then show only small amounts of ketones.

ADULT DIABETIC KETOACIDOSIS REGIMEN

INSULIN REGIMEN

50 units Human Actrapid insulin made up to 50 mls with Normal Saline solution

Blood glucose ≥ 15 mmol/l:	6 units / hour
Blood glucose < 15 mmol/l:	3 units / hour

1st syringe:	insulin:	saline:	Sign:	
2nd syringe:	insulin:	saline:	Sign:	

Patient Name:..

Hospital Number:....................

Date........................ Ward.....................

Patient label

for children: If hyperosmolar use this chart for monitoring. Refer to wall chart/formulary for insulin and fluid

Date:... Day on IV insulin.................

FLUID REGIMEN (convert to or add glucose solution once blood glucose < 15 mmol/l)

FLUID*	VOLUME	RATE	KCl in mmol	Dr signature	Time started and batch	Time finished	Nurse signature
0.9% NaCl	**1 litre**	**30 min**	*Day one only*	*delete*	*if regimen*	*continued*	
0.9% NaCl	**1 litre**	**1 hour**	*Day one only*	*delete*	*if regimen*	*continued*	

- use 0.9% saline till plasma glucose < 15 mmol/l, then convert to or add 5% or 10% glucose to maintain plasma glucose 7 – 11 mmol/l
- consider half normal saline if measured (uncorrected) plasma sodium rises above 150 mmol/l

Protocol time	Clock Time	Neuro score	Urine ketones	Glucose mm	Insulin U/hr	pH	K+ mm	Fluid in mls/hr	Fluid in mls/hr	Fluid out mls/hr	Fluid out mls/hr	Cumulative fluid balance
0												
1												
2												
3												
4												
5												
6												
7												
8												
9												
10												
11												
12												

When urine ketones 1+ or less, convert to IV sliding scale or subcut insulin if patient eating.
If converting to subcut, give premeal subcut soluble dose, then meal, then discontinue IV insulin
See over page for 13-24 hour observation chart plus neurological assessment score

Figure 10.1 The King's College Hospital DKA treatment and monitoring chart.

Hyperosmolar non-ketotic coma

The other hyperglycaemic emergency in diabetes is hyperosmolar non-ketotic coma (HONK). This occurs in Type 2 patients, classically as a presenting condition in an older person who has been drinking large volumes of sugary fluids (such as Lucozade or Coca-Cola) in response to malaise, thirst or sometimes weight loss. In this way the patient replaces water with glucose and plasma glucose levels may be very high indeed (up to 40–80 mmol/L). Because there is residual insulin secretion, sufficient to stop lipolysis and ketogenesis if not to control glucose metabolism, these patients are not significantly acidotic. However, they are invariably very dehydrated and often elderly and frail, so they present a major management problem.

As with DKA, the initial treatment is by rehydration and insulin. These patients, lacking ketosis, are more insulin-sensitive than the classical DKA patients, so 3 units/h (0.05 units/kg body weight/h) is usually adequate. These patients are also very hyperosmolar and this may show as high plasma sodium. Initial replacement with normal saline as for DKA is appropriate (it is rare to receive the laboratory measurement of the plasma sodium before this has been instigated) and this fluid will be hypotonic compared to the patient's plasma anyway, but if the plasma sodium rises after intial therapy or is over 150 mmol/L (corrected) replacing half the prescribed saline with 5% glucose or using half normal saline becomes appropriate. These patients are at higher risk of cerebral oedema than patients in DKA and caution should be exercised to reduce their glucose concentrations at the same rate — no more than 5 mmol/L/h. They are also more likely to experience thrombotic complications and should normally receive prophylactic anticoagulation.

Treatment of cerebral oedema

Cerebral oedema should be suspected if the patient complains of headache and the conscious level begins to fall after initial recovery as the metabolic situation is corrected. Associated signs include bradycardia and hypotension. Diagnosis is established by computed tomography (CT) scanning and treatment is with mannitol (2.5 mL/kg/min over 15 min and repeat if necessary), with referral to neurosurgery for placement of an intracerebral pressure monitor and consideration of further intervention. This is not an easy complication to treat. It is thought to be less likely to occur if the total fluid deficit anticipated for the patient is replaced over not less than 48 h.

Lactic acidosis

This is an extremely rare metabolic emergency for the diabetologist to manage but it may become more common with the growing popularity of metformin. Outside diabetes, lactic acidosis occurs as a complication of major illness (hypovolaemia, profound hypotension and circulatory failure, sepsis) as the circulation fails to maintain adequate oxygen supply to the peripheral tissues and anaerobic metabolism results in rising lactate levels. In diabetes, lactic acidosis was a recognized complication of therapy with the early biguanide phenformin. Its successor, metformin, is intrinsically safer and scarcely raises lactate levels in health or in healthy people with diabetes. However, metformin can be associated with raised lactate levels in renal failure (when the metformin is not cleared) or hepatic failure when lactate clearance is impaired and occasional cases are reported where the drug has been started in a patient already in renal failure; where a patient on metformin has gone into renal failure as a result of severe dehydration or hypovolaemia following a myocardial infarct or other insult; and, very rarely, when hypertonic radiodense dyes have precipitated renal failure during X-ray procedures. Provided the recommended precautions are taken when prescribing metformin (page 65), lactic acidosis in diabetes will remain a rarity. However, it is in the differential diagnosis for DKA and can be identified after clinical suspicion and if the anion gap at presentation of the acidosis is too great to be accounted for by ketones. Lactate can be measured in plasma and should be in any case of doubt.

Treatment is as for DKA but in lactic acidosis the acidosis requires correction with bicarbonate. This is given more aggressively than in DKA, where it should hardly be used at all (page 90).

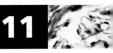

Management of Diabetes During Surgery and Other Illnesses

Summary

- Surgery and other acute illness damage diabetes control because of the associated stress and reduced mobility

- Poor glycaemic control impairs a person's ability to heal

- Diabetic complications may increase the risk of a surgical procedure

- Glycaemic control should be maintained by intravenous insulin in a patient who cannot eat and who is sick

- The insulin is usually accompanied by a glucose infusion to minimize catabolism during the period of fasting and stress

- Once the sick person is eating again, the route of insulin administration can revert to subcutaneous, but close monitoring and the administration of supplemental insulin doses to maintain normoglycaemia are essential

- Close monitoring of any insulin regimen is essential

- Type 2 patients can revert to oral therapies when recovered from the acute episode, except after myocardial infarction where there is evidence that continuing intensive insulin therapy for at least 3 months provides added benefit

Patients with diabetes are not protected from the other ills that beset mankind. They are more, rather than less, likely to find themselves in need of other medical attention. The diabetic patient undergoing surgery needs particular attention, because:
- the circumstances of the surgery upset diabetes control;
- poor diabetes control increases the risks complicating recovery; and
- chronic complications of diabetes carry additional risk of the surgery and its management for the patient.

Effects of surgery on diabetes control
(Box 11.1)

The patient undergoing surgery is in a catabolic state because of the requirement for prolonged fasting and because of associated stress. Surgery induces an insulin resistance that is measurable 24 h later and is related to the hyperglycaemic effects of the stress response (stress hormone secretion and activation of the sympathetic nervous system) and the release of cytokines. Emotional as well as physical stress related to the primary pathology requiring surgery may con-

---

Box 11.1 **Contributors to metabolic decompensation in surgery**

Stress hormone release
    Adrenaline (epinephrine)
    Noradrenaline (norepinephrine)
    Cortisol
    Growth hormone
Sympathetic nervous system activation
Bed-rest and reduced activity
Cytokine release

Net result: insulin resistance and hyperglycaemia

Box 11.2 **Complications of diabetes to be considered in surgery**

Metabolic
Hyperglycaemia
    Dehydration
    Potassium loss
    Impaired leucocyte function + glucose in
        secretions = increased risk of infection
Hypoinsulinaemia
    Proteolysis
        catabolic state
        poor wound healing
    Lipolysis
    Ketogenesis
        dehydration
        nausea
        acidosis

Chronic complications
Autonomic neuropathy
    Cardiac arrythmias
    Respiratory arrest
    Incomplete gastric emptying
    Blood pressure anomalies
Renal impairment
    Drug clearance
    Fluid balance problems
Peripheral vascular disease
    Heel skin breakdown
Cardiovascular disease
    Increased risk of infarction

---

tribute and other factors such as bed-rest and reduced physical activity levels exacerbate the tendency to hyperglycaemia. Unchecked, the hyperglycaemia will lead via glycosuria to an osmotic diuresis, dehydration and impaired leucocyte function, with increased risk of infection and delayed wound healing.

The interaction of modern anaesthetic drugs with metabolic control is not an enormous issue but should be considered. Isoflurane has been reported as causing a greater rise in plasma glucose than fentanyl and midazolam for example but the effects are transient and easily controlled with insulin. Of more concern is the difficulty in detecting fluctuations of blood glucose in the anaesthetized or muscle-relaxed patient. Efficient and regular blood glucose monitoring is essential during anaesthesia and perioperative management.

Effects of uncontrolled diabetes in surgery
(Box 11.2)

As in any setting, inadequate insulinization will result in excess catabolism—hyperglycaemia exceeding the renal threshold (usually ~ 10 mmol/L) may lead to excess loss of body water and potassium. Leucocyte function is impaired at glucose levels of 15 mmol/L or more; lipolysis and ketogenesis start at insulin levels of less than 10 µU/ml and proteolysis slightly earlier. Thus, plasma glucose during and after surgery should be maintained at 4–9 mmol/L, and 7–

9 mmol/L during anaesthesia to minimize risk of undetected hypoglycaemia.

Non-metabolic complications of diabetes in surgery (Box 11.2)

The diabetic patient is at increased risk of cardiovascular disease, neuropathy and renal impairment, all of which may impact upon surgical management. These implications should be assessed prior to surgery. Particular care should be observed in patients with peripheral vascular disease to prevent heel ulceration by prolonged contact of the heels with hard surfaces such as trolleys, operating tables and mattresses. The heels of the diabetic patient must be lifted off the bed if there is to be prolonged immobilization and assessed at regular intervals for evidence of breakdown of the skin. Patients with neuropathy may have an associated autonomic neuropathy with cardiac denervation and require scrupulous cardiovascular monitoring throughout anaesthesia because of increased risk of respiratory arrest or arrythmias. In advanced autonomic neuropathy, the possibility of excess residual gastric contents secondary to gastroparesis must be considered because of the risk of aspiration.

Insulin replacement for surgery in Type 1 diabetes

The patient requires active management of insulin replacement and glycaemic and metabolic control from the moment he/she stops eating until eating is re-established. In all except the most minor procedures, this is best managed with intravenous glucose and insulin. It is traditional to run an insulin infusion in parallel with a glucose infusion, with 10% glucose solutions being preferred in order to deliver *at least* 150 g carbohydrate in 24 h to minimize catabolism without excessive fluid replacement. Apart from the associated volume of water, this glucose infusion is best considered separate from the other fluid and electrolyte replacement requirements of the patient, which should be run in parallel with it. This allows a stable glucose supply against which to run the insulin. Insulin and glucose infusion requires potassium supplementation. Outside the setting of diabetic ketoacidosis, we do not recommend altering glucose infusion during intravenous insulin administration. If the blood glucose concentration rises the insulin dose is increased and vice versa. Rapidly switching between glucose and saline because the blood glucose is lower or higher — at the same time as adjusting the insulin infusion rate — is a recipe for confusion.

It is important to recognize that intravenous insulin infusions mandate hourly blood glucose monitoring. In circumstances where the regimen has been

> **Box 11.3 Insulin requirements in special settings**
>
> Increase by 30–50% in
>   Obesity
>   Liver disease
>   Steroid therapy
> Increase by 50–100% in sepsis
> Increase by up to 500% in cardiopulmonary bypass

well established and the rate of insulin administration has remained constant over many hours, it may be permissible to reduce monitoring to 2- or even up to 4-hourly but any change in insulin regimen thereafter requires resumption of hourly monitoring.

Patients on intravenous glucose and insulin regimens require regular monitoring of potassium, at least daily or more frequently if the patient's condition is unstable.

A critical point about intravenous insulin in Type 1 diabetes is the transient duration of action of the insulin (half-life 7 min). If the insulin infusion is interrupted, hyperglycaemia and then ketosis will rapidly ensue. Because of this, it is traditional to forbid the turning off of intravenous insulin regimens at any time. In practice, an insulin infusion can be interrupted if the patient is persistently hypoglycaemic but for no longer than 30 min without repeat blood glucose monitoring. Note that certain conditions dramatically increase insulin requirements (Box 11.3).

Managing intravenous insulin

Intravenous sliding scale (Box 11.4)
This regimen is based on the patient's normal requirements. Background infusion of intravenous glucose at a fixed rate is established (e.g. 10% glucose at 62 mL/h) and a dilute solution of insulin is infused via a programmable syringe pump at a rate based on the patient's usual 24 h insulin requirement and adjusted according to hourly bedside blood glucose monitoring. Potassium is added to the glucose (e.g. 20 mmol/0.5L). Note that this does not replace the full fluid requirements of the patient and these should be added and run in parallel.

Box 11.4 Writing up an intravenous sliding scale

Glucose
10% glucose 62 mL/h

Potassium
20 mmol/0.5 L

Insulin
50 units soluble insulin made up to 50 mL in normal saline = 1 unit/mL

Calculate patient's total daily insulin dose (all short- and intermediate-acting insulins taken in a day), or take it as 48 units/24 h if unknown

Set insulin rate for plasma glucose range 7–9 mmol/L at 1/24 total daily dose

Prescribe higher doses for higher ranges, lower doses for lower ranges (Table 11.1)

Make sure prescription shows no duplication, e.g. ranges of 7.1–9.0 and 9.1–11.0 rather than 7–9, 9–11

Allow insulin to be turned off only if plasma glucose <3.5 mmol/L on two successive occasions despite reduction of insulin rate. Monitor every 30 min till insulin infusion resumed

Measure plasma glucose hourly and adjust insulin according to prescribed scale

Check progress at 2 h and 4-hourly to see if insulin doses need adjustment

Check potassium 4–8-hourly

Do not stop intravenous insulin until subcutaneous regimen begun

Table 11.1 An example of an intravenous insulin infusion regimen (based on a patient with a total daily insulin requirement of 48 units/day). Ten per cent glucose 0.5 L + 20 mmol/L KCl, 62 mL/h. Fifty units human soluble insulin made up to 50 mL with normal saline = 1 unit/mL.

Blood glucose mmol/L (hourly)	Insulin Units/h	Insulin mL/h
If blood glucose <3.5mmol/L on two consecutive occasions, turn insulin off and recheck glucose in 30 min		
< 4.0	0.5	0.5
4.0–7.0	1.0	1.0
7.1–9.0*	2.0	2.0
9.1–11.0	3.0	3.0
11.1–14.0	4.0	4.0
14.1–17.0	5.0	5.0
> 17.0	6.0	6.0

*For this level, dose in units/h = total daily dose if known ÷ 24.

The insulin infusion rate then prescribed for near-normal glycaemia (e.g. when plasma glucose is in the range 7–9 mmol/L) is 1/24th the patient's total daily insulin requirement. For patients where this is not known, an assumption of a requirement of 48 units/24 h (2 units/h) is reasonable. Less insulin is prescribed if the plasma glucose is falling and more if it is rising. Once the regimen is started, it should be inspected after 2 h, and 4-hourly thereafter, to make sure that the dose ranges do not need changing. An example for such a regimen is given in Table 11.1.

Glucose, potassium and insulin infusion (Box 11.5)
An alternative regimen puts the insulin and potassium and glucose into a single container and infuses them at a fixed rate based on general principles. A starting regimen is 15 units soluble insulin in 0.5 L 10% glucose with 10 mmol potassium chloride given at 100 mL/h. Hourly blood glucose monitoring is started and if the blood glucose rises above 10 mmol/L or falls below 4.4 mmol/L, the infusion needs to be replaced with a mixture containing more or less insulin, respectively (Box 11.5). The advantage of this regimen is that glucose can never be given without insulin and vice versa. However, a disadvantage is the waste and inconvenience of replacing full bags when the blood glucose concentration drifts out of the desired range. In one study the regimen provided acceptable control in 82% of patients and it has the advantage of simplicity.

When to start an intravenous insulin regimen

For a well-controlled patient undergoing surgery on a given day, it is reasonable to start the intravenous insulin early on the morning of the operation. There is no reason to alter the insulin regimen prior to this as it is not until the patient misses breakfast that his/her insulin requirements are significantly altered. If the patient is already in hospital, it is reasonable to measure the plasma glucose at 3 a.m. and start the intravenous insulin then if >9 mmol/L, as it is likely to continue to rise as morning approaches. For the pa-

Box 11.5 **Glucose, potassium and insulin (GKI) regimen**

Glucose
10% glucose 0.5 L

Potassium
10 mmol per half-litre bag of 10% glucose

Insulin
15 units soluble insulin per half-litre bag of 10% glucose

Run at 100 mL/h
If plasma glucose < 6.6 mmol/L remake with 25 units insulin/L
If plasma glucose < 4.4 mmol/L remake with 20 units insulin/L
If plasma glucose > 10.0 mmol/L remake with 35 units insulin/L
If plasma glucose > 11.1 mmol/L remake with 40 units insulin/L

Do not stop intravenous insulin until subcutaneous regimen begun

tient at home, he/she can be told to check the glucose at this time and take a small dose of soluble insulin (e.g. 10% of his/her total 24 h insulin requirement) if high to avoid presenting with unacceptable hyperglycaemia in the morning. Otherwise, it is usual to start the intravenous glucose and insulin infusion at 6 a.m. This allows time to establish a respectable glucose level and to adjust the regimen if necessary on the basis of the first 2 h of blood glucose monitoring prior to any anaesthetic intervention.

How to finish intravenous insulin infusions

Because of the rapidity with which the action of intravenous insulin dissipates, it is essential that an intravenous insulin regimen in a person with Type 1 diabetes is not stopped until the subcutaneous insulin regimen has been resumed. Once a decision to recommence feeding in the postoperative state is made, the intravenous insulin infusion should be continued until the end of the first meal. An appro-

priate dose of soluble insulin should be given before that meal (e.g. one-quarter of the intravenous requirement of the previous day, or the patient's usual pre-meal soluble insulin dose) and the intravenous insulin may be discontinued on conclusion of the meal.

It is important to note that while 150 g glucose infused over a 24-h period may limit catabolism, it is not a replacement for feeding. Patients whose clinical condition requires them to remain nil by mouth for more than 48 h should be considered for full parental nutrition therapy and an insulin regimen should be constructed specifically for this.

Insulin administration during parenteral nutrition

There are few studies on which to base advice for insulin administration during parenteral nutrition. However, it should be self-evident that if the patient's plasma glucose concentration is running over the renal glucose threshold (usually 10 mmol/L) much of the energy content of the expensive nutritional preparations will be lost in the urine. It is therefore essential to control blood glucose in patients with diabetes during parenteral nutrition. An intravenous regimen such as that described for surgery with significantly higher doses would be ideal but would require almost continuous hourly blood glucose monitoring which is probably unreasonable for both the patient and the hospital staff. Some authorities cover the feed with an initial dose of a mixed insulin, expecting the soluble component of the insulin to provide rapid insulinization as the intravenous foods are administered and the delayed-acting component to continue insulinization for the duration of the administration. A second dose of an intermediate-acting insulin alone is given exactly 12 h later. Insulin dose adjustments are made on the basis of regular blood glucose monitoring but, once a regimen is established, it is probably adequate to revert to 4-hourly testing, with a prescribed option for a small dose of soluble insulin to be given if the plasma glucose on any occasion is > 10 mmol/L (e.g. 10% total daily dose for 10–15 mmol/L; 20% total daily dose if > 15 mmol/L). If supplemental doses are given, the standard doses should be increased by appropriate amounts the next day.

Subcutaneous insulin regimens in sick patients with diabetes (Box 11.6)

Effective insulin replacement—and good glucose control—can be difficult when intercurrent illness and/or diminished appetite make insulin requirements unpredictable. The immediate postoperative period is a case in point but the same is true for any significant illness where good control is required. Intravenous insulin will work, but once the patient is eating it is unkind to both the patient and the staff to continue this because of the requirement for hourly blood glucose monitoring. In this setting it is most appropriate to administer soluble insulin subcuta-

neously half an hour before each meal (if it is a fast-acting analogue, immediately before each meal) with an intermediate-acting insulin given at bedtime. Blood glucose monitoring should be performed before each meal, 2 h after completion of each meal, at bedtime and at 3 a.m. A good starting dose would be one-quarter (25%) of the patient's previous 24 h insulin requirement or, if this is unknown, 0.1 unit/kg body weight. If the plasma glucose is high 2 h after meals, at bedtime or at 3 a.m., or times when the action of the most recent insulin injection will be at its peak, a supplemental dose can be given. As a guide, if very tight control is required, an additional 10% of the total daily dose (or, alternatively, one-quarter to one-third of the usual of the prescribed meal dose) can be administered if the plasma glucose is over 9 mmol/L, for all patients if the value is over 13 mmol/L, an additional 20% of the total daily dose or half of a meal dose should be given.

Later inspection of the patient's insulin administration will allow supplemental doses to be added to the preceding meal or bedtime dose so that within 24–48 h normoglycaemia should be achieved with only four injections. An example of this is given in Fig. 11.1. It is desirable to run the plasma glucose between 7 and 9 mmol/L; this is slightly above true normoglycaemia, providing some protection against sudden hypoglycaemia, but is below the usual renal threshold for glycosuria, minimizing the risk of dehydration from hyperglycaemia.

When these regimens are used in patients who are sick (e.g. during sepsis) the prescribing physician should be aware of the rapid fall in insulin requirement that may occur as the primary problem resolves. The insulin regimen requires daily revision until the patient is medically stable. Care should be taken to watch and provide for hypoglycaemia.

Treatment of hypoglycaemia is best given orally (see Chapter 9) but glucagon (1 mg intramuscularly) should be available for the nurses to use if blood glucose falls below 3 mmol/L and the patient cannot be treated orally. After treatment of a hypoglycaemic episode, the blood glucose should be checked (e.g. at 30 min) to ensure it has risen above 4 mmol/L.

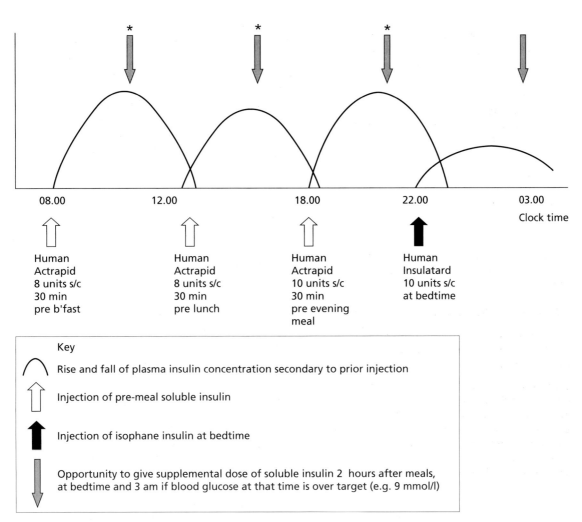

Figure 11.1 Subcutaneous insulin for a sick patient who is eating. *Give 2 units Human Actrapid 2 h post meals, bedtime or 3 a.m. if blood glucose > 9mmol/L; or give 4 units Human Actrapid 2 h post meals, bedtime and 3 a.m. of blood glucose > 13 mmol/L.

Surgery in patients with Type 2 diabetes mellitus

Patients well managed on diet, exercise ± insulin sensitizing agents

It is likely that these patients will tolerate a period of fasting with no rise in plasma glucose concentration, and possibly even a fall. Although plasma glucose should be monitored prior to surgery, at 2- and then 4-hourly intervals during recovery, no specific addi-tional action need be taken if the glucose remains less than 10 mmol/L. Glucose-containing infusion fluids may cause hyperglycaemia, in which case intra-venous insulin will be required and a regimen similar to that for Type 1 diabetic patients should be instituted.

Patients on insulin secretagogues

Here the risk is both of hypoglycaemia, particularly with long-acting insulin secretagogues such as glibenclamide, as the sulphonylurea continues its action and the patient ceases to eat; or, conversely, hyperglycaemia as the immobility and stress around the operation increase the insulin requirements for the patient. In general, these patients should stop their oral agents on the morning of surgery (the night before for long-acting agents) and glucose monitoring should start. Intravenous glucose and insulin infusion as for Type 1 patients should be started if the plasma glucose rises above 10 mmol/L. Glucose infusion alone should be started if the plasma glucose is 4 mmol/L or less with the introduction of insulin at appropriate rates as the glucose rises above 9 mmol/L.

Minor surgery

Very minor procedures where the patient is expected only to miss breakfast for patients with Type 2 diabetes can be carried out as in the non-diabetic with the avoidance of insulin secretagogues that morning. For Type 1 diabetic patients this is not best practice although if the procedure is very minor and only requires a late breakfast, it is acceptable simply to delay the morning insulin injection until the first meal. It should be realized that it is likely that the patient will become hyperglycaemic and possibly ketotic if this insulin administration is significantly delayed and blood glucose monitoring is therefore mandatory.

Day surgery

Increasingly, attempts are being made to carry out surgical procedures requiring general anaesthesia without overnight admission. Little has been done to assess how best to manage diabetes in these circumstances. We have developed the following pragmatic schemes. For patients in poor control, e.g. HbA_{1c} > 9%, day case surgery involving general anaesthesia is probably not recommended.

Day surgery for patients on oral medication
Surgery should be scheduled for the morning, as early as possible. Patients will be asked to stop eating and drinking at midnight on the evening prior to the procedure. Patients on oral medication, metformin and long-acting sulphonylureas such as glibenclamide

and chlorpropamide should stop the medication 24 h prior to the procedure; thiazolidinediones, tolbutamide, glipizide, gliclazide, glimepiride, natiglinide and repaglinide can be stopped that morning. If on bedtime insulin only, this may be continued as the glucose control overnight should not be affected if only breakfast is to be missed.

Once the patient is admitted for the procedure and made nil by mouth, 2-hourly blood glucose monitoring is mandated. Intravenous glucose should be started if blood glucose is < 5 mmol/L, a standard intravenous insulin and glucose regimen if blood glucose > 11 mmol/L. Once using intravenous solutions, hourly blood glucose testing at least is required and suitable adjustment of the regimens to keep blood glucose between 7 and 11 mmol/L.

Intravenous insulin should be continued until the patient is able to eat, when it can be discontinued. Type 1 patients should receive a dose of subcutaneous insulin just before the meal based on their usual meal requirement. If plasma glucose is > 5 and < 15 mmol/L 2 h post meal, the patient can be discharged, to resume the usual medications at the next dose time. Patients on chlorpropamide and glibenclamide should be kept under observation until the evening, to guard against late hypoglycaemia. Metformin should only be resumed once it is known that the patient is renally and haemodynamically stable.

Type 1 patients should arrive for the procedure as early as possible, having checked that they are not hypoglycaemic before leaving home. Hourly blood glucose monitoring and intravenous insulin should be started on arrival at the day surgery centre and continued until after the first meal taken postoperatively, which should be covered by an appropriate dose of soluble or fast-acting insulin, according to the patient's usual dosage. If blood glucose is between 5 and 15 mmol/L 2 h post meal and the patient can monitor his/her blood glucose at home and is aware of 'sick day' rules, he/she can be discharged.

Home management of illness

The management of illness at home is always complicated by the difficulty in management of the diabetes. This is probably most true for insulin-treated diabetes, where the illness tends to elevate blood glucose and any associated anorexia risks hypoglycaemia.

For a Type 1 diabetic patient the first rule of self-management of illness is *not to stop taking insulin even if not eating*. Cessation of insulin therapy because of anorexia is a common cause of diabetic ketoacidosis. For this reason, ill, anorexic and particularly vomiting patients who have Type 1 diabetes may need admission to hospital but much minor illness can be managed at home, provided the patient or someone staying with the patient can measure blood glucose and urinary ketones accurately and is confident that, with some help, he/she can manage.

For a day of illness with hyperglycaemia and anorexia, we recommend the following.

1 Drink plenty of fluids.

2 If not eating, sip steadily on sugary fluids at mealtimes.

3 Measure blood glucose 2 hourly.

4 If initial blood glucose > 13 mmol/L take 20% total daily insulin dose as fast-acting injection. Thereafter, measure blood glucose 2 hourly and:

  • if ketostix negative or + but blood glucose high (> 13 mmol/L) take 10% total daily insulin dose 2 hourly, until levels start to fall;

  • if ketonuria present as ++ or +++, and blood glucose high (> 13 mmol/L) take 20% of total daily insulin dose 2 hourly until blood glucose levels start to fall.

5 Take usual dose of evening intermediate-acting insulin but check blood glucose at bedtime and at 3 a.m. to see if additional fast-acting insulin is needed.

6 When ketonuria has resolved, return to usual regimen.

For a day of illness where appetite is maintained but blood glucose is running high, continue usual dosage of insulin through the day but take additional fast-acting insulins pre-meals and 2 h after meals if blood glucose is > 13 mmol/L. The extra insulin should be omitted if the blood glucose is < 13 mmol/L or over 13 mmol/L but falling from a higher value. The rule of thumb to use supplemental doses of half the usual pre-meal dose or 10–20% of the total daily dose, according to the presence or absence of ketonuria, can be used.

Patients should be encouraged to seek telephone advice from their diabetes care team when managing illness at home and they must be admitted to hospital for intravenous rehydration and insulin if they are very nauseated, vomiting, experiencing deteriorating symptoms or if the hyperglycaemia, or more worryingly the ketonuria, does not begin to resolve.

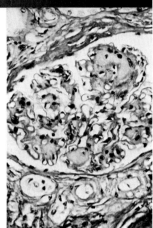

Special
Situations

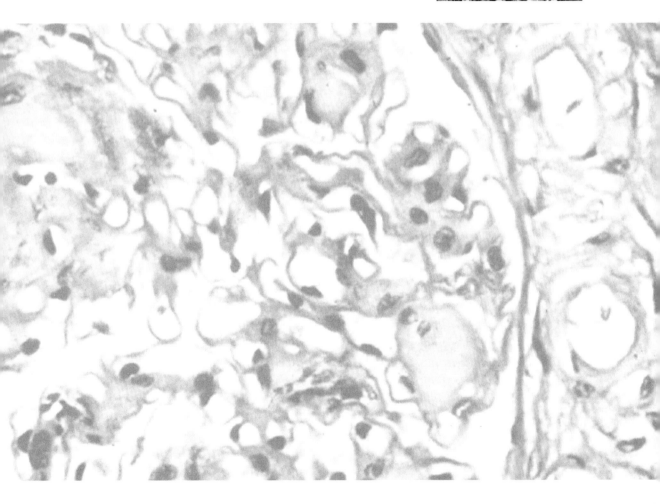

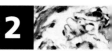

Pregnancy and Diabetes

Summary

- The diabetic woman has a higher risk of complicated pregnancy and fetal loss than her non-diabetic peers

- This risk is substantially reduced by proper diabetic and obstetric management

- Good glycaemic control is essential at conception and in early pregnancy to minimize risk of congenital abnormality

- Good glycaemic control is essential through pregnancy to minimize risk of fetal hyperinsulinism and macrosomia

- Good glycaemic control is essential in labour to minimize risk of neonatal hypoglycaemia

- Modern fetal monitoring reduces the risk associated with continuation of pregnancy in diabetic women to term

- The diabetic woman desirous of pregnancy is best managed in a combined specialist clinic, where obstetric and diabetic care can be delivered simultaneously — both for the convenience of the woman and to facilitate communication between the disciplines

- Hypoglycaemia is a risk for the mother, especially in the first few weeks of pregnancy, but not for the fetus

- Insulin is the appropriate hypoglycaemic agent for use in pregnancy, although insulin-resistant women (including those with Type 2 diabetes) may use metformin to achieve pregnancy and in the first few weeks of pregnancy

- Insulin requirements rise in the 2nd and 3rd trimesters, but fall to pre-pregnancy levels immediately upon delivery of the placenta

- All fertile women with diabetes should be aware of the risk of unplanned pregnancy and given adequate family planning advice

- All pregnancies should be screened for gestational diabetes which should be managed actively to reduce risk of macrosomia and neonatal hypoglycaemia, and which offers an early warning of later Type 2 diabetes in the mother

The UK, in common with all other countries, reports worse outcome for pregnancy in diabetic women than in their non-diabetic peers, although much has improved since the early days of insulin therapy when fetal loss was >35%. Perinatal mortality currently runs as high as 5% and major congenital abnormalities at 8–9% (Table 12.1). These figures remain higher than those of the background population,

Table 12.1 Pregnancy outcomes in the UK expressed as percentage of pregnancies. (*British Medical Journal*, 1997; **315**: 275–281, with permission from the BMJ Publishing Group.)

	Hawthorne *et al.*			Casson *et al.*		
	Perinatal mortality	Neonatal mortality	Congenital malformations	Stillbirths	Infant mortality	Congenital malformations
Diabetic	4.8	5.9	8.1	2.5	1.99	9.4
Background population	0.89	0.39	2.13	0.5	0.68	0.97

Table 12.2 Fetal outcome by HbA_1 at booking.

HbA_1	Spontaneous abortion	Major congenital abnormality	Normal live birth
<11%	8	3	89
11–14%	21	15	64
>14%*	33	33	33
GDM		As control population	

* Non-diabetic mean + 9 standard deviations, equivalent to approximately 10% in a DCCT aligned HbA_{1c} assay.
DCCT, Diabetes Control and Complications Trial; GDM, gestational diabetes mellitus.

interventional delivery is much more common and large-for-dates babies, although usually healthy, remain common.

Types of pregnancy in diabetes

Three separate scenarios exist and require distinct management.
1 *Type 1 diabetes* predating pregnancy.
2 *Type 2 diabetes* predating pregnancy.
3 *Diabetes* arising for the first time in pregnancy.

Diabetes that predates pregnancy should be strictly controlled prior to conception and all fertile diabetic female patients should be advised about pregnancy planning. They should be encouraged to use contraception, prior to making a deliberate decision to embark upon a pregnancy, at which time diabetes control should be tightened and contraception discontinued once treatment goals established. This is to avoid the increased risk of poor fetal outcome (spontaneous abortion and congenital malformation) with rising HbA_{1c} (Table 12.2).

Diabetes diagnosed for the first time in pregnancy may be the coincidental first presentation of Type 1 or Type 2 disease, in which case it can arise at any stage in the pregnancy. It may also be gestational diabetes, a condition related to the insulin resistance of later pregnancy and a predictor of Type 2 diabetes in later life, which resolves after delivery. Typically, this type of gestational diabetes arises at around the 28th week of pregnancy. Because there is no hyperglycaemia during organogenesis, and in contrast to pregnancy in coincidental diabetes, there is no increased risk of fetal malformation. The metabolic abnormalities of later pregnancy are associated with accelerated fetal growth and macrosomia in all diabetes. All these fetal risks can be greatly reduced by strict glycaemic control throughout the pregnancy.

The diagnosis of diabetes in pregnancy is associated with increased operative intervention. There is dispute about whether this is always clinically indicated or whether the professional awareness of increased risk to the mother and baby by itself increases risk of intervention.

Gestational diabetes mellitus

Any diabetes newly diagnosed in pregnancy is strictly 'gestational' but the term is often reserved for patients developing glucose intolerance in association with the insulin resistance of later pregnancy, with the expectation of resolution of the metabolic abnormality post-partum. The condition is most common in populations with a high prevalence of Type 2 diabetes, which gestational diabetes mellitus (GDM) indeed predicts. Pregnant women should be screened for diabetes around the 28th week. The precise timing of the test is controversial as active management after this time may be too late to alter the fetal growth pattern, especially if the disease did appear earlier. Screening earlier in the course of the pregnancy will miss the women who develop the condition more typically at the 28th week.

There is still no consensus about the appropriate way to screen for GDM. Screening based on risk factors such as obesity, history of previous large baby, polyhydramnios, current large baby, is considered too insensitive and all pregnant women should be screened. The gold standard would be an oral glucose tolerance test for all, but this is not always feasible. Our practice is a random plasma glucose at 26–28 weeks with a formal oral glucose tolerance test arranged immediately if a non-fasting plasma glucose value is >6.7 mmol/L (Box 12.1).

The diagnostic criteria recommended by the World Health Organization (WHO) are that any glucose intolerance in pregnancy is regarded as GDM. Thus, the 2-h glucose of 75 g oral glucose tolerance test of ≥7.8 mmol/L is considered diagnostic.

Women with newly diagnosed GDM should have a complication screen if the 2-h blood glucose is >11.1 mmol/L because they may have pre-exisiting late diagnosed Type 1 or Type 2 diabetes. Women whose 2-h plasma glucose is between 7.8 and 11 mmol/L probably do not require complication screening. Women with Type 1 or Type 2 diabetes should have a retinal examination in each trimester if there is no retinopathy at the onset of pregnancy, or monthly in the presence of retinopathy at conception, as pregnancy itself carries a risk of rapid deterioration, and this is made worse if a women, unexpectedly pregnant, suddenly improves previously poor glycaemic control for the sake of her baby.

Management

Women should be given dietary advice and taught to monitor fasting and postprandial glucose levels. Insulin therapy is started if the former exceeds 5.5 mmol/L or the latter 7 mmol/L. The timing of the postprandial test is currently controversial, many adhering to the usual 90-min postprandial test. However, there is evidence from a practice in California that keeping the 1-h postprandial glucose test under 7 mmol/L is associated with a very low incidence of macrosomia.

Insulin should be started rapidly and it is our current practice to use soluble insulin 30 min before meals to control postprandial hyperglycaemia and bedtime isophane insulin to control fasting glucose levels. Targets for therapy, based on the Californian experience, are 3.5–5.5 mmol/L before meals and 4–7 mmol/L postprandially (Box 12.2). The risk of significant hypoglycaemia in gestational diabetes, where insulin resistance is prevalent, is surprisingly low but women may need very high insulin doses in the last trimester.

Exercise should be encouraged. Labour is managed as for any insulin-treated diabetic woman (see below).

Post-partum, these women should be checked for resolution of their glucose tolerance. Immediately on completion of delivery, all insulin can be discontinued. Maternal plasma glucose can be checked at 2 and 4 h post-partum to ensure that the GDM was not in fact coincidental new Type 1 or Type 2 diabetes. If the fasting blood glucose the next day is <6 mmol/L

Box 12.1 **Screening for diabetes in pregnancy**

Random plasma glucose at 26–28 weeks
If 6.8 mmol/L or more → oral glucose tolerance test
Fasting plasma glucose >7.0, 2 h >7.8 = gestational diabetes mellitus
Diet, exercise, home blood glucose monitoring
If pre meal >5.5 or 1 h post meal >7 mmol/L → insulin

---

and a single 90-min postprandial level is <7 mmol/L, no further action need be taken at that time. A formal oral glucose tolerance test should be arranged for 3 months post delivery—this test is commonly carried out at 6 weeks because it is convenient to arrange it to coincide with other appointments but new cases of diabetes will be missed as the effect of the previous treatment programme may persist at this time (Box 12.3).

Women whose oral glucose tolerance has reverted to normal are warned that they have increased risk of GDM recurring in subsequent pregnancies and they should be tested for this early in the pregnancy (20 weeks and onwards); they are also at higher risk of developing Type 2 diabetes as they get older and should be given lifestyle advice to help prevent this. It is advisable to ask their primary care physician to check a fasting plasma glucose annually thereafter to ensure early diagnosis. Women who remain obese after GDM have approximately 65% risk of developing Type 2 diabetes over 15 years. In normal weight women, the risk falls to 38%.

This advice is given even more strongly to women who have impaired glucose tolerance post-partum, where it may be considered advisable to arrange annual glucose tolerance testing. Women with persistent diabetes should be treated as having Type 2 diabetes (see page 111).

Type 1 diabetes and pregnancy

Type 1 diabetic women who wish to become pregnant should be encouraged to plan their pregnancies carefully and take adequate contraception until their plasma glucose is optimal. We use the same treatment targets for Type 1 diabetes as for GDM, although the evidence base for this in Type 1 is lacking. During pre-pregnancy counselling, the usual glucose targets are intensified, and intensified insulin therapy is suggested. Some are ideally achieving an HbA_{1c} of <6.5%, with no problematic hypoglycaemia, prior to discontinuing contraception. However, women who have major problems improving glycaemic control to this degree should be encouraged to achieve the best results possible for them and then be supported in pregnancy. All women should be encouraged to use multiple daily injection therapy prior to pregnancy to establish their requirements. It is unlikely that good control will be established in a Type 1 patient with twice daily mixed insulins and premixed insulins are likely to cause a problem as the increase in insulin requirement in the latter half of pregnancy is often very large. The absorption of large doses of insulin is very slow compared to absorption of smaller doses.

We traditionally use pre-meal soluble insulin with isophane insulin either at bedtime alone or twice daily to provide background glucose control. Women already using fast-acting analogues are permitted to remain on them, especially if the use of the analogue was indicated for clinical reasons (such as nocturnal hypoglycaemia or marked postprandial hyperglycaemia). The safety of these insulins in pregnancy has not yet been established, but where they are successfully improving glycaemic control, any potential risk of the new insulin is likely to be significantly less than the known risk of hyperglycaemia to the fetus. Care is needed to check that the insulin action does not 'run out' between injections, as it is likely that recurrent transient hyperglycaemia is damaging to fetal development. Small doses of isophane insulin can be added to the analogue to extend the insulin action if necessary. A particular problem may occur between the cessation of action of the pre-evening meal analogue injection and the onset of action of the bedtime isophane. If this happens, the evening isophane may be given earlier in the evening (3 h after the evening meal) or, as with other times of day, a small additional dose of isophane can be added to the analogue before the evening meal.

Women with Type 1 diabetes need to undertake 4–7 blood glucose tests daily in the run up to pregnancy and through the pregnancy. Ideally, they test pre- and postprandially daily but it is more practical to suggest alternate days of pre- and post-prandial testing.

Insulin requirements may fall in very early pregnancy and hypoglycaemia can be a particular problem at this time. Hypoglycaemia is not thought to damage fetal development but can be problematic for the mother.

Hypoglycaemia remains a major problem for Type 1 diabetic women throughout pregnancy. The very strict glucose control required for optimal fetal development is difficult to maintain with currently available exogenous insulins without increasing hypoglycaemia. The reader is referred to Chapter 9 for a further discussion of this topic and strategies for prevention but it is important to note here that hypoglycaemia without symptoms and sudden severe hypoglycaemia is a risk for pregnant Type 1 diabetic women and, if these are suspected, very careful advice must be given about undertaking potentially dangerous activities such as driving.

Blood glucose control should be managed by intravenous insulin infusion during labour (see below) and the infusion rate should be halved on delivery of the placenta. The pre-pregnancy dose or the dose used in early pregnancy should be resumed post-partum, once the woman is eating again, but it must be recognized that breast-feeding is a significant exercise. Care should be taken to avoid hypoglycaemia, particularly at night, and women can be encouraged to eat more. A reduction in overnight insulin dose may also be needed.

Type 2 diabetes and pregnancy

Until recently it was considered that all hypoglycaemic agents should not be used before and during pregnancy and this is still a rule we follow with one exception (see below). Type 2 diabetic women planning pregnancy should be converted to daily injection therapy with insulin; this is to achieve the precision of control that pregnancy requires, establish the woman's likely insulin needs before the pregnancy and allow the rapid increase in insulin requirement that is likely in the second and third trimester. Hypoglycaemia is a relatively small risk for these women but the insulin doses required can be extremely large.

Diet and exercise are obviously particularly important in the run up to pregnancy and during the pregnancy itself.

We use the same treatment targets for Type 2 diabetic women as for other pregnant women with diabetes.

There has been a recent publication suggesting equivalent pregnancy outcome for women managed on sulphonylureas through pregnancy. While this is reassuring for women who become pregnant while still taking oral medication, the outcome of both groups in the study was not ideal. There are data suggesting that metformin is associated with worse perinatal outcome. Metformin may be useful to encourage fertility in insulin-resistant Type 2 diabetic women with polycystic ovarian syndrome and it is our policy to continue metformin in such women in association with insulin therapy, discontinuing the drug once pregnancy is established.

Management of diabetes in labour

Exposure to a maternal blood glucose of over 7 mmol/L during labour increases the risk of neonatal hypoglycaemia. We therefore recommend intravenous insulin therapy during labour, using the insulin dosage the mother is taking towards the end of the pregnancy as a guide to the appropriate doses she will need during labour. Apart from the significantly higher insulin doses this predicates, the regimen can be as for surgery (Chapter 11). Because the insulin resistance of pregnancy disappears on delivery of the placenta, the insulin infusion rate should be halved when delivery is complete. Insulin can be stopped altogether in women whose diabetes is thought to be strictly gestational.

In Type 1 diabetic women, intravenous insulin must be continued until the woman is eating again and established on subcutaneous injection therapy.

The target for plasma glucose during labour should be 4–7 mmol/L. Other intravenous insulin regimens are acceptable, provided they can deliver the required degree of glycaemic control.

The intravenous insulin regimen should be started once the woman stops eating for obstetric reasons during labour. For women being prepared for Caesarian section, the intravenous insulin can be started just before breakfast on the day, although a check of the blood glucose at 3 a.m. should be made and the insulin infusion started then if the blood glucose is over 5 mmol/L, as the prediction would be that the level will continue to rise thereafter as the bedtime isophane effect wanes.

Hypertension in diabetic pregnancy

Diabetic women with coexisting hypertension can have additional problems in pregnancy, as the blood pressure medication commonly requires intensifying as pregnancy progresses and this can interfere with placental blood flow. Angiotensin-converting enzyme (ACE) inhibitors should be stopped by the 12th week of pregnancy. It is customary to control blood pressure in pregnancy with old-fashioned and trusted agents such as alpha methyldopa, with labetalol and nifedipine as second- and third-line agents.

Risk to the mother in pregnancy

Microvascular complications commonly progress during pregnancy, partly, it is believed, because of the vascular changes of normal pregnancy and partly because for some women there needs to be a rapid intensification of glycaemic control. The latter can exacerbate microvascular complications, particularly if rapid improvement from previously very poor control is established. Women with advanced background or preproliferative retinopathy should be observed very closely by an experienced ophthalmologist and laser therapy applied if the retinopathy deteriorates. Microalbuminuria commonly becomes worse and may progress into full proteinuria. This may be partly related to the withdrawal of ACE inhibitor therapy in previously stable microalbuminuric women but was clearly recognized before these drugs were in use. The only treatment is to try to keep the blood pressure no higher than 120/80 mmHg. Women with microalbuminuria or established proteinuria, particularly if there is associated hypertension, should be warned about the risk of their pregnancy becoming complicated, with strong probability for inpatient care for observation, blood pressure control and rest and, frequently, early delivery of very small infants in more advanced cases.

The progression of microvascular disease reverts to its previous pattern post-partum but this will be no consolation to a woman who loses vision or develops nephrotic syndrome during her pregnancy.

Scanning the baby during pregnancy

Ultrasound is used to follow fetal development during pregnancy (Table 12.3). Our policy is for a viability scan at 8 weeks and a scan to check nuchal translucency at 12 weeks, the latter to screen for aneuploidy and cardiac defects. A further cardiac scan is performed at 21 weeks and a fetal anomaly screen at 23 weeks, at which time the first of monthly Doppler studies of the uterine and placental arteries is performed to assess placental function. Increased resistance to flow in the uterine arteries is evidence of increased risk of intrauterine growth retardation

Table 12.3 Monitoring pregnancy in diabetes.

Week	Visits*	HbA$_{1c}$	Retinal screen	Microalbuminuria	Fetal ultrasound
8	+	+	+ Monthly thereafter if retinopathy present	+ Monthly thereafter if retinopathy present	+ For viability
12	2–4 weekly	+	+	+	+ Nuchal translucency
21	2–4 weekly				Cardiac
23	2–4 weekly				Fetal anomaly and Doppler
24	2–4 weekly	+	+	+	Ultrasound and Doppler
28	2–4 weekly				Ultrasound and Doppler
32	1–2 weekly				Ultrasound and Doppler
36	1 weekly	+	+	+	Ultrasound and Doppler
40	Term				Ultrasound and Doppler

*Where ranges are suggested the choice is made based on individual patient needs. Women with problematic control may need more regular visits, and/or telephone consultations in between scheduled visits. Women with stable control and good understanding of the way to adjust their insulin can be reviewed less often.

(IUGR) and pre-eclampsic toxaemia (PET). After 28 weeks, monthly ultrasound scans, with Doppler studies, allow monitoring of fetal growth and obesity and liquor volume. Fetal growth commonly accelerates towards higher centiles after the 28th week, especially in gestational diabetes. In contrast, if the mother has extensive microvascular disease or is requiring vigorous treatment of hypertension, IUGR is a greater risk and regular scans allow identification of those fetuses with <50th centile growth, who are growth restricted.

Early delivery and the use of dexamethasone

If an obstetric decision is made that the baby is likely to be delivered prematurely (up to 34 weeks), the babies of diabetic mothers should not be denied the benefits of dexamethsone to mature the fetal lungs. We admit diabetic women for dexamethasone treatment, because of the acute and sometimes severe loss of glucose control that ensues. It lasts about 48 h. We use the usual calculation to establish a sliding scale for

intravenous insulin, adjusting the dose of insulin infused on the basis of hourly blood glucose monitoring but, as the woman is still eating normally, we do not use intravenous glucose. We add, to the full sliding scale dose, the woman's usual pre-meal subcutaneous insulin boluses. This avoids exposing the baby to the postprandial rise in blood glucose after a meal, before the intravenous insulin is adjusted to compensate, and means the woman gets 50–150% extra insulin in the 24-h period.

Breast-feeding

Breast-feeding should be encouraged as with any mother and baby. It is usual to use insulin rather than sulphonylureas in Type 2 diabetes to control hyperglycaemia during breast-feeding to avoid any risk of contamination of the breast milk. Breast-feeding has a similar effect to exercise and great care should be taken to avoid hypoglycaemia, particularly overnight. Many women choose to run their blood glucose slightly high post-partum to reduce this risk.

Manufacturers of newer ACE inhibitors suggest

avoiding their use during lactation but the penetration of the drugs into breast milk is low and enalapril or captopril can be restarted if needed to control microalbuminuria or blood pressure. The continued use of alpha methyldopa is possible but has been associated with depression.

Risks of maternal diabetes to the baby

The major problems of maternal diabetes to the baby are as follows.
• Increased risk of congenital malformation related to maternal hyperglycaemia during organogenesis. Although sacral agenesis and cardiac malformations are cited particularly, there are no truly diabetes-specific malformations. The use of folic acid in the first 14 weeks of pregnancy is important to reduce risk of abnormalities of the central nervous system, as the background risk for these is higher in diabetes but there are no data to indicate whether the conventional 400 µg dose or a higher dose of 5 mg offer different benefits.
• Risk of macrosomia is thought to be related to maternal hyperglycaemia in mid to late pregnancy and is reduced by tight glycaemic control in later pregnancy.
• Increased risk of intrauterine death, partly also related to glycaemic control.
• Increased risk of premature delivery, in part secondary to macrosomia but arguably also related to the greater monitoring and higher levels of professional anxiety engendered by a diagnosis of maternal diabetes.
• Risk of neonatal hypoglycaemia, thought to relate to persistent hyperinsulinaemia secondary to maternal hyperglycaemia. If blood glucose is managed appropriately during late pregnancy and delivery, the risk of clinically significant neonatal hypoglycaemia is thought to be reduced.

The baby of a diabetic mother has a 2–4% risk of developing Type 1 diabetes. Interestingly, the baby of a Type 1 diabetic father has a risk of 4–6% and a child with a diabetic sibling has a 6–8% risk. Nevertheless, the diabetes almost never develops in the neonatal period. Only 10% of Type 1 diabetes arises in people with a positive family history.

Box 12.4 Contraceptive options for women with diabetes

Women under 30 years
• Combined oral contraceptive with 30–35 µg oestrogen, e.g. Microgynon, Ovysmen
• Depot progestogen, e.g. Depo-Provera, Noristerat
• Progestogen-only pill, e.g. Micronor, Microval
• Etonogestrel implant, Implanon

Women over 30 years
• Depot progestogen
• Etonogestrel implant, Implanon
• Progestogen-only pill, e.g. Micronor, Microval
• Copper-containing intrauterine device
• Progestogen-releasing interuterine system, e.g. Mirena
• May use combined pill up to age 35 if non-smoker with no other cardiovascular risk factors, (see text)

Pregnancy planning

If diabetic pregnancy is to be managed appropriately, the woman needs to plan her pregnancy so that she can optimize her diabetes control before and during conception, organogenesis and fetal development. Appropriate contraceptive advice is an essential part of this (Box 12.4). Because of the vascular risk of diabetes itself, the ideal medical contraception would be a progestogen-only preparation such as the 'mini-pill' or depot injections, or slow-release progestogen implants. However, the mini-pill becomes significantly less effective if not taken regularly at 24-h intervals and so is often not appropriate for young women with hectic lifestyles. Some women are reluctant to use the depot preparations which cannot be stopped at will. All can be associated with weight gain and initially erratic vaginal bleeding, although this commonly settles into prolonged amenorrhoea. Depo-Provera, unlike the mini-pill, suppresses oestrogen levels and the patient's oestradiol level should be checked after 5 years' use. If the level is less than 100, a 6-month course of oestrogen replacement therapy is thought to be beneficial to reduce the risk of osteoporosis, although the evidence for this is anecdotal. For many women with uncomplicated Type 1 diabetes who do not smoke, have no additional cardiovascular risk factors (such as family history, obesity, hypertension or hyperlipidaemia) and especially if they are under 30 years old, the best option may be the common combined oral contraceptive, which will give a regular withdrawal bleed. Modern contraceptives do not exceed an oestrogen dose of 35 μg/day.

Barrier contraception using condoms offers additional protection against infection but is less reliable than the pill, with which they may be used. Modern intrauterine devices, including those releasing progestogens, are another good option for the diabetic woman, although in general best reserved for women who have had at least one previous pregnancy and are in monogamous relationships.

13

Diabetes in Children

Summary

■ Diabetes in children is most commonly Type 1 although with the rising tide of obesity, Type 2 diabetes is now well described in adolescents

■ Very poor glycaemic control in children limits linear growth and in the long term, poor glycaemic control is associated with increased risk of complications

■ Severe hypoglycaemia in the under 7s has been associated with intellectual impairment later, and avoidance of severe hypoglycaemia is a particularly important aim of therapy in this age group

■ The principles of diabetes management are similar for children as for adults but the effects of diabetes on physical, social and emotional growth must be considered and managed actively

■ The child with diabetes and his/her family both need professional support

Nature of the problem

Until recently, diabetes in children was almost exclusively Type 1, with a small number of single-gene diseases causing diabetes also described (Tables 13.1 and 13.2). However, with the rapid increase in obesity and inactivity rates in children, Type 2 diabetes is increasingly seen in adolescents and even some prepubertal children; particularly, but not exclusively, in populations with high background rates of Type 2 diabetes, which include most non-European ethnic groups.

The principles of management of diabetes in children are not different from those discussed in the appropriate chapters, but the importance of ensuring normal growth and development (both physical and emotional) takes equal priority with the aims of preventing long-term complications. The former is best carried out by experienced paediatric teams but this is sometimes at the expense of the latter and close re-

lationships between paediatric and adult services benefit the child with diabetes enormously. This is particularly true during adolescence when the transition of management of the child's care from paediatric to adult health services must be done carefully and sensitively. However, it is true for all stages of the child's life, as the paediatric team needs to keep in mind the long-term consequences of poor control which they will not see in their patients and the adult diabetes team needs to be very aware of the difficulties young patients and their families will have had managing diabetes through childhood.

Diagnosis

The diagnostic criteria in children are as in adults. As with adults, the most common childhood form, Type 1 diabetes, will be recognized by a shorter history, the associated malaise and weight loss and the

Table 13.1 Diabetes in children.

Type 1 diabetes mellitus
Autoimmune
Not autoimmune (no known markers)

Other specific types of diabetes
1 Single gene defects of insulin secretion:
Maturity onset diabetes of youth (MODY; Table 13.2)
Other
  Mitochondrial DNA 3423 mutations
  Wolfram syndrome

2 Genetic disorders of insulin action
Type A insulin resistance
Leprechaunism
Rabson–Mendenhall syndrome
Congenital lipoatrophy

3 Secondary to other pancreatic disease
Especially in children:
  Beta thalassaemia
  Cystic fibrosis
  Alpha antitrypsin deficiency
  Congenital absence of pancreas or islets

4 Secondary to other endocrine disease
Cushing's syndrome; gigantism

5 Secondary to drugs or toxins
Glucocorticoids
Asparaginase

6 Secondary to infection
Congenital rubella

7 Other forms of immune disorder
Polyglandular syndrome
APECED
Stiff man

8 Rare genetic disorders
Down's syndrome
Klinefelter's syndrome
Prader–Willi syndrome
Turner's syndrome
Laurence–Moon–Biedl syndrome
Myotonic dystrophy
Ataxia telangiectasia
Porphyria

Type 2 diabetes

presence of ketones in the urine. Non-Type 1 diabetes in childhood is probably still likely to be Maturity Onset Diabetes of Youth (MODY). This was first described in the 1960s at King's College Hospital. It is a type of diabetes occurring in children which, apart from the age of onset, appears to have much more in common with adult Type 2 disease. It is now known that MODY is caused by one of a series of single-gene defects (Table 13.2) and should be suspected when a child presents with non-insulin dependent diabetes mellitus with a strong family history coming from one side of the family only, in which the age or diagnosis of the disease has become progressively younger with successive generations. It has recently been suggested that a significant number of children who present with hyperglycaemia during an acute illness should be investigated for MODY once the acute episode has resolved.

There is a high incidence of diabetes in children with Down's syndrome (usually Type 1) and that and Wolfram syndrome (diabetes insipidus, diabetes mellitus, optic atrophy and deafness: DIDMOAD) are insulin-deficiency diseases. Congenital insulin resistance is seen as Type A in association with acanthosis nigricans and hyperandrogenism, most easily recognized in girls because of the associated hirsutism and polycystic ovarian syndrome. Type B insulin resistance is more rare and is associated with insulin receptor antibodies. Lephrechaunism and Rabson–Mendenhall syndrome relate to abnormalities of the insulin receptor and childhood obesity syndromes such as Prader–Willi, Alström's, and Laurence–Moon–Biedl are rare causes of obesity with diabetes. The increasing prevalence of obesity is making 'simple' Type 2 diabetes a force to be reckoned with in this age group. Werner's syndrome is a rare cause of premature ageing and diabetes can also occur with severe insulin resistance in different congenital lipodystrophies. Finally, non-insulin dependent diabetes can be inherited from maternal mitochondrial DNA in relatively uncommon syndromes such as maternally inherited diabetes in deafness (MIDD) and mitochondrial myopathy, encepelopathy, lactic acidosis and stroke-like episodes (MELAS).

In paediatrics, diabetes is also seen secondary to pancreatic damage in cystic fibrosis and beta thalassaemia. With true Type 1 diabetes in children, the doctor should beware of the risk of other associated autoimmune diseases. Coeliac disease in particular has been reported in up to 8% of children attending a diabetic clinic. It is our policy to screen for coeliac disease, using blood tests, at diagnosis and after 5 years,

Table 13.2 Maturity onset diabetes of youth (MODY).

Name	Gene	Course	Susceptibility to complications
MODY 1	HNF4α	Progressive insulin deficiency	High risk
MODY 2	Glucokinase	Stable mild hyperglycaemia	Low risk
MODY 3	HNF1α	Progressive insulin deficiency	High risk
MODY 4	Insulin promoter Factor 1		
MODY 5			
MODY 6			

or if diabetic control is very unstable and the child has suggestive symptoms.

Type 1 diabetes remains the most common and is the almost invariable cause of diabetes pre puberty. Although Type 1 diabetes depends on inheriting specific genes and tissues types, these confer only a susceptibility to diabetes rather than the diabetes itself. Other, presumably environmental, factors trigger the disease. Only 10% of Type 1 diabetes arises in families with a history of the disease but a child has a 2–3% risk of diabetes if his/her mother has diabetes, 4–6% if his/her father has diabetes and 5–10% if a sibling has diabetes.

Type 1 diabetes can occur at any age in childhood but there is a peak incidence of new cases during the teenage years, possibly related to the insulin resistance of puberty making obvious a pre-existing insulin secretory defect. Pubertal insulin resistance is physiological and specific for carbohydrate metabolism. In healthy children with a fully functional pancreas, this insulin resistance results in hyperinsulinaemia, which stimulates protein anabolism as protein and fat metabolism remain normally insulin-sensitive. This is presumably an important contributor to growth. In the child with Type 1 diabetes, the insulin resistance of puberty is associated with a dramatic rise in insulin requirements often leading to a rapid loss of previously stable glycaemic control. Clearly, emotional and sociological factors can also interfere with diabetes control in adolescence but the insulin requirement of puberty, even in the most compliant and nonrebellious teenager, can reach 2 units/kg/day. The natural increase in insulin resistance of puberty is made worse by any period of sustained poor control, an effect known as 'glucose toxicity'.

Management of Type 1 diabetes in childhood

Management is with insulin injections. This can be difficult in very small children, who can require very small doses of insulin and in whom changes of 1 or even 0.5 unit can swing them from hyperglycaemia to hypoglycaemia. Some very young children may need to be managed on small doses, or once or twice daily background insulin only but, in general, children will need fast-acting insulins for meals and some background insulin to cover the between meal periods and night time.

We start school-aged children on a mixture of a short- and intermediate-acting insulin before breakfast (commonly using a premixed insulin for convenience) with a soluble insulin before the evening meal and an intermediate-acting insulin given at the child's bedtime or, in cases of extreme difficulty with overnight control (nocturnal hypoglycaemia and/or resistant morning hyperglycaemia), the parents' bedtime. This can allow adequate intermediate-acting insulin to be given in the evening to control fasting blood glucose with diminished risk of hypoglycaemia in the middle of the night. The evidence suggests that over 30% of children using twice daily mixed insulins will experience significant and prolonged but usually asymptomatic hypoglycaemia in the night. The use of a split evening regimen has not been demonstrated to improve this situation in children as it has in adults. Subcutaneous insulin infusions at night only have been used for children with difficult overnight glycaemic control and there is evidence that older children can also manage pump therapy well. The use of the new genetically modified insulin analogues has obvious attraction in children—the fast short action of NovoRapid or Humalog is associated with less nocturnal hypoglycaemia, albeit at the expense of some hyperglycaemia in the early part of the night. Their fast action profiles also mean that they are reasonably efficacious if given immediately after eating, which can be helpful in the management of the very young child who is a fussy or unpredictable eater. Likewise, the newly available long-acting insulin analogue Glargine (Lantus), by providing a peakless background insulin, may offer advantages for the diabetes control of children going to bed early and rising late. However, this author has reservations about the use of these very new genetically modified insulins in children, simply because they do have slightly different receptor-binding characteristics from human insulin and their long-term safety, while not in question, has not been proven. We use these insulins where there is a clear clinical problem that we expect these insulins to solve, after discussion with the child and his/her parents.

Very close watch needs to be kept on children approaching puberty. Sudden dramatic loss of control may occur as insulin requirements rise. Up to 2 units/kg body weight is probably quite normal for these children.

Treatment of MODY

Sulphonylureas can be very effective in the treatment of MODY and, as with adults, we generally recommend the use of shorter acting agents such as glipizides. All of these agents stimulate insulin secretion via specific receptors associated with the beta-cell potassium channel and they work well in MODY where the main problem is a molecular failure to recognize plasma glucose levels. Metformin may have an increasing role in the management of obesity-related diabetes where insulin resistance is a major feature

and non-metformin insulin sensitizers, such as the thiazolidinediones, may also be useful, although experience in children with these agents is lacking and we do not use them as first line. With metformin (and alpha glucosidase inhibitors if used) in children, care should be taken to ensure no malabsorption of other substances such as vitamin B_{12}.

Diet and exercise in children with diabetes

Dietary management has to be prescribed for the Type 1 diabetic child, as there is no experience in teaching children the sort of dietary principles that an adult can learn to help them eat flexibly and use flexible insulin regimens. For children therefore it is still usual to prescribe a diet pattern of three meals a day, containing equivalent amounts of starchy carbohydrates for meals at the same time of day, with snacks between the meals and at bedtime. The family is taught equivalent values of different carbohydrate sources so they can vary the diet while maintaining insulin requirements at a reasonably stable level. The problem for children is their desire to eat as their peer group and also the unpredictable but often very vigorous nature of their exercise. Parents, school staff and children need to be advised about the requirement for extra carbohydrate between meals and to cover exercise, and the need for less background insulin if unexpectedly vigorous exercise is undertaken.

During adolescence, children and their families need a lot of support to help them avoid dietary habits that play havoc with diabetes control and focus on replacement of popular dietary items such as fizzy drinks with their diet equivalents can be very important. Fatty fast foods, while no healthier in the diabetic child than in anyone else, may not necessarily damage diabetes control, although the fat slows the absorption of any associated carbohydrate. High-fat diets, including crisps and fried foods, are particularly damaging to children with diabetes.

In Type 2 diabetes, dietary and lifestyle change is mandatory. Here high-calorie fatty meals are to be avoided and caloric restriction is needed. The main aim of therapy, however, should be to increase exercise levels—not an easy task for an overweight child to undertake, but essential. Strategies to help families, particularly low income families where both parents may be working, to help them support their child in exercising and avoiding fast foods need to be developed. One region in the USA has just achieved the banning of soft drinks machines in schools—a policy the UK would do well to ponder!

Targets for glycaemic control in children

Hypoglycaemia is probably the major anxiety for the parents of a young child with Type 1 diabetes. There are concerns that recurrent severe hypoglycaemia, from which a full recovery is almost invariably made at the time, may have cumulative effects on cortical function. The data collected so far are, in general, reassuring and certainly there does not appear to be a major effect of recurrent hypoglycaemia in children on long-term cognitive ability. The exception is in children under the age of 7. These children are at a stage of brain development and recurrent severe hypoglycaemia, particularly if associated with frequent seizures, can be associated with a degree of impaired intellectual performance when tested in the teenage years. On the other hand, very poor diabetes control can be associated with delayed linear growth and the skill is to walk a path between the two extremes. For children under 7, the avoidance of severe hypoglycaemia is particularly important and the lower end of the glucose target range should be no less than 5 mmol/L and may even be higher. Care should then be taken that the upper limit of the target glucose range is not set too high (no more than 9 mmol/L pre meal). Glycated haemoglobin of 8% in a Diabetes Control and Complications Trial (DCCT) aligned assay running up to 6.1% in non-diabetic children is a satisfactory compromise treatment goal for the under-7s.

Above the age of 7, attempts can be made to bring the diabetes into closer control if the child and his/her family are interested and willing to undertake at least two blood tests a day and preferably three insulin injections.

At around the time of puberty, a close watch should be kept on the HbA_{1c}, which can rise dramatically between clinic visits, if these are more than 3 months apart. Where children cannot be seen so regularly, arrangements can be made for them to have the HbA_{1c} tested—provided they and their parents are aware to seek advice if it has begun to rise.

The paediatric diabetes clinic

A paediatric diabetes clinic should include a paediatrician with an interest in diabetes; a dietitian with paediatric experience; a paediatric diabetes specialist nurse who has understanding of the social security provisions for children and their families and can liaise meaningfully with schools and other children's institutions. For older children, an ideal clinic will also include an adult diabetologist. In addition to examining the glycaemic control and enquiring about problematic hypoglycaemia, the paediatric diabetes clinic should measure height and weight and ensure that children with diabetes are growing appropriately along their centile lines. Periods of loss of glycaemic control are often associated with a slowing in linear growth which catches up as the diabetes control is improved. It is also important to observe the development of puberty, to ensure that development is proceeding normally and to be forewarned about the probable onset of the insulin resistance associated with this life stage. Physical examination of the children should also include regular inspection of injection sites as lipohypertrophy and other problems are more common in children than in adults, partly perhaps because of inexperience or nervousness in the insulin administrator and partly because of the smaller surface area available for injection.

Screening for complications in children with diabetes should start in children with Type 1 diabetes at the onset of puberty or after 5 years, whichever is sooner, and should include annual screening for microalbuminuria and retinopathy, inspection of the feet (if only to encourage proper care of the feet in the child for the future) and measurement of blood pressure.

Microalbuminuria remains rare in the prepubertal child. In puberty, 10–20% of diabetic children may show microalbuminuria. However, about 2% of non-diabetic children may exhibit at least transient microalbuminuria and microalbuminuria of uncertain significance can also be seen in very poor glycaemic control. For these reasons, the use of angiotensin-converting enzyme (ACE) inhibitors in diabetic children with microalbuminuria is not usual. However, in a teenager with persistent microalbuminuria, ACE inhibition should be considered and discussed with the child and parents.

Hyperlipidaemia in diabetic children should be treated with diet and exercise and by optimizing glycaemic control. Outside the setting of familial hypocholesterolaemia, however, it is reasonable to defer checking lipids until after puberty.

Social problems for children with diabetes

Having diabetes is not easy for anyone but it is particularly difficult for the young child and his/her family. Where diabetes has developed in early childhood, parents manage the disease for the child. Later, problems may arise during the teenage years, as the child is struggling for independence and the parent is afraid to let go. In general, most families manage extremely well but they may need additional support.

Because of the tight relationship between insulin administration, food intake and glycaemic control, meals can often become a focus of stress between the child with diabetes and his/her family. The evidence suggests that eating disorders are more common in children, particularly girls, with diabetes. In any event, the coexistence of diabetes, particularly insulin-dependent diabetes, and an eating disorder creates enormous difficulties in management. The ability to lose weight (through glycosuria) while eating freely by underinsulinization presents a real temptation to the diabetic child, particularly one who is a little overweight and perhaps particularly for girls. Omission of insulin injections and insulin avoidance is an extremely common method of controlling weight which is often associated with very poor glycaemic control. Attempts to improve glycaemic control with insulin alone are associated with weight gain as the glycosuria stops and this can make it very difficult for the child to follow the prescribed

regimens. Eating disorders and insulin omission should be considered in any child presenting with persistent very poor control (glycated haemoglobins of 11% or over) and often need prolonged and sensitive management, with the involvement of family and child psychiatry.

Children with diabetes can feel very isolated, commonly not knowing any other children with diabetes. This can be particularly problematic when the family experience of diabetes is of long duration, poorly controlled Type 2 diabetes with complications. Need for blood testing and self-injection can cause problems in today's needle conscious society and few children like to be different from their peers. Professional support for families but also for school teachers in dealing with these issues is very important and here there is a need for a diabetes specialist nurse with experience in these matters.

Parents of young children with diabetes should be aware that they are entitled to some financial support as it is assumed that the child with diabetes needs greater parental attention and more time than the healthy child. These additional sources of income can be very useful.

Later, as the child grows, practical arrangements for advising about social life, sexual encounters and employment opportunities become important. It is recommended that formal protocols are put in place for the transition of the child with diabetes from paediatric to adult services, with clear guidance for the child, his/her family and the clinical services involved as to when and where this happens and who is responsible for steering the child through the process. Children mature at different rates, so an age cut-off is probably unhelpful. Some clinics continue to provide outpatient care until formal education is complete, although that can be at very variable ages. Transition clinics, 'young adult' clinics and joint management between paediatricians and adult diabetologists have all been tried and it is not yet clear that there is any particularly appropriate model. The main concern is to avoid uncertainty for the child and ensure that there is at least one health care professional nominated to whom the child can turn if necessary.

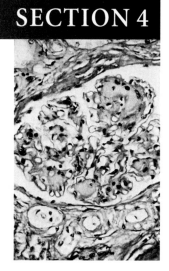

Diabetic Complications

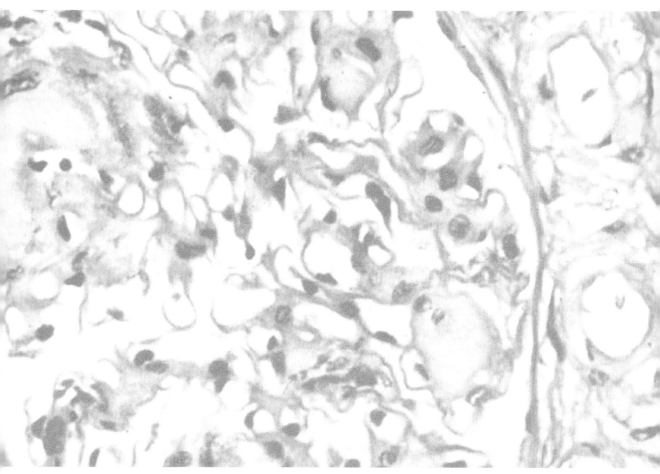

An Overview of Microvascular Complications

Summary

- Microvascular complications of diabetes affect the eyes (retinopathy), kidneys (nephropathy) and peripheral nerves (neuropathy)

- They develop with increasing duration of diabetes, although some patients are spared even after many decades

- Microvascular complications are sometimes present at diagnosis of Type 2 diabetes which has often been undiscovered for several years

- Poor glycaemic control over many years increases the risk of microvascular complications

- The incidence of microvascular complications is reduced, and their onset delayed, by tight glycaemic control

- Hypertension contributes to the progression of both retinopathy and nephropathy, and its control has beneficial effects in both of these situations

- Early detection of microvascular complications by regular (usually annual) screening is essential in order to introduce appropriate and timely treatments

An overview of microvascular complications

The complications of diabetes are greatly feared by patients, parents and other family members. The ever-present threats of blindness and amputations can cause lifelong anxiety: a blemish on a toe or painful loins are often equated with the prospect of amputation or transplantation. Many patients will know others with diabetic complications and will assume that these are inevitable. Complications must be discussed with patients and placed in their correct perspective to remove needless anxiety.

The scale of the chronic complications of diabetes became clear in the late 1920s and 1930s when detailed descriptions of the syndromes were first made. There are microvascular complications specific to diabetes, and other non-specific problems, which occur with increased frequency in diabetes, notably cardiovascular disease (Table 14.1). The epidemiology of the individual complications is discussed in the relevant chapters.

There is encouraging evidence in Type 1 diabetes of a reduction in the incidence of diabetic nephropathy. The results of the Diabetes Control and Complications Trial (DCCT) for Type 1 diabetes and the UK Prospective Diabetes Survey (UKPDS) for Type 2 diabetes show clearly that the development of nephropathy and retinopathy, and also neuropathy, can be delayed and their progression retarded by intensified diabetes therapy. UKPDS has also demonstrated the benefits to be obtained from tight blood pressure control, particularly on the evolution of both nephropathy and retinopathy. There are now specific treatments to slow the progression of established nephropathy, preserve vision in those with

Table 14.1 Major complications of diabetes.

Microvascular complications	Increased frequency of other diseases
Diabetic nephropathy	*Macrovascular disease*
Retinopathy	Coronary heart disease
Peripheral neuropathies	Peripheral vascular disease
Autonomic neuropathy	Strokes
Skin	*Nerves*
Necrobiosis lipoidica	Carpal tunnel syndrome
	Cranial nerve palsies
Joints	Mononeuropathies
Diabetic cheiroarthropathy	

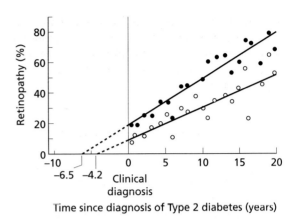

Figure 14.1 Presence of any retinopathy according to years since clinical diagnosis of Type 2 diabetes among patients in southern Wisconsin (●) and in rural Western Australia (○). Solid lines represent data fitted by weighted regression; lines are extrapolated to indicate the time at which onset of observable retinopathy is estimated to have occurred. (After Harris, M.I. *et al. Diabetes Care* 1992; **15**: 815–821.)

established retinopathy, and decrease the chance of neuropathy leading to foot damage.

Macrovascular disease affecting the coronary arteries, cerebral circulation and peripheral vessels is considerably increased in patients with diabetes, and associated with substantial morbidity and mortality. The evolution of these disorders in relation to hyperglycaemia, hypertension and hyperlipidaemia, and their amelioration in response to adequate treatment measures is described in Chapter 19.

Duration of diabetes and complications

The chronic microvascular complications of diabetes—retinopathy, nephropathy and autonomic and peripheral neuropathy—are rarely seen before 5–7 years' duration of diabetes in Type 1 diabetes and evolve most commonly after 10–20 years. However, Type 2 diabetic patients not infrequently present with retinopathy, neuropathy or foot ulceration and sometimes proteinuria as well. More than one-quarter of these patients have retinopathy at the time of diagnosis. This is because Type 2 diabetes has almost always been present for several years before presentation (Fig. 14.1). Patients with Type 2 diabetes must be screened for complications from the time of presentation, as these patients are already at risk. Prevalence and severity of complications continue to increase as duration of diabetes lengthens, but after 30 years their annual incidence appears to decrease. Some people with diabetes are free from complica-

tions even after 60 years or more. Indeed, we know one patient who developed Type 1 diabetes when she was 10 years old in 1932, treated by Dr R.D. Lawrence, who is free of all complications after 70 years of indifferently controlled diabetes and is now exceptionally fit aged 80 years. Her records at King's College Hospital are complete from diagnosis in 1932 to the present day!

Association of complications

Microvascular complications often develop in parallel with each other and with increasing duration of diabetes. Retinopathy generally occurs first and is not infrequently the only microvascular complication. It is quite possible for some patients with advanced proliferative retinopathy to be entirely free from any traces of nephropathy. In contrast, almost all patients (over 95%) with nephropathy have background or proliferative retinopathy and the absence of retinopathy in a proteinuric patient should stimulate a search for other causes of the nephropathy. Neuropathy can develop in patients without nephropathy and sometimes even with negligible retinopathy but is likely to be present in those with established nephropathy. Patients with proteinuria are at very high risk of developing macrovascular and especially coronary artery disease with its attendant high mortality (Chapters 15 and 19).

Pathogenesis of diabetic complications

The major organs most affected by microvascular damage are the eye, the kidney and peripheral nerves, but no single explanation of the pathogenesis of these complications affecting different tissues is possible.

The theories regarding the development of complications involve metabolic and vascular abnormalities; these are not mutually exclusive because metabolic changes can cause structural changes in the microvascular circulation. The effects of persistent hyperglycaemia and hypertension in causing microvascular damage are described in more detail below.

Ultrastructural basement membrane thickening in small blood vessels is the hallmark of long-standing diabetes; it is seen in many tissues including the kidney, retina, nerve, skin, muscle and adipose tissue. It is closely related to the duration of diabetes, but its relationship to functional abnormalities is less clear.

While there are known familial trends in the development of some diabetic complications, notably nephropathy, the many attempts to discover genetic markers of susceptibility to particular complications have so far failed to identify any specific variants to help patients or clinicians.

Glycation of proteins

Glucose binds to many proteins, mainly linking to lysine residues, and the extent of the reaction depends upon the prevailing glucose concentration. This initial reaction is followed by a rearrangement to form a more permanent product. Glycation products formed on collagen, DNA and some long-lived macromolecules may undergo irreversible chemical rearrangements to form advanced glycation end products (AGE) which accumulate throughout life. Both function and structure of some tissues can be altered as a result of glycation: thus, activity of some enzymes may change, physical properties of, for example, collagen may be altered, or cell rigidity may increase as it does in the Schwann cell basal lamina in peripheral nerves. Glycation is proportional to the prevailing blood glucose over the life of the glycated substrate, glycated haemoglobin (HbA_{1c} or HbA_1) is used to provide a measure of long-term glycaemic control.

More detailed consideration of the pathogenesis of individual complications will be found in the relevant chapters.

Aldose reductase pathway

In the presence of hyperglycaemia, the metabolism of glucose is to some extent diverted by the aldose reductase pathway to the production of sorbitol (Chapter 17). Because sorbitol does not readily pass out of cells, it may accumulate in the lens of the eye, brain and nerves. Whether or not this contributes to the development of diabetic neuropathy remains contentious, although it is likely that premature cataract formation in diabetes is related to the accumulation of sorbitol. However, it is disappointing that the development of drugs inhibiting the action of aldose reductase have had no significant clinical impact.

Role of vascular endothelial cells

Understanding of the role of vascular endothelial cells in the generation of microvascular disease is gradually evolving. Vascular endothelium produces vasoactive mediators including nitric oxide, endothelins and prostanoids. The mechanism of production of nitric oxide, which to a considerable extent regulates vasomotor tone, is known to be defective in diabetes. The precise way in which this may lead to microvascular disease is not entirely clear at present. However, the haemodynamic hypothesis proposes that capillary pressure and blood flow are increased early in the course of diabetes, stimulating basement membrane thickening and arteriolar sclerosis, which are characteristic of long-standing diabetes, leading eventually to malfunction of vascular autoregulation.

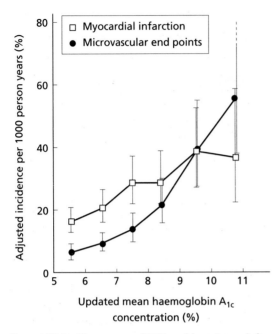

Figure 14.2 Incidence rates and 95% confidence intervals for myocardial infarction and microvascular complications by category of HbA$_{1c}$ concentration, adjusted for age, sex and ethnic group, expressed for white men aged 50–54 years at diagnosis and with mean duration of diabetes of 10 years. (From Stratton, I.M. *et al. British Medical Journal* 2000; **321**: 405–412, with permission from the BMJ Publishing Group.)

Damaging effects of persistent hyperglycaemia

Persistent hyperglycaemia over many years is the principal underlying cause of the microvascular complications of diabetes. It is also an independent risk factor for the development of macrovascular coronary artery disease and cataract formation. The UKPDS study of Type 2 diabetes showed precisely the increasing hazard in relation to continuously rising HbA$_{1c}$ levels (Fig. 14.2), without any specific threshold point, and then demonstrated the benefits of tight control.

For every 1% increase in HbA$_{1c}$:

1 microvascular* complications were increased by 37%;

---

* Microvascular complications are here defined as retinopathy requiring photocoagulation, vitreous haemorrhage, and fatal or non-fatal renal failure.

2 any diabetes-related endpoint (micro- and macrovascular) was increased by 21%; and

3 deaths related to diabetes were increased by 21%.

Damaging effects of hypertension

Hypertension is a major risk factor for the development of coronary artery disease leading to myocardial infarction, and increases the risk of strokes and heart failure. It also exacerbates the progression of retinopathy, the evolution of proteinuria and probably the deterioration of nerve function.

The UKPDS study of Type 2 diabetes (page 129) has shown, for every 10 mmHg increase in systolic blood pressure:

1 any complication related to diabetes was increased by 12%;

2 deaths related to diabetes were increased by 15%;

3 myocardial infarction was increased by 11%; and

4 microvascular complications were increased by 14%.

Prevention of complications

Major advances in recent years have resulted in a decrease in incidence of some complications, most notably nephropathy. Delaying diabetic complications, together with retardation of their progression when they occur, is now possible, chiefly by tight control of the diabetes and of hypertension, together with reduction of other 'risk factors' (page 186). Even when the complications are established, their progression to cause serious damage can be either delayed or avoided.

1 *Patients* should be supported to give up smoking, which has been clearly shown to accelerate progression of both nephropathy and retinopathy.

2 *Treatment* of hyperlipidaemia is also of importance in reducing the development of macrovascular disease (page 187).

Non-attendance at clinics, especially in socially deprived populations, greatly increases the risk of complications and indeed premature mortality. Such observations emphasize the need to adopt a broader view of complication prevention which extends beyond the deceptively simple concept of 'tight glycaemic control'.

Benefits of tight glycaemic and blood pressure control on diabetic complications

Sustained optimal diabetic control delays the onset and retards the progression of diabetic complications, while good antihypertensive treatment also retards the development of exudative retinopathy and slows the progression of nephropathy. These observations result principally from two recent major trials, DCCT for Type 1 diabetes, and UK PDS for Type 2 diabetes which reported in 1993 and 1998, respectively. Their results have given enormous encouragement to patients, nurses and physicians by demonstrating that efforts to improve control can be highly effective.

Diabetes Control and Complications Trial for Type 1 diabetes (DCCT)

This trial was conducted in the USA and involved 1441 patients, half within 5 years of diagnosis with no complications, and half with 5–15 years' duration and early microvascular complications, randomized to intensified or conventional insulin therapy over 9 years. The trial was ended prematurely because of its results. It reported in 1993 that intensified insulin therapy was associated with reductions in retinopathy, nephropathy and neuropathy by 35–70% (Fig. 14.3).

Five years after termination of the DCCT, the benefits with regard to amelioration of complications have persisted, despite lapse of the previously tight blood glucose control in the intensively treated group, to levels of HbA_{1c} indistinguishable from those in the now better controlled conventionally treated patients.

UK Prospective Diabetes Study of Type 2 diabetes (UKPDS)

This multicentre study of 5102 Type 2 diabetic patients was coordinated from Oxford, UK and published its conclusions in 1998. The trial assessed

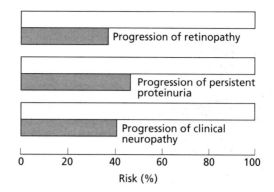

Figure 14.3 Risk reduction for complications in young Type 1 diabetic patients under intensive therapy. (After Diabetic Control and Complications Research Group (DCCT) 1993.)

both the effects of persistent hyperglycaemia and hypertension on the development of micro- and macrovascular complications, and also demonstrated the benefits of 10 years of better compared to less satisfactory control of both glycaemia and blood pressure. Benefits were achieved regardless of the drugs used to reach the required standards of either blood glucose or blood pressure control.

The effect of better blood glucose control on microvascular complications was as follows.
1 *Reduction of microvascular complications* (chiefly the need for photocoagulation) by 25%.
2 *Reduction of any diabetes endpoint* by 12%.
3 *Reduction of any diabetes-related death* by 10%.

Glycaemic control was also shown to reduce the evolution of microalbuminuria after 9 years, and of vibration perception after 15 years of the study. There was also a reduction in of the incidence of myocardial infarction, although the *P*-value for the comparison with the control group was only 0.056. The effect on overall diabetes-related mortality did not achieve statistical significance.

The UKPDS also showed the considerable benefits of tight blood pressure control (Fig. 14.4). By achieving a mean blood pressure of 144/82 mmHg, representing a reduction of systolic BP of 10 mmHg compared to the less intensively treated group, microvascular endpoints (chiefly the need for photocoagulation) were reduced by 37%; and risk of vision declining by three lines on the Snellen chart was reduced by 47%, chiefly by protection from the development of macular disease. Better control of

129

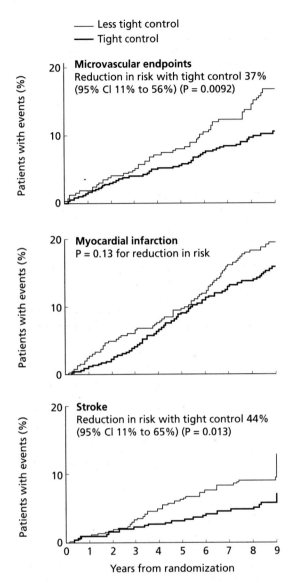

Figure 14.4 Kaplan–Meier plots of proportion of patients who developed microvascular endpoints (mostly retinal photocoagulation), fatal or non-fatal myocardial infarction or sudden death, and fatal or non-fatal strokes following tight control or less tight control of blood pressure. (From UK Prospective Diabetes Study Group (UKPDS); *British Medical Journal* 1998; **317**: 703–713, with permission from the BMJ Publishing Group.)

blood pressure also resulted in a 32% reduction in deaths related to diabetes, and a 44% reduction in strokes; there was a non-significant reduction in myocardial infarction. Further details on the benefits of good blood pressure control in general and on established nephropathy in particular are described in Chapters 19 and 15.

The benefits of controlling glycaemia required persistently good control over a decade; while benefits of successful blood pressure control were witnessed after approximately 4–5 years. Targets for control of blood glucose, HbA_{1c}, blood pressure, weight and lipids are described on pages 131 and 191.

Pharmacological agents and prevention of complications

Over several decades, there have been many trials of various pharmacological agents to discover whether any of them can effectively reduce the development of diabetic complications. Unfortunately, none so far has been shown to have sufficient clinical efficacy to recommend their use in clinical practice. Aldose reductase inhibitors underwent trials over some 25 years without gaining a place in the management of diabetic complications. Drugs which cleave the protein–glucose links of AGEs are still under investigation, and there is now considerable interest in inhibitors of protein kinase C (PKC inhibitors) which, by reducing the intracellular accumulation of diacylglycerol, may prevent damage to endothelial cells. Gamma linolenic acid (evening primrose oil), which had shown some promise in slowing the progression of neuropathy has not been shown to be sufficiently effective to recommend its use.

Early detection of diabetic complications: annual screening procedures

Detection of the earliest signs of diabetic complications is an essential requirement of diabetes care leading to early preventive and treatment strategies that can abort progression of some of the most serious consequences.

Screening is ideally performed as a structured service undertaken by nurses and technicians outside the process of medical consultations, which should themselves be informed by the results from the screening programme. It should be performed at

Table 14.2 Targets for control of diabetes.

	Very good	Acceptable	Less than ideal
Body mass index (kg/m^2)	<25	<27	>27
HbA$_{1c}$(%) (non-diabetic 4.0–6.0%)	<6.5	6.5–7.5	>7.5

Targets for blood pressure and serum lipid levels are described in Chapters 19 and 20.
Individual targets should be established for each patient.

onset and then annually and from the onset of diabetes in all Type 2 diabetic patients. Complications in Type 1 diabetes, however, are unlikely to develop during the first 5 years after diagnosis, so that the complete annual screening protocol can be deferred for a short time. The screening programme can be performed wherever appropriate facilities exist. Once complications are present and established, more frequent screening and/or treatment may be needed (Table 14.2).

Eye screening requires specialist equipment and is often undertaken as a community responsibility, and there are strong representations that there should be a national screening programme. Detection and prevention of foot problems linked to delivery of adequate community podiatry services is also crucial and highly effective in preventing serious foot disorders.

The annual complications screening programme comprises the following (Box 14.1).

Subsequent chapters deal with each complication in turn, and include a description of modern strategies for the early detection of these complications.

Box 14.1 **Annual complications screening programme**

Weight (height): body mass index.
Blood pressure.
Eye examination: visual acuity, fundoscopy and photography through dilated pupils.
Foot examination: check for deformities, abrasions and ulcers; sensation (monofilament tests, and other sensory modalities if available); palpate foot pulses.
Blood tests: HbA$_{1c}$; lipid profile; creatinine.
Urine tests: tests for proteinuria or microalbuminuria. Ideally, microalbuminuria should be assessed in an early morning urine sample. If proteinuria is detected, total 24 h proteinuria (or the albumin/creatinine ratio (ACR)) and assessment of renal function are indicated.

Important questions at the annual review include the following.
1 Assessment of smoking status.
2 Symptoms of neuropathy.
3 History of angina or claudication.
4 Discussion of family planning.
5 Questions about hypoglycaemia.
6 New medications and coexisting medical conditions.

15

Diabetes and the Kidney

Summary

■ Diabetic nephropathy represents specific renal damage affecting overall between 10% and 20% of diabetic patients

■ Microalbuminuria is its earliest manifestation: its progression occurs insidiously over many years, although a few cases regress towards normal

■ Once persistent proteinuria is established, glomerular filtration rate slowly decreases albeit at variable rates

■ Early detection of nephropathy by discovery of microalbuminuria is essential in order to institute early protective treatment with angiotensin converting enzyme inhibitors (ACEI) or angiotensin 2 receptor inhibitors (AT2 receptor inhibitors)

■ In those with established proteinuria, tight blood pressure control is highly effective in retarding the decline of renal function, using ACE inhibitors or AT2 receptor inhibitors as agents of first choice, combined with other agents as required

■ Morbidity and mortality from cardiovascular disease are considerably increased in patients with either microalbuminuria or proteinuria

■ Diabetic nephropathy is the commonest single cause of renal failure, which can be effectively managed by either transplantation or dialysis

Diabetic nephropathy is a specific renal disease affecting a significant proportion of all diabetic patients. In most developed countries, diabetes is now the most common single cause of end-stage renal failure, accounting for almost one-third of patients needing renal support treatments. While Type 1 diabetes is responsible for the majority of cases in patients aged under 50 years, there are now more patients with Type 2 diabetes and end-stage renal failure, especially among non-white populations (notably Asians, Africans and Caribbeans) who appear particularly prone to this complication.

The development of proteinuria indicative of nephropathy in a diabetic patient is a serious prognostic marker, accompanied by progressive retinopathy and often neuropathy. It not only portends a decline of renal function, but it is also associated with a major increase in the tendency to cardiovascular disease such that most Type 2 diabetic patients with proteinuria, and many of those with Type 1 diabetes, die from myocardial infarction. Notwithstanding, recent advances have led to the means for substantially retarding the progression of the disease, and delaying or even eliminating the development of end-stage renal failure.

Pathology (Fig. 15.1)

Kidney volume is enlarged at a very early stage of Type 1 diabetes, and this involves both expansion of

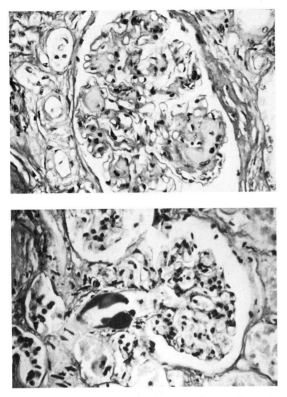

Figure 15.1 Microscopic appearances of diabetic nephropathy showing glomerulosclerosis, including mesangial thickening, nodular changes, closed glomerular capillaries and arteriolar hyalinization.

glomeruli as well as some expansion of tubular tissue. The kidneys remain either enlarged or at least normal in size throughout and characteristically are not diminished in size even in advanced renal failure, in distinction from other causes of end-stage disease. Structural changes in the kidney are detectable at an early stage, and thickening of the basement membrane has been recorded after only 2 years of Type 1 diabetes. Diffuse mesangial enlargement can also be detected after as little as 2 years. Basement membrane thickening increases with increasing age and duration of diabetes, but mesangial thickening is not necessarily progressive and may still be normal after as many as 25 years of diabetes. However, patients with established disease (proteinuria) have marked mesangial expansion. The expanding mesangium reduces the filtration surface area and the number of

closed capillaries and is thus associated with a fall in glomerular filtration. Nodular lesions, as originally described by P. Kimmelstiel and C. Wilson (1936), are sometimes present and are pathognomonic for diabetes (the changes of diffuse glomerular lesions are not): they comprise accumulations of para-aminosalicylic (PAS)-positive material often in the central mesangium of a lobule. Eventually, many glomeruli become completely sclerosed. Hyaline lesions are sometimes seen on the inside of Bowman's capsule ('capsular drop') or as a 'fibrin cap' within a capillary loop, but these changes are not specific for diabetes.

Hyalinization of the glomerular afferent arterioles is common but non-specific, although hyalinization of the efferent arterioles is probably pathognomonic for diabetes. Tubular basement membrane width also increases and there may be some tubular atrophy.

Differences between the structural changes in Type 1 diabetes and Type 2 diabetes have been described, notably striking interstitial changes in Type 2 diabetes sometimes associated with minimal glomerular changes. Whether these account for lower rates of progression in Type 2 diabetes is not known. Approximately 20% of patients with Type 2 diabetes and renal disease have a non-diabetic form of kidney damage. Renal ischaemic changes have a more important role in Type 2 diabetes.

Renal lesions in diabetes progress slowly over many years and more rapidly in the presence of poor diabetic control and hypertension. Reversal of both basement membrane and mesangial thickening has been demonstrated only after 10 years of normoglycaemia achieved following successful pancreas transplantation.

Causes of nephropathy

Poor glycaemic control of diabetes is now established as the predominant factor in the genesis of diabetic nephropathy as with other microvascular complications. Hyperglycaemia increases the expression of matrix by mesangial cells. The benefits of tight diabetic control in delaying the onset and retarding the progression of nephropathy have been demonstrated in Type 1 diabetes by the Diabetes Control and Complications Trial (DCCT) study in the USA (page 129), and in Type 2 diabetes by the UK Prospective Diabetes Study (UKPDS) (page 129).

Hypertension, especially common at the onset of Type 2 diabetes, increases the rate of evolution of all microvascular diabetic complications including proteinuria. Furthermore, parents of patients with Type 1 diabetes developing nephropathy have a higher arterial blood pressure than parents of patients who have no nephropathy. Nephropathy is also known to have a familial tendency: thus, in families with two or more Type 1 diabetic siblings, when one sibling develops nephropathy, the other has a four-fold risk of developing nephropathy compared with a sibling of a diabetic patient without nephropathy. Some racial groups with Type 2 diabetes have a substantially increased risk of developing nephropathy, especially those of Asian origin as well as Africans and Caribbeans, black and Hispanic Americans and Polynesians. Genetic factors are almost certainly important in the development of diabetic nephropathy, although the precise genetic basis for this complication has not been elucidated: most of the interest has centred on the gene encoding the angiotensin-converting enzyme (ACE), and there has been some suggestion of a positive association with a base pair deletion (the DD genotype), and it is also this genotype which is associated with a more rapid progression of the treated disease.

Molecular mechanisms by which hypertension exacerbates the development of nephropathy are increasingly understood. Transforming growth factor beta (TGFβ), vascular endothelial growth factor (VEGF, a permeability factor) and epidermal growth factor (EGF) may be involved, are increased by mechanical stretching of mesangial cells, and known to increase elements of human matrix component such as fibrinonectin. Mesangial stretch also increases the activity of protein kinase C (PKC) which in turn activates p38 mitogen activated protein kinase (MAP kinase). Growth hormone and insulin-like growth factor (IGF) may be involved. Current investigations involve the development of antagonists to many of these factors in an attempt to determine whether matrix accumulation and fibrosis can be reduced, and the course of nephropathy can be ameliorated.

A high intraglomerular pressure is an important determinant of the development of nephropathy.

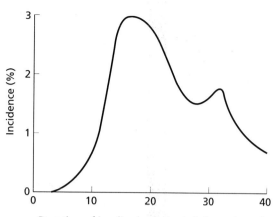

Figure 15.2 The incidence of diabetic nephropathy with increasing duration of Type 1 diabetes. The second peak is not confirmed in all studies. (After Andersen A.R *et al.* *Diabetologia* 1983; 25: 496–501.)

Patients with a single kidney have an increased risk of nephropathy, and renal artery stenosis gives protection. The role of hyperfiltration as a predisposing factor is uncertain.

Epidemiology

There is an increasing incidence of nephropathy after 7–10 years of Type 1 diabetes, rising to a peak at 10–25 years, later falling considerably (Fig. 15.2); few patients develop it *de novo* after 30 years of diabetes. There is an increased incidence in those diagnosed before age 20 and in males, as for other renal diseases. In recent years there appears to be a fall in the proportion of those developing nephropathy; while previously between 30 and 50% of Type 1 diabetic patients developed nephropathy, this is now much diminished and may be no more than 10–20% when good control and high quality care are attained (Fig. 15.3). Fortunately, the majority of patients never develop nephropathy. In Type 2 diabetes, the cumulative incidence of persistent proteinuria is similar to that in Type 1 diabetes: it is commonly present at diagnosis (as is retinopathy) indicating the presence of undiagnosed diabetes for some years.

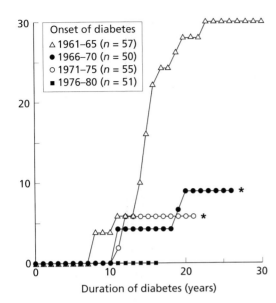

Figure 15.3 Cumulative incidence of clinical nephropathy in Type 1 diabetic patients divided into four cohorts according to year of onset, and in whom diabetes began before the age of 15 years. Asterisks denote significant difference in incidence between the indicated group and the cohort with onset of diabetes in 1961–65. From Bojestig M *et al. New Eng J Med* 1994; **330**: 15–18. Copyright © 1994 Massachusetts Medical Society.

Initiating factors and progression promoters in diabetic nephropathy

Factors leading to initiation and those determining rate of progression of diabetic renal disease are gaining increasing recognition (Table 15.1).

Natural history of diabetic nephropathy

Early physiological changes

During the early years of diabetes, hyperfiltration is common and associated with overall renal enlargement. Filtration is returned towards normal by tight glycaemic control, although even then the kidneys often remain enlarged. Protein excretion at this stage is normal. Type 2 diabetic patients tend not to have hyperfiltration or renal enlargement at diagnosis of diabetes, although duration of diabetes itself is seldom defined and it may have been present for many years.

Table 15.1 Initiating factors and progression promoters in diabetic nephropathy.

Initiation of nephropathy	Progression promoters
Persistently poorer diabetic control	Blood pressure
Hypertension in Type 2 diabetes	Proteinuria
Genetic factors	Persistently poorer diabetic control
	Genetic factors
	Smaller kidneys (or glomeruli)
	Smoking
	High dietary protein

Incipient nephropathy

The development of microalbuminuria may occur after a minimum of 5 years of Type 1 diabetes and heralds the onset of diabetic renal disease indicating 'incipient nephropathy' (Table 15.2). Approximately 80% of those with microalbuminuria show progression of the disease with increasing duration of diabetes and, if inadequately treated, some 10–20% each year develop persistent proteinuria. Microalbuminuria in the remaining one-fifth of patients either remains stable or may even regress. Renal function is normally stable in patients with the microalbuminuria of incipient nephropathy. Blood pressure gradually increases from the stage of microalbuminuria, although patients at this stage are not generally hypertensive. Both microalbuminuria and proteinuria resulting from nephropathy are not uncommonly present at diagnosis of Type 2 diabetes, and retinopathy is also present in more than one-quarter of patients at this time. Proteinuria is more likely to have a non-diabetic cause in Type 2 diabetes than in Type 1 diabetes and is often the consequence of long-standing hypertension.

Persistent proteinuria

Proteinuria, once present, slowly increases although it does not generally exceed 5 g/day and true nephrotic syndrome is rare. Proteinuria may decline as end-stage renal failure develops. Glomerular filtration rate (GFR) falls progressively and relentlessly in untreated patients such that end-stage renal failure

Table 15.2 Microalbuminuria and diabetic nephropathy stages in diabetic renal involvement and nephropathy. (From Mogensen, C.E. (2000) Definition of diabetic renal disease in insulin dependent diabetes mellitus based on renal function tests. In: *The Kidney and Hypertension in Diabetes Mellitus* (ed. C.E. Mogensen), 5th edn, pp. 13–28. Kluwer Academic Publishers, Boston.)

Stage	Designation	Main characteristics	Main structural changes	GFR (mL/min)	UAE	Blood pressure	Suggested main pathophysiological change
Stage I	Hyperfunction /hypertrophy	Glomerular hyperfiltration	Glomerular hypertrophy	≈150	May be increased	N	Glomerular volume and pressure increase
Stage II	Normoalbuminuria	Normal UAE	Increasing basal membrane (bm) thickness	hyperfiltration	N (high in stress situations)	N	Changes as indicated above but quite variable
Transition from I→II	Transition phase	High normal UAE	Not known	Hyperfiltration	Increasing	Increasing	Somewhat poor metabolic control
Stage III	Incipient DN microalbuminuria	Elevated UAE	UAE correlated to structural damage	Still high GFR	20→200 µg/min	Elevated compared to stage II	Advancing glomerular lesions. Permeability defect not located
Stage IV	Overt DN	Clinical proteinuria or UAE >200 µg/min	Advanced structural damage	Decreasing	>200 µg/min	Often frank hypertension increases by ≈5% yearly	High rate of glomerular closure advancing and severe mesangial expansion
Stage V	End stage renal disease						

Stage V is ESRD. GFR, glomerular filtration rate; UAE, urinary albumin excretion; DN, diabetic nephropathy; N, normal.

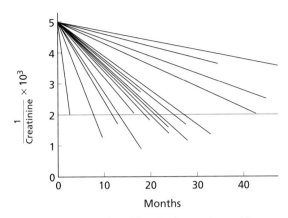

Figure 15.4 Decline of renal function in 16 patients with nephropathy.

is reached in an average of 7–10 years. However, individuals vary widely in the rate of decline of GFR (Fig. 15.4) which may be as much as 8–12 mL/min/year. Blood pressure also increases, and the severity of the hypertension influences the rate of decline. Most of these patients develop coronary artery disease, and have left ventricular hypertrophy on echocardiogram as well as increased lipid levels. Retinopathy is almost invariably present in these patients with a 10-fold increased risk of blindness, but the reverse is not true; it is quite possible to have advanced retinopathy without any renal abnormality. Patients with proteinuria also have a considerably increased risk of neuropathy, autonomic neuropathy, peripheral vascular disease and diabetic foot disease.

Progressive renal impairment does not always follow in Type 2 diabetic patients, and when renal function does decline it often does so more slowly. The risk of cardiovascular events and premature death is very high.

Early renal impairment

When the serum creatinine exceeds 150 mmol/L, renal impairment is clearly present and around this time liaison with a nephrologist is desirable. Serum creatinine may increase from 200 mmol/L to end-stage renal failure in as little as 12 months or may take many years.

Nephropathy is normally asymptomatic until it is advanced, when oedema and breathlessness develop.

Anaemia often occurs relatively early in the course of the disease before renal failure is established, and much sooner than in non-diabetic renal disease, as a result of diminished erythropoietin (EPO) production which can be corrected by injections of EPO, sometimes with considerable clinical benefit.

Detection and investigation

It is vital to detect diabetic nephropathy as early as possible in order to start treatment before there is loss of renal function.

Testing urine samples for the presence of protein and microalbuminuria should be routine practice at every clinic visit and is obligatory at the annual review. If proteinuria develops it is important to distinguish the onset of nephropathy from other causes of renal disease.

Microalbuminuria is detected by measurement of the albumin:creatinine ratio (ACR) or urinary albumin concentration. The test is best performed on a first morning urine sample. If microalbuminuria is detected, it should be confirmed by repeat sampling within the ensuing months. If macroalbuminuria suddenly occurs, diagnoses other than diabetes should be considered. Laboratory and near patient commercial tests specifically designed for microalbuminuria should have a sensitivity >80% and specificity >90%.

Diagnostic categories

Microalbuminuria
ACR >2.5 mg/mmol/L (men); >3.5 mg/mmol/L (women)
Albumin concentration >20 mg/L
Urinary albumin excretion rate 20–300 mg/24 h or 20–200 µg/min in an overnight specimen.

Proteinuria
ACR >30 mg/mmol/L
Albumin concentration >200 mg/L
Urinary albumin excretion rate >300 mg/24 h
Urinary protein excretion >500 mg/24 h

If albuminuria is detected, the following investigations are recommended.

1 Check the history for evidence of other renal disease.

2 A midstream urine specimen should be sent for culture and microscopy and detection of red blood cells.

3 Ultrasound examination of the kidneys (size, shape, stones, obstruction).

4 Measurement of serum creatinine, and comparison with previous levels.

5 Blood pressure measurement and chest X-ray if raised, electrocardiogram (ECG).

6 A 24-h or timed overnight urine collection (single sample not adequate).

7 Careful retinal examination.

If proteinuria has evolved gradually over several years in the presence of retinopathy, and there are no unusual features such as haematuria, unequal size kidneys or a history of urinary tract complaints, then extensive investigation is not necessary. In Type 2 diabetes, however, there is a greater chance of non-diabetic renal disease being present, and renal biopsy may be needed especially if there are atypical features. In both Type 1 diabetes and Type 2 diabetes, the absence of retinopathy should make one suspect other causes of renal disease. Rapid onset of proteinuria is never caused by diabetes and should always be fully investigated, including assessment of antinuclear factor and complement levels, as well as a renal biopsy. Diabetic nephropathy can coexist with other renal diseases, and in most diabetic subjects of more then 10 years standing there will be some arteriolar hyalinization and glomerulosclerosis. Expert histological assessment is needed to confirm the mesangial expansion and other changes that together characterize diabetic glomerulosclerosis (Fig. 15.1).

Management

Glycaemic control and blood pressure levels are important in determining the rate of deterioration. While blood pressure control is the most important determinant, the benefits of good glycaemic and blood pressure control are additive. Overall management is multifactorial and also comprises control of dyslipidaemia, discouragement of smoking and restriction of excessively high protein intake.

Glycaemic control

Microalbuminuria is reduced by good glycaemic control, which also reduces the chances of progression to clinical nephropathy. However, once nephropathy is established and the GFR is declining, control of blood pressure becomes the first priority. Improving diabetic control can be seen to make a significant further impression once blood pressure control is established.

Blood pressure management

Established microalbuminuria (at least two out of three positive samples) is managed with ACE inhibitors.

1 In Type 1 diabetes, treatment is started regardless of blood pressure. If raised, blood pressure should be reduced to < 135/75 mmHg but ACE inhibitor treatment should be given even to normotensive patients (see below for suggested doses).

2 In Type 2 diabetes, treatment aims to maintain a blood pressure of < 135/75 mmHg.

ACE inhibitors and angiotensin 2 (AT2) receptor antagonists reduce microalbuminuria and delay the onset of established proteinuria.

Established proteinuria is defined as proteinuria > 500 mg/24 h or albuminuria > 300 mg/24 h. This phase is always managed by vigorous hypotensive treatment, aiming where possible for a blood pressure < 135/75 mmHg. This both reduces (or occasionally eliminates) proteinuria and slows progression of the declining GFR best demonstrated in Type 1 diabetes. It is also protective of some aspects of cardiovascular disease (see below). Again, there is apparent added benefit of using ACE inhibitors as the first-line agent.

There are many measurable benefits of tight blood pressure control. Reduction of blood pressure reduces proteinuria. The most important measure is reduction in blood pressure with any effective agent but there are potential added benefits from the use of ACE inhibitors or AT2 receptor antagonists, which may reduce proteinuria independently of the reduction of blood pressure. Patients may even be rendered free from proteinuria when they are effectively treated. Decline of the GFR is effectively retarded following rigorous blood pressure control such that a decrease of >6 mL/min/year can be reduced to as little as 2 mL/min/year, while the decrease can be reduced to a virtually normal decline of <1 mL/min/year in some patients with optimal blood pressure control. Thus, the development of end-stage renal failure may be delayed sometimes by several years, and there is evidence that at least in Type 1 diabetes the numbers needing a kidney transplant are decreasing. As the life expectancy of the diabetic patient on dialysis is relatively short compared to non-diabetic renal failure patients, prolonging the time taken to progress to end-stage renal failure translates into years of added life, although renal transplantation does give major benefit to diabetic patients.

Choice of antihypertensive agent

ACE inhibitors or AT2 receptor antagonists are the agents of choice for diabetic nephropathy patients at any stage. They provide benefits both in reducing proteinuria and retarding decline of glomerular filtration over and above their blood pressure lowering effects in comparison to other agents. However, the overriding need is to maintain good blood pressure control in all those with nephropathy using any hypotensive agent to suit the individual patient. In Type 2 diabetes, UK PDS demonstrated that no drug gave a preferential benefit (comparing atenolol and an ACE inhibitor) but the study was not really designed to assess this. Combinations of drugs are almost always required, especially in overweight Type 2 diabetic individuals where more than two drugs are often needed; the ideal BP of <135/75 mmHg may be difficult to achieve and some compromise following informed discussion with patients may be necessary. Tight blood pressure control may induce or exacerbate postural hypotension, which should be avoided (Table 15.3). Fluid retention is often a problem and diuretics are therefore frequently needed. For Africans and Caribbeans, probably the best second-line agent is a calcium-channel blocker such as verapamil. In very severe hypertension in such patients, the order may be reversed to ensure rapid control of blood pressure.

Creatinine should be checked within 1 week of starting ACE inhibitor or AT2 receptor antagonist

Table 15.3 Antihypertensive agents for diabetic patients.

For microalbuminuria (recommended doses in normotensive patients)
ACE inhibitors*
    enalapril 10 mg b.d.
    lisinopril 20 mg/day
    ramipril initially 2.5 mg/day, titrated to 10 mg if blood pressure does not fall too low

Angiotensin 2 (AT2) receptor antagonists*†
    irbesartan 300 mg/day
    losartan 50 mg/day

For albuminuria with hypertension
ACE inhibitors (or AT2 antagonists) to which may be added:
    calcium-channel blockers (not nifedipine)
    diuretics
    beta-blockers
    others

*Only some of the longest established and therefore most studied agents are mentioned here by name. Many others are available and can be found in the *British National Formulary*.
†AT2 antagonists do not cause the cough often induced by ACE inhibitors, but are more expensive than the latter.

treatment in case a rapid rise occurs in patients with renal artery stenosis. They should be changed to another agent, and appropriate investigations undertaken. This is particularly important in patients with impalpable foot pulses, who are obviously at higher risk. For further information on treatment of hypertension, specific indications and contraindications to individual drugs see Chapter 20.

Monitoring renal function

Regular assessment of renal function is required in order to monitor the progress of patients with diabetic nephropathy.

Serum creatinine should be measured regularly. Approximations of GFR are useful, notably by calculation of the inverse creatinine (1/serum creatinine; Fig. 15.4) or the use of the Cockroft–Gault formula:

[88 (145 – age in years)/(serum creatinine in mmol/L) – 3] for men;

[75 (145 – age in years)/(serum creatinine in mmol/L) – 3] for women.

Routine isotopic measurement of GFR is not practicable and is a research procedure.

Other measures

1 Dyslipidaemia. Detection and management of hyperlipidaemias is important because of the huge increase in cardiovascular disease in those with nephropathy. However, the idea that reducing lipidaemia slows the progression of the renal disease is unproven.

2 Restricting protein intake has a small beneficial effect on the decline of GFR, but unless the intake is very high (>1 g/kg/day) restriction is not normally advised.

3 Some patients, especially those on ACE inhibitors, may need a reduced potassium intake to avoid hyperkalaemia.

4 Drugs used in advancing renal failure need careful consideration. Fibrates and non-steroidals may worsen renal function; metformin should be stopped and non-renally excreted sulphonylureas used (page 60). Insulin doses often need to be reduced because of diminished renal degradation.

5 Normochronic anaemia due to diminished EPO production occurs relatively early in the course of the disease. EPO injections can bring about considerable clinical improvement.

6 When the serum creatinine exceeds 150 mmol/L, patients are best managed in a specialist joint renal–diabetic clinic, where appropriate education and counselling are provided. Considerable fear is generated when patients are told that they have 'kidney damage' with visions of dialysis and transplantation. This may encourage compliance with therapy but must be handled sensitively and carefully, to avoid damage to patient well-being. The proper context of the disease must be presented by physicians and nurse educators, knowing that with good treatment the majority with proteinuria will not go on to end-stage renal failure.

Mortality

Diabetic patients with proteinuria from nephropathy have a high mortality, chiefly as a result of exten-

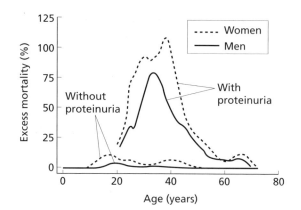

Figure 15.5 Relative mortality of diabetic patients with and without the system proteinuria in men and women as a function of age. Mortality is greatly increased at all ages in proteinuric patients. From Borch-Johnsson K *et al. Diabetologie* 1985;**28**:590–596.

sive cardiovascular disease leading to myocardial infarction. While Type 1 diabetic patients without proteinuria have a mortality rate of about twice that of a non-diabetic population, those with proteinuria have relative mortality rates of more than 50-fold compared to those of a non-diabetic population (Fig. 15.5). Thus, about 25% of Type 1 diabetic patients with nephropathy die from myocardial infarction before reaching end-stage renal failure. The majority of the older Type 2 diabetic patients with nephropathy die from this cause, with only 1–2% of all patients reaching end-stage renal failure needing treatment. There are several theories explaining the link between nephropathy and cardiovascular disease and it is likely that a shared pathway, possibly involving endothelial dysfunction, is common to both. Microalbuminuria in Type 2 diabetes is as much a predictor of cardiovascular disease as of renal disease.

Complications

The risk of all complications including cardiovascular disease, retinopathy and associated blindness, and neuropathy is particularly high in diabetic patients with nephropathy. Detection and appropriate management thus remain of the greatest importance in the management of this vulnerable group.

Cardiac disease in diabetic nephropathy

Coronary arteriograms in Type 1 diabetic patients reaching end-stage renal failure show that 25–40% have severe coronary disease, 20% are known to have had myocardial infarcts and over 50% have abnormal electrocardiograms. Thus, as renal failure advances, detailed cardiac assessment and treatment must be undertaken, preferably before renal transplantation is needed.

Cerebrovascular and peripheral vascular disease

As many as 10% of patients, especially those with Type 2 diabetes, who develop renal failure, have had disabling strokes, and about 5% have had amputations. Arterial calcification is common and extensive, and gangrene develops in toes and occasionally fingers.

Renal artery stenosis

Renal artery stenosis caused by atheroma may be more common in diabetic than non-diabetic patients. Its presence may be made manifest either by the acute deterioration of renal function especially after starting treatment with ACE inhibitors, or the demonstration of kidneys of unequal size. Isotopic diethylene triamine penta-acetic acid (DTPA) investigation can indicate the presence of this disease. If angioplasty is envisaged, arteriography is needed, but the benefits of angioplasty in diabetic nephropathy are still uncertain.

Angiography

Coronary, renal or femoral arteriography are often needed to determine whether angioplasty or arterial surgery are required. Dye injection often precipitates acute renal failure in those whose renal function is already impaired (serum creatinine 130 mmol/L). Measures to protect renal function are therefore essential; patients must be kept well hydrated using intravenous fluids (for full details of management in this situation see page 180).

Retinopathy

Retinopathy precedes proteinuria in most patients, and the absence of retinopathy should prompt reconsideration of the diagnosis. Over 75% of patients with advanced renal failure have proliferative retinopathy and 25–30% are blind. Retinopathy continues to progress even after successful dialysis or transplantation, with continuing neovascularization; frequent examination and energetic photocoagulation for new lesions are necessary.

Neuropathy

Diabetic neuropathy is present in most patients reaching advanced nephropathy, although the severity varies considerably from those without symptoms to those devastated by the problems of peripheral or autonomic neuropathy. The chief problems are the development of foot ulcers, sepsis and digital gangrene. Charcot neuroarthropathic joints and neuropathic oedema also occur. Foot problems are much more serious in the presence of peripheral vascular disease which must be actively treated.

Autonomic neuropathy is almost universally detectable in advanced nephropathy patients. Gustatory sweating is common, and sometimes remits after transplantation. The reasons for this are obscure. Serious problems from postural hypotension and failure of bladder emptying are fortunately rare, but disabling when they occur.

End-stage renal failure and renal support

Diabetes is now the most common single cause of end-stage renal failure in most developed countries and accounts for 25–35% of patients needing renal support. All diabetic patients at this stage should be considered for renal support and over 80% are suitable. Blindness alone is not a contraindication and many patients who appear to have poor prospects manage extremely well. Overwhelming diseases such as carcinomatosis, advancing dementia or other disabling manifestations of cerebrovascular disease are contraindications to starting renal support treatment; prognosis in those with very severe ischaemic heart disease is poor. A few individual patients may choose not to proceed with the treatment.

Indications for starting renal support treatment

Decline of health with malaise, fluid retention and dyspnoea, in the presence of advanced renal failure indicate the need to start treatment. This is often at an earlier stage than in non-diabetic patients; before serious nausea, anorexia or generalized pruritus develop and when serum creatinine is in the range 450–550 µmol/L or when GFR is < 20 mL/min. Treatment should not be delayed as nutrition and well-being often deteriorate rapidly.

Mode of treatment

Renal transplantation is the treatment of choice, although in practice most patients undergo a period on continuous ambulatory peritoneal dialysis (CAPD) first. Prognosis and quality of life on these treatments are now very good, although mortality is approximately 10% higher than for non-diabetic patients, chiefly because of coronary artery disease.

Patients always undergo full clinical assessment while on CAPD regarding their physical and psychological fitness to undergo renal transplantation. Cardiac function requires special attention, while treatment for retinopathy, peripheral vascular disease and problems in the feet must all be fully assessed.

Haemodialysis is generally advised for patients who are both unsuitable for transplantation and unable to cope with CAPD, and as a result the outcome is often less satisfactory.

Continuous ambulatory peritoneal dialysis

CAPD is relatively simple and can be used either to maintain health until transplantation is possible or as a definitive therapy. Two-year survival is now comparable to that for transplantation and is about 75% for both Type 1 and Type 2 diabetic patients. One advantage of CAPD is the facility for intraperitoneal insulin

administration: soluble insulin is added to each bag, initially using the existing total daily dose in divided amounts, often giving less at night. The dose may eventually be quite different from that given subcutaneously. The technique is often satisfactory and excellent control can be achieved without hypoglycaemia. Glucose absorption and hyperglycaemia are considerable when bags containing 3.86% glucose are used and more insulin is needed than in those with 1.36% glucose.

Peritonitis is an added hazard for diabetic patients; intraperitoneal insulin should not be used in those who are not capable of the stringent aseptic techniques that are needed. If peritonitis or other intercurrent illness develops, uncontrolled diabetes is best treated by intravenous insulin infusion.

Transplantation

The outcome for renal transplantation has progressively improved during the last decade, although even now mortality remains some 10% higher than among those without diabetes. More than 85% of patients are alive 2 years after kidney transplantation, 60–80% of them with satisfactory renal function. Diabetic complications, especially vascular disease, account for the poorer results for people with diabetes; mortality rates are much higher when there is severe ischaemic heart disease or heart failure. After transplantation, myocardial infarction is responsible for 30–50% of deaths, significantly more than amongst non-diabetic recipients. While the remainder of early deaths are mainly from infection, deaths beyond 2 years after transplantation are mostly from heart disease. Ten years after transplantation 20% have suffered myocardial infarction, 15% strokes and 30% amputations.

Management of diabetes during transplantation surgery is always undertaken by intravenous insulin infusion. When intercurrent infections develop, intravenous insulin is also needed in addition to subcutaneous insulin. If rejection episodes require high-dose steroids, very high insulin infusion rates up to 20 units/h are required. Routine treatment after recovery is best undertaken using a short-acting insulin preparation before each main meal, and medium-acting insulin at bedtime (for full details see page 95). Diabetic complications continue to develop after successful transplantation, and joint care by renal and diabetic physicians is essential.

Recurrence of diabetic glomerulosclerosis

Mesangial expansion and basement membrane thickening recur after renal transplantation but the rate of their evolution varies substantially from one patient to another, and in many it is very slow indeed. A few of the survivors for more than 10 years have undergone a second transplant for a recurrence of diabetic nephropathy. There is anecdotal evidence that diabetic renal pathology regresses when the diabetic kidney is transplanted into a non-diabetic recipient.

Pancreas transplantation

Combined kidney and pancreas transplantation is undertaken at some major centres; patient survival is similar to that for renal transplantation alone. The procedure aims to eliminate diabetes and with it the need for insulin injections, and about 50% of patients continue to have a functioning pancreas with insulin independence 5 years after transplantation. Patients who are liberated from decades of restrictions and self-discipline imposed by diabetes experience a joy and happiness rarely witnessed in medical practice. This is the prime reason for offering combined transplantation. Other benefits derive from slowing the redevelopment of glomerulosclerosis in the transplanted kidney, and halting the progression of neuropathy. Even reversal of glomerular lesions in the native kidney has been described 10 years after transplantation (page 133). Retinopathy, which by this stage has almost always been laser treated, is unaffected. The future potential for islet cell transplantation is briefly described on page 74.

Non-diabetic renal disease

Some patients, especially those with Type 2 diabetes, develop unrelated non-diabetic renal disorders. Clues to their presence have been presented above, but renal artery stenosis should be particularly mentioned. This is most common in Type 2 diabetic patients with hypertension and peripheral vascular disease. Full renal assessment including ultrasound examination is essential and renal arteriography is often required to confirm or exclude the diagnosis. The distinction is vital as ACE inhibitors and AT2 receptor antagonists may provoke considerable deterioration in renal function or even precipitate renal failure in the presence of bilateral disease.

Glomerulonephritis and other renal disorders can occur in diabetic patients and require renal biopsy for diagnosis and treatment in their own right.

Urinary tract infections

Urinary tract infections occur in people with diabetes with the same frequency as in those without diabetes, but they are sometimes exceptionally severe and (rarely) may cause the renal papillae to slough, giving rise to necrotizing papillitis or, more rarely, emphysematous cystitis with air in the bladder wall. The infection is particularly troublesome in the rare patient with urinary retention from neurogenic bladder. Diabetic control is easily disturbed by urinary infection, and as with any infection must be regained quickly, with insulin if necessary, while the infection is treated with antibiotics.

Pyelonephritis with septicaemia is not uncommon in diabetes, with occasional formation of perinephric abscesses. The source of the infection may not be immediately apparent and patients sometimes present in profound shock without an obvious site of infection.

Conclusions

It is now possible to delay diabetic nephropathy by good glycaemic control, to slow or halt its progression by blood pressure control especially with ACE inhibitors or AT2 receptor antagonists, and to provide renal support treatment for those developing end-stage renal failure. Patients with nephropathy usually have other complications and are at high risk for cardiovascular disease, which must also be managed actively. Screening and energetic treatment to prevent the disease should now be available for everyone with diabetes.

Diabetic Eye Disease

Summary

- The occurrence of diabetic retinopathy increases with lengthening duration of diabetes and is present in the majority of patients after 30 years

- Its course is significantly retarded by tight glycaemic and blood pressure control

- Regular (annual) eye examination is essential to detect early treatable changes before visual acuity is reduced

- Referral to an ophthalmologist is required urgently if vision is declining and for several other specific indications

- Timely treatment by laser photocoagulation preserves vision

- Blindness due to diabetes may result either from the consequences of retinopathy itself, cataract (which is increased in diabetes), or rarely rubeotic glaucoma

Blindness is one of the most feared complications of diabetes. It is either caused by a specific retinopathy causing haemorrhage and scarring; maculopathy; cataract formation; or, most rarely, by rubeotic glaucoma. In Type 1 diabetes, retinopathy, with or without cataracts/glaucoma and other eye disease, accounts for nearly 90% of all visual impairment. In Type 2 diabetes, diabetic retinopathy accounts for only about one-third of all visual impairment, 50% being caused by cataracts, glaucoma or macular degeneration. While retinopathy develops in most, although not all, patients with diabetes of long duration, blindness occurs in up to 12% of Type 1 diabetic patients and 5% of Type 2 diabetic patients after 30 years of diabetes. Because diabetes is very common, however, diabetic retinopathy is one of the four most common causes of blindness in the community, the others being cataract, glaucoma and senile macular degeneration. Most blind diabetic patients are over 60 years of age.

Patients fear greatly for their eyesight and some-times panic in response to inconsequential visual symptoms. They can gain considerable encouragement from the knowledge that good control retards the development of retinopathy and other diabetic complications, although even that may have its own problems when anxious patients equate transient hyperglycaemia with potential loss of sight. Those undergoing laser treatment and who are losing sight live in a minefield of uncertainty, and may become agitated or depressed. They need much attention at such difficult times.

Retinopathy

Pathophysiology

Capillary abnormalities are the earliest changes to occur in diabetes; small areas of capillary closure with associated retinal non-perfusion can be seen using fluorescein angiography with retinal photography

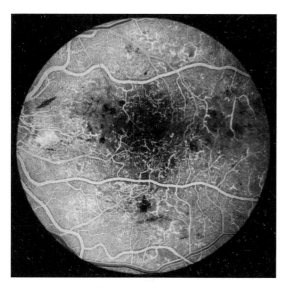

Figure 16.1 Retinal fluorescein angiogram showing areas of capillary closure, capillary leakage and microaneurysms.

(Fig. 16.1). The areas of non-perfusion increase in size until lesions visible on ophthalmoscopy appear. Subsequently, arteriolar and arterial occlusion may develop and areas of non-perfusion increase.

The cause of these early abnormalities is not well understood. Endothelial cell proliferation and then degeneration occur; capillary closure is associated with disappearance of the endothelial cells. The underlying abnormalities are numerous. There may be an early increase of retinal blood flow, and there are numerous coagulation and biochemical abnormalities with, for example, an accumulation of sorbitol in the vessel wall.

Capillary closure and retinal ischaemia result in excessive leakage from diseased capillaries, visualized using fluorescein angiography. When this is severe, maculopathy and macular oedema can occur. Ischaemic areas, seen as cotton wool spots, provide the stimulus to the growth of new vessels. These new vessels are fragile and may bleed, healing with scarring and permanent damage to the retina.

Numerous angiogenic factors have been implicated. Prominent among these is vascular endothelial growth factor (VEGF), and there is also evidence for involvement of transforming growth factor beta (TGFβ), insulin-like growth factor-1 (IGF-1) and others. The theoretical basis for laser photocoagulation treatment in proliferative retinopathy is the destruction of ischaemic retina thereby reducing the release of angiogenic factors.

Early changes

There are unconfirmed observations suggesting an early breakdown of the blood–retinal barrier with leakage of fluorescein into the vitreous. Increased retinal blood flow may also be an early feature of diabetes and is exaggerated by hyperglycaemia. Retinal blood flow falls as diabetic control is improved.

Background retinopathy

Microaneurysms (Plate 1, facing page 148)

These are the earliest recognizable abnormalities of diabetic retinopathy. They represent minute bulges or dilations of retinal capillaries. They appear as tiny red dots; more of them are seen using the technique of fluorescein angiography. They are abnormally permeable but by themselves not harmful. They come and go over time.

'Hard' exudates

These are yellow-white discrete patches of lipid which often occur in rings around leaking capillaries (Plate 1). They may coalesce to form extensive sheets of exudate. They cause blindness only when they develop on the macula.

Haemorrhages

These appear as small (dot) and large (blot) red spots on the retina (Plate 1). They harm vision when they appear on the macula. Flame-shaped haemorrhages may occur but are more characteristic of hypertension.

Preproliferative retinopathy

Ischaemia of the retina predisposes to development of the dangerous formation of new vessels, probably in response to release of angiogenic factors, as described above. Lesions indicating an ischaemic and therefore 'preproliferative' retina are as follows.

1   Multiple dot and blot haemorrhages.

2 Cotton wool spots (previously 'soft exudates'); these are small zones of intracellular oedema in the retinal nerve fibre layer developing in an area of ischaemia from capillary closure. They are indistinct, large (disc size) and pale. The greater the number of cotton wool spots, especially when there are more than five, the more serious the implications.

3 Venous beading, loops and reduplication (Plate 2, facing page 148).

4 Arterial streaking manifested by parallel white streaks on either side of the arteries.

5 Intraretinal microvascular abnormalities (IRMAs) are fine vascular loops lying within the retina, probably representing true intraretinal neovascularization (Plate 2).

6 Retinal atrophy.

Proliferative retinopathy

New vessel formation occurs either on the optic disc (new vessels on the disc, NVD) or in the periphery of the retina (new vessels elsewhere, NVE) (Plates 3 and 4, facing page 148). NVD may grow forward into the vitreous and the risk of vitreous haemorrhage is very great, resulting in blindness in about 30% of cases after 3 years if untreated. The hazard is less for NVE although they often precede the development of NVD and may eventually cause retinal traction and detachment.

New vessels may bleed. Large preretinal haemorrhages may occur, not always affecting vision, but vitreous haemorrhages are more serious, causing blindness rapidly, painlessly and without warning. The vitreous usually clears after some weeks with some recovery of vision, but with repeated haemorrhages vision deteriorates permanently.

Advanced diabetic eye disease

New vessel formation and haemorrhage lead to the development of fibroglial proliferation, which appears as white fibrous strands which contract and cause severe retinal detachment and tears (Plate 4).

When new vessel formation occurs in the anterior chamber and on the iris (rubeosis iridis) a particularly painful and intractable form of glaucoma may develop (rubeotic glaucoma). When conservative management for this condition fails, enucleation is sometimes needed for the relief of pain.

Maculopathy

Disease at the macula is one of the causes of blindness in diabetes. It occurs in several forms and is more common in Type 2 than in Type 1 patients.

Macular oedema

This is a thickening or swelling of the macular portion of the retina. It occurs both in the presence of hard exudates and, less commonly, in their absence. It is very difficult to visualize by direct ophthalmoscopy and is better detected by loss of visual acuity, exacerbated by focusing the image on the macula by the use of a pinhole. On inspection, the macular region appears indistinct and has a subtle grey discoloration. Fluorescein angiography reveals extensive capillary leakage. It may progress rapidly so that early recognition and treatment (laser photocoagulation) are required; even then vision is threatened.

Exudative maculopathy

Hard exudates, when they encroach or surround the macula, threaten vision. This can be treated with laser therapy.

Ischaemic maculopathy

This is caused by occlusion of the supplying blood vessels and may be associated with cluster haemorrhages, pale blood vessels and cloudy swelling of the retina. Visual acuity is severely diminished and treatment is not very effective.

Natural history of retinopathy

Retinopathy usually develops insidiously over many years. It is infrequently present before 5–10 years' duration in Type 1 diabetes, although in Type 2 diabetes it is not uncommon at diagnosis, especially in older patients, when more than one-quarter of patients have visible retinopathy. After 20 years of diabetes, more than 80% of Type 1 diabetic patients have some degree of retinopathy and almost half of all patients with Type 2 diabetes show changes after 15 years. In many cases this is a mild background retinopathy

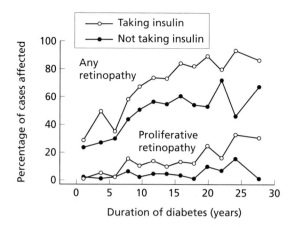

Figure 16.2 Frequency of retinopathy (any degree) and proliferative retinopathy by duration of diabetes in people receiving or not receiving insulin and who were diagnosed to have diabetes at or after 30 years of age. From Klein R *et al. Arch Ophthalmol* 1984; **102**: 527–532.

which changes little over many years. Rather unpredictably, however, changes may develop which threaten vision, either from macular disease or from vitreous haemorrhage in proliferative retinopathy. Maculopathy develops insidiously and is predominantly a disease of Type 2 diabetes, while proliferative retinopathy occurs more frequently in people with Type 1 diabetes, up to half developing this form of disease after 30 years compared with only 20% of Type 2 diabetic patients (Fig. 16.2).

It is not known why progression is very slow in some cases and in others fast. It is not simply the result of poor diabetic control. Paradoxically, retinopathy can deteriorate in association with the institution of strict glycaemic control, especially if started after long periods of poor control. In many cases, where the eyes are initially healthy, cotton wool spots (microinfarcts) appear but these usually disappear with time. In patients with more advanced background retinopathy, very rapid progression of proliferative retinopathy may occur. Accelerated retinopathy occasionally occurs during pregnancy, associated with rapid improvements in glucose control.

Management of retinopathy and prevention of blindness

Prevention, screening and active treatment for established retinopathy are the three principal approaches to the management of diabetic retinopathy.

Prevention

The benefits of tight blood glucose and blood pressure control in retarding the development of retinopathy are described on page 128. No drug therapy has yet been confirmed as offering clinically useful amelioration of either retinopathy or any of the other diabetic complications, although trials of new agents continue. Potential candidates included are antiangiogenesis factors from the world of oncology, protein kinase C (PKC) inhibitors and growth factor inhibitors.

Screening

Screening for retinopathy in order to prevent blindness has become a major part of diabetes care and any system must be carefully organized. It is important because retinopathy needing treatment by photocoagulation must be detected before vision has deteriorated, otherwise improvement is unlikely. In general, laser therapy cannot restore vision that has been lost.

The eyes of all adult new diabetic patients should be examined at diagnosis and annually thereafter, or more often if advancing changes are observed. In children, screening can be delayed until the onset of puberty, or after 5 years' duration of diabetes, whichever is sooner.

Vision-threatening retinopathy may be present at diagnosis in Type 2 diabetes, but rarely occurs in Type 1 diabetes in the first 5 years after diagnosis or before puberty. While an annual examination is recommended, screening may need to be more frequent when retinopathy is established, especially when pre-proliferative changes are present, or if the macula is threatened. Collaboration with an ophthalmologist then becomes essential.

Visual acuity
Facilities for testing visual acuity using a Snellen

chart should be routine in diabetic clinics. The best corrected vision should be recorded, using either the patient's own glasses, or by optical correction using a 'pinhole' held in front of the eye. Patients whose visual acuity is poor, or those in whom it is found to decline, should be referred to an ophthalmologist for proper diagnosis and treatment without delay. However, normal visual acuity does *not* exclude serious retinopathy.

Collaboration with selected and informed local optometrists in some areas can be valuable; a form of cooperation card recording visual acuity as measured by the optometrist can be held by the patient and brought to the clinic. Many appropriately trained optometrists will also be able to assist by recording the presence of retinopathy.

Fundus examination

This should be undertaken through dilated pupils in a darkened room, and these facilities should be available in diabetic clinics. Tropicamide (1% Mydriacyl) eye drops are the best for dilating the pupils; they have a rapid action and reversal takes place spontaneously and rapidly in 2–3 h without the need for reversal with pilocarpine eye drops, which in any case do not reverse the effects on accommodation. Patients should be warned not to drive home until their vision is clear again after dilation. They should also be warned to present urgently if pain develops after dilation, as this may indicate precipitation of acute glaucoma. This is a very rare occurrence even in populations with higher risk of glaucoma, such as the African and Caribbean populations, but it is sensible to be cautious.

Physicians caring for people with diabetes should be trained to examine fundi properly and be able to detect lesions needing more specialized care from ophthalmologists, and in particular those likely to need laser photocoagulation. It is not practicable for routine screening to be undertaken by ophthalmologists themselves.

Retinal photography

Retinal photography, preferably with ophthalmoscopy, is the screening method of choice. It is undertaken by retinal cameras which are either sited at geographically accessible locations, or in rural areas by mobile cameras. The pupils should be dilated. The preferred method uses digital photography which yields suitable images which can be electronically stored making them easily available for consultation, review and teaching. Programmes are being developed that can assess the photographic for lesions. Conventional colour photographs also provide good images, while the quality of Polaroid photographs is less than ideal.

It is ideal to provide both conventional funduscopic and photographic screening procedures, and there is evidence that the combined screening procedure reduces the failure rate. A national screening programme has been proposed and should be adopted. Photographs should be reported by a trained professional using strict criteria for review by an ophthalmologist who decides on the need for ophthalmological referral. The appropriate consultation must then be arranged without delay and before deterioration of vision resulting from delayed treatment occurs, often leading to expensive litigation. Schemes such as the excellent Diabetes Eye Complication Screen (DECS) developed at St Thomas's Hospital, and now extended to most of south London, includes a visual acuity test, glaucoma screen, digital eye photograph and often fundoscopy as well, all concisely reported to the general practitioner and with a direct referral route to ophthalmology for serious disease.

Diabetes UK have indicated that the standard for retinopathy screening should achieve a sensitivity >80%: this can be reached by digital retinal photography with sensitivity levels between 81 and 97% and a specificity of 97–99%. Provided that mydriasis is used, the failure rate is less than the 5% level set by Diabetes UK.

Fluorescein angiography

Fluorescein angiography is useful in detecting exudation from intraretinal vascular abnormalities and in detecting areas of ischaemia in the capillary bed, with resulting 'non-perfusion'. It will also confirm the presence of neovascularization if there is any doubt. Positive findings may indicate the need for laser therapy. The detection of the source and extent of macular oedema and the extent of areas of non-perfusion are the main indications for fluorescein angiography,

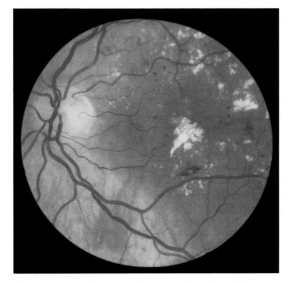

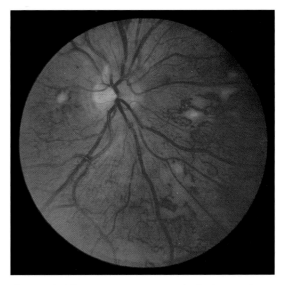

Plate 1 Extensive background retinopathy with multiple microaneurysms (dots), blot haemorrhages and many hard exudates, especially in the ring surrounding the macula. This is especially common in Type 2 diabetes and is often associated with macular oedema; it presents a major hazard to vision.

Plate 2 This illustrates extensive intraretinal microvascular abnormalities (IRMA) with some new vessel formation elsewhere (NVE) and cotton wool spots, best seen at 9 o'clock to the disc. There are also extensive microaneurysms and blot haemorrhages.

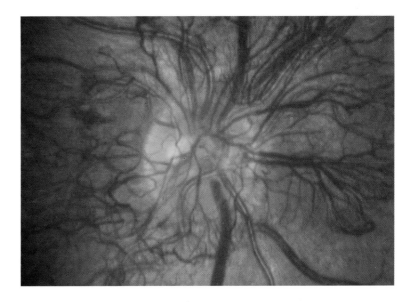

Plate 3 Extensive new vessels arising from the disc.

[Facing p. 148]

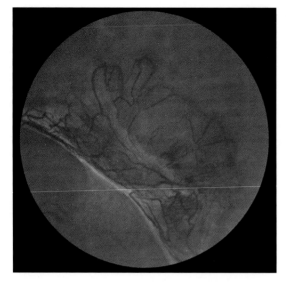

Plate 4 This shows extensive new vessel formation (retinitis proliferans) growing forward into the vitreous and subsequent fibrosis, the crescentric line, which has pulled the retina away.

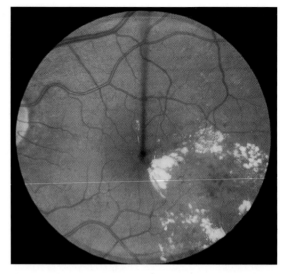

Plate 5(a) Successful treatment with photocoagulation—the appearances of active background retinopathy before (a) and after (b) photocoagulation. In (b) pigmented scars in the areas of retinal ablation can be seen.

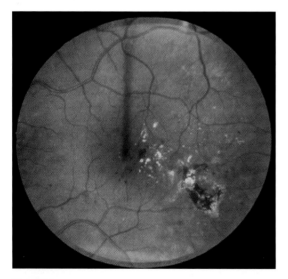

Plate 5(b)

Assessment of absolute risk of cardiovascular disease over 5 years

WOMEN

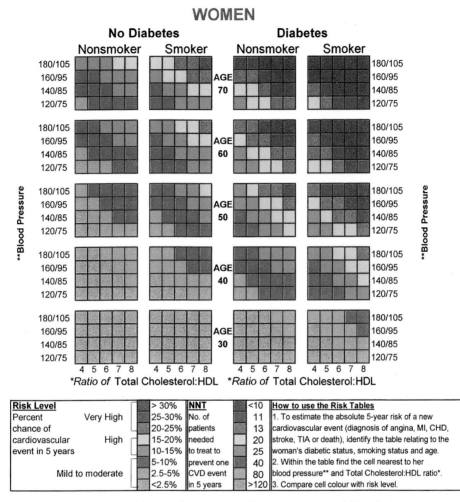

Risk Level			> 30%	NNT	<10	How to use the Risk Tables
Percent	Very High		25-30%	No. of	11	1. To estimate the absolute 5-year risk of a new
chance of			20-25%	patients	13	cardiovascular event (diagnosis of angina, MI, CHD,
cardiovascular	High		15-20%	needed	20	stroke, TIA or death), identify the table relating to the
event in 5 years			10-15%	to treat to	25	woman's diabetic status, smoking status and age.
			5-10%	prevent one	40	2. Within the table find the cell nearest to her
	Mild to moderate		2.5-5%	CVD event	80	blood pressure** and Total Cholesterol:HDL ratio*.
			<2.5%	in 5 years	>120	3. Compare cell colour with risk level.

Patients should be offered advice on reducing their cardiovascular risk through lifestyle changes
Smoking cessation   *Physical activity / exercise*
Cholesterol reduction / low fat diet   *Weight reduction*

A possible threshold of risk for starting discussion of drug treatment
For patients with raised blood pressure: 10% CVD risk over 5 years
For patients with raised cholesterol: 20% CVD risk over 5 years (patients<70 years)

Patients with symptomatic CVD are assumed to have a CVD risk of > 20% over 5 years
Patients with diabetes AND either CHD or proteinuria are at very high risk and should be fast tracked onto treatment
Patients with BMI>30, family history of CHD in relatives <55 years are at greater absolute risk, consider increasing
*   by one risk category (one colour change)*

Notes
*Ratio of total cholesterol :HDL: If HDL is not available, dummy HDL values of 1.2 for men and 1.4 for women
        can be used to calculate the ratio
**BP: Where systolic and diastolic values do not correspond to the table, take the value which gives the higher risk

Plate 6(a)   Assessment of absolute risk of cardiovascular disease over 5 years in (a) women and (b) men. East London Raised Blood Pressure Guidelines 1996.

Assessment of absolute risk of cardiovascular disease over 5 years

MEN

No Diabetes — Nonsmoker / Smoker

Diabetes — Nonsmoker / Smoker

**Blood Pressure (left and right axes): 180/105, 160/95, 140/85, 120/75 (repeated for AGE 70, 60, 50, 40, 30)

AGE 70 / AGE 60 / AGE 50 / AGE 40 / AGE 30

Ratio of Total Cholesterol:HDL — 4 5 6 7 8   4 5 6 7 8   4 5 6 7 8   4 5 6 7 8

Risk Level			NNT		How to use the Risk Tables
Percent	Very High	> 30%	NNT	<10	How to use the Risk Tables
chance of		25–30%	No. of	11	1. To estimate the absolute 5-year risk of a new
cardiovascular		20–25%	patients	13	cardiovascular event (diagnosis of angina, MI, CHD,
event in 5 years	High	15–20%	needed	20	stroke, TIA or death), identify the table relating to the
		10–15%	to treat to	25	man's diabetic status, smoking status and age.
		5–10%	prevent one	40	2. Within the table find the cell nearest to his
	Mild to moderate	2.5–5%	CVD event	80	blood pressure** and Total Cholesterol:HDL ratio*.
		<2.5%	in 5 years	>120	3. Compare cell colour with risk level.

Patients should be offered advice on reducing their cardiovascular risk through lifestyle changes

Smoking cessation   Physical activity / exercise

Cholesterol reduction / low fat diet   Weight reduction

A possible threshold of risk for starting discussion of drug treatment

For patients with raised blood pressure: 10% CVD risk over 5 years

For patients with raised cholesterol: 20% CVD risk over 5 years (patients<70 years)

Patients with symptomatic CVD are assumed to have a CVD risk of > 20% over 5 years
Patients with diabetes AND either CHD or proteinuria are at very high risk and should be fast tracked onto treatment
Patients with BMI>30, family history of CHD in relatives <55 years are at greater absolute risk, consider increasing
by one risk category (one colour change)

Notes

*Ratio of total cholesterol :HDL: If HDL is not available, dummy HDL values of 1.2 for men and 1.4 for women
can be used to calculate the ratio

**BP: Where systolic and diastolic values do not correspond to the table, take the value which gives the higher risk

Adapted from 'Guidelines for the management of mildly raised blood pressure in New Zealand 1994'
Full reference in 'East London Raised Blood Pressure Guidelines 1996'.

Plate 6(b)

because these abnormalities cannot be assessed by ophthalmoscopy. This method of investigation is also useful in cases of unexplained loss of central vision when the shutdown of capillaries or cystic changes at the fovea may be the cause of poor visual acuity.

Screening by optometrists

Regular screening by optometrists provides an additional resource for the extended care of the diabetic patient. Agreed local standards are essential to maintain the highest quality. These include compulsory training days; the routine dilation of the pupils; efficient reporting to the general practitioner and to the hospital clinic attended by the patient; and a recall system, reminding patients to attend for annual examination. A record held by the patient especially of visual acuity readings can be very valuable.

With these different mechanisms available for eye screening, it is important that overlap and duplication should be avoided. This requires careful local organization.

Indications for referral to an ophthalmologist

Referrals to an ophthalmologist should be undertaken without delay, and frequently with a sense of urgency. The indications include the following.
Urgent (within 1 day to 1 week):
- declining vision;
- proliferative retinopathy with vitreous haemorrhage; or
- presence of clinically significant macular oedema.
Referrals within approximately 1 month:
- proliferative retinopathy without vitreous haemorrhage;
- presence of preproliferative lesions;
- presence of any form of progressing or extensive diabetic retinopathy, especially when the lesions are near the macula;
- presence of hard exudates near the macula; or
- other lesions which herald the development of maculopathy.

Treatment by laser photocoagulation

The prevention of blindness requires treatment of appropriate lesions by photocoagulation before vision has deteriorated and before vitreous haemorrhage has occurred (Plate 5a,b, facing page 148). The indications for this treatment are as follows.

1 *New vessels on the optic disc.* Peripheral ablative photocoagulation causes regression of these vessels presumably by removal of the angiogenic stimulus, thus preventing vitreous haemorrhage; treatment should not be delayed. Laser treatment is most effective in this situation, especially if it is undertaken before haemorrhage or any deterioration of vision has occurred.

2 *Peripheral new vessels.* These are treated directly by laser burns, destroying the vessels and preventing bleeding. Treatment is less urgent than for NVD.

3 *Exudative retinopathy.* This should be treated, especially when circinate exudates develop near the macula. Photocoagulation is indicated when visual acuity begins to deteriorate by one or two lines on the Snellen chart. Leaking blood vessels at the centre of the rings of exudate are treated by photocoagulation to prevent further leakage.

4 *Maculopathy* (described on page 146).

Laser treatment is usually an outpatient procedure; its availability will be greatly enhanced with the recent development of portable laser equipment. Some patients find the procedure painful, although very few patients require anaesthetizing. Serious side-effects of treatment occur relatively infrequently. They include restriction of visual fields, especially after peripheral ablative photocoagulation; relative night blindness; transiently reduced visual acuity from mild macular oedema; and, occasionally, a post-treatment bleed. Inadvertent macular burns are, fortunately, very rare.

Vitreous haemorrhage

Photocoagulation should be performed after the vitreous has cleared. If bilateral vitreous haemorrhages have occurred, patients should be admitted for complete bed-rest so that vitreous clearing is accelerated and early laser treatment can be performed. If the vitreous becomes permanently opaque after repeated haemorrhages, then vitrectomy can be performed; its success is limited by the existence of retinopathy, but it often helps those who have been completely blind to obtain some navigational vision or better. The procedure of vitrectomy can also be used to remove some preretinal fibroglial membranes and relieve traction detachments of the retina.

The lens: refractive changes and cataract

Refractive changes

The development of myopia (2–3 dioptres) is common in uncontrolled diabetes; it is occasionally the presenting symptom and may be diagnosed as such by an astute optician. This refractive shift is caused by osmotic changes in the lens and possibly to factors involving ionic pumps as well. The refractive change is reversed after starting insulin (and, much more rarely, after starting tablets) and patients become hypermetropic for a time, perhaps 2 or 3 weeks, during which they experience difficulty with reading. They are sometimes alarmed unless warned. Those experiencing this problem should not at this stage obtain new glasses because the problem resolves spontaneously. The use of temporary glasses at this time can be helpful.

The onset of cataract formation is sometimes accompanied by the development of myopia while blurred vision and diplopia are common symptoms during hypoglycaemia.

Cataract

Cataract formation in people with diabetes is one of the most frequently observed problems and is more common than in non-diabetic people. Cataracts have an increased prevalance in adults with diabetes with a 3–4-fold increased risk in the age range 50–64 years, this excess risk decreasing in later years. Activation of the polyol pathway (not necessarily leading to an accumulation of sorbitol) may amplify oxidative mechanisms already important for senile cataract development while glycation or carbamylation of lens proteins could play a further part in the process.

Cataract takes various forms. It can appear as the dots, flakes, spokes or subcapsular opacities ('snowstorm') of cortical cataract; or with nuclear sclerosis in which opacities are dense, central and may have yellow-brown discoloration. The rate of progress of lens opacities is difficult to predict. It is usually slow

and, as interference with vision is usually late and treatment often effective, it is justifiable to be reasonably optimistic to the patient. The word 'cataract' may be frightening and is better avoided in describing the minor lens opacities which are so often seen in elderly people.

Juvenile diabetic cataract is a very rare but distinctive form of cataract that develops acutely in young Type 1 diabetic patients. A dense subcapsular or floccular cataract forms at the posterior pole of the lens in just a few weeks or months, leading to blindness in that eye. It is usually bilateral and irreversible, requiring surgical treatment. Its cause is unknown and it is not particularly associated with poor diabetic control.

Treatment for mature cataract is by surgical extraction followed by lens implant, contact lens application or the provision of spectacles. A high success rate is expected, although occasional disappointments occur if extensive retinopathy has been hidden by the presence of lens opacities.

Glaucoma

Glaucoma occurs in people with diabetes as in others; evidence of an increased prevalence is weak and a reported association with autonomic neuropathy has not been confirmed. The association of proliferative retinopathy with rubeosis iridis and intractable glaucoma has been discussed on page 146. The presence of glaucoma usually means that the eyes should not be dilated for retinal examination except by an experienced ophthalmologist in patients with chronic open angle glaucoma. However, the examination is required, or retinopathy may be missed.

The iris

The iris is occasionally affected in diabetes in several ways:
1 new vessel formation, i.e. rubeosis iridis (page 146);
2 reduction in pupillary size and light reaction, especially in relation to autonomic neuropathy, where it has been used as a diagnostic test;

3 iritis occurs in a small number of patients in relation to autonomic neuropathy (page 157); or

4 loss of pigment can occur.

Ocular palsies

Diplopia of sudden onset can be caused by acute, reversible ocular palsies, notably of the IIIrd and VIth nerves which occur in diabetes as 'mononeuropathies' and are described in detail on page 162. Transient diplopia can occur during hypoglycaemia. Diplopia can also herald the onset of myasthenia gravis, a rare association with diabetes.

The optic disc

Optic atrophy is not a feature of diabetic retinopathy. There is an association in the rare DIDMOAD syndrome (diabetes insipidus, diabetes mellitus, optic atrophy and deafness; page 14) and patients with some but not all of these features have been described. Optic atrophy also occurs in some of the neurological conditions associated with Type 2 diabetes (page 14).

Papilloedema is not a feature of diabetic retinopathy.

The blind diabetic patient

Blindness may develop suddenly following vitreous haemorrhage from new vessels, or insidiously over weeks or months as exudative maculopathy or macular oedema gradually progress. Rubeotic glaucoma is particularly painful and disagreeable although relatively uncommon. Retinal detachment may occur and may cause blindness. Cataract formation is common but relatively easy to treat.

Once blind, the patient should register with the local authority because some amenities are available. Rehabilitation is available for suitable patients at the Royal National Institute for the Blind Centre, Torquay. Reading Braille is a valuable asset but some people with diabetes have a subtle sensory neuropathy affecting the fingers that prevents them doing so.

Management of diabetes may be made complicated by significant visual loss. Pen devices that indicate doses as dialled with an audible click may help patients retain their independence. Speaking meters for home blood glucose measurement were abandoned because of fears of inaccurate readings resulting from poor technique but should be revisited as a matter of urgency, with modern meters that require very small amounts of blood.

17

Diabetic Neuropathies

Summary

■ The neuropathies of diabetes comprise principally a slowly progressive distal symmetrical sensory polyneuropathy associated with autonomic dysfunction and other long-term microvascular complications in stark contrast to a diverse group of mononeuropathies which have a specific course generally leading to complete resolution

■ Sensory impairment is predominant and frequently symptomless

■ Symptoms from neuropathy include numbness, paraesthesiae and sometimes pain

■ Severe neuropathic pain and can occur: it normally resolves in 6 to 24 months but requires much supportive treatment

■ The hands are rarely clinically affected by diabetic neuropathy, although symptoms from carpal tunnel compression are common

■ Symptomatic autonomic neuropathy is relatively rare, and when it does occur comprises diarrhoea, gastroparesis, postural hypotension, neurogenic bladder and erectile dysfunction

■ Mononeuropathies include proximal motor (femoral) neuropathy, various radiculopathies and cranial nerve palsies.

Peripheral nerves are prone to damage in patients with diabetes. Nerve function deteriorates in response to pressure, ischaemia or metabolic abnormalities and these are the chief causes of neuropathies in diabetes. Alcohol, which can itself cause neuropathy, tends to make diabetic neuropathies worse. Different patterns of the neuropathies therefore exist; there are pressure palsies, mononeuropathies (probably ischaemic in origin) and diffuse sensory and autonomic polyneuropathy (probably both metabolic and ischaemic in origin). Only the last is related to duration of diabetes, is progressive and occurs in long-duration diabetes, often alongside other diabetic complications. Pressure palsies and mononeuropathies are not specific for diabetes, unrelated to diabetes duration or other complications, and often recover. Painful neuropathies develop either in association with established neuropathies or independently and are poorly understood. A suggested classification for diabetic neuropathies is shown in Table 17.1.

Distal symmetrical polyneuropathy with accompanying evidence of autonomic dysfunction is extremely common amongst diabetic patients. Lack of precise diagnostic criteria leads to difficulties in determining the overall prevalence, which is, however, estimated as affecting approximately 25–30% of both Type 1 and Type 2 diabetic patients increasing to over 40% in the elderly. As with other diabetic complications, many are spared, even after many years of diabetes. While abnormal cardiovascular autonomic function tests can be shown to be abnormal in as

Table 17.1 Clinical classification of neuropathies.

Classification	Characteristics
Progressive neuropathy	
Symmetrical sensory neuropathy	Gradual onset associated with duration of diabetes and other complications. No recovery
Autonomic neuropathy	
Reversible neuropathies	
Mononeuropathies	Rapid onset, no association with duration of diabetes or other complications. Recovery usual
Femoral radiculopathy	
Truncal radiculopathies	
Cranial nerve palsies	
Pressure palsies	
Carpal tunnel syndrome	Not specific for diabetes
Ulnar nerve compression	
Lateral popliteal compression (foot drop)	

many as 16–40% of patients, the unpleasant symptomatic features of autonomic neuropathy remain uncommon, affecting perhaps no more than 0.5–1% of diabetic patients, the majority of whom are female Type 1 diabetic subjects.

Vascular, metabolic and structural changes

Diabetes and its associated metabolic changes in peripheral nerves combine to cause endothelial dysfunction in their associated vascular supply, leading to a decrease of nitric oxide production and diminished nerve blood flow, although there is still controversy regarding the role of ischaemia as a cause of diabetic neuropathy. Nevertheless, small vessel changes in peripheral nerve have been described, and *in vivo* studies have clearly demonstrated a reduction in sural nerve endoneurial oxygen tension, oxygen saturation and nerve blood flow in diabetic patients with neuropathy.

Metabolic changes, notably changes of the redox potentials are probably equally important. A hypothetical scheme is shown in Fig. 17.1. Nerve conduction in experimental and, to some extent, human diabetes improves in response to many agents which include prostacyclin, various other vasodilators (notably calcium-channel blockers and angiotensin-

converting enzyme inhibitors), aldose reductase inhibitors, alpha lipoic acid and gamma linolenic acid (evening primrose oil), although there are no available agents known to modify the development of neuropathy to any clinically significant extent.

Biochemical changes

Poor glycaemic control over several years without doubt accelerates the development of neuropathy, as it does the evolution of other diabetic complications (page 127). Advanced glycosylated end products (AGEs) can be demonstrated in various components of diabetic nerve. Those with optimal metabolic control develop neuropathy at a much slower rate and progression in those with established disease is retarded. Near normalization of metabolism following pancreatic transplantation halts the progression of neuropathy and may even result in some improvement in nerve conduction velocity.

Biochemical changes have been demonstrated in peripheral nerves from diabetic patients as well as in animal models. Schwann cells and endoneurial capillaries contain the enzyme aldose reductase which converts glucose to the sugar alcohol sorbitol, which is in turn metabolized to fructose. Thus, nerves from patients with diabetes contain increased amounts of glucose, sorbitol and fructose. An activated polyol pathway disturbs redox potentials, reducing the production of nitric oxide.

Deficient neurotrophic growth factors, notably nerve growth factor (NGF), may have a role in the pathogenesis of diabetic neuropathy as such growth factors are required for development and maintenance of several nerve fibre types. Unfortunately, trials of treatment with NGF have not so far benefited diabetic patients with neuropathy and have demonstrated significant side-effects.

The presence of autoantibodies to some neural tissues has been demonstrated in Type 1 diabetic patients, and the concept that autoimmunity may contribute to the development particularly of symptomatic autonomic neuropathy has been suggested. However, the correlation between the presence of these autoantibodies and the development of various neuropathies has not been convincingly demonstrated, and further research in this field is required.

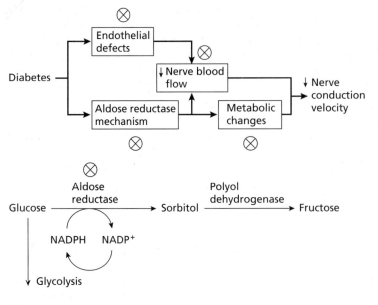

⊗ Indicates the points at which pharmacological intervention can lead to improvements in nerve conduction velocity

Figure 17.1 Hypothetical scheme of vascular and metabolic changes in diabetic neuropathy.

Symmetrical sensory neuropathy

Axon degeneration of both myelinated and unmyelinated fibres is demonstrable, although there is a spectrum of disease ranging from predominantly small fibre loss (representing pain and temperature sensory modalities and autonomic fibres) to a major loss of all fibre types. There is also evidence of axonal regeneration in most nerve biopsies taken from diabetic patients, even when the neuropathy is clinically very mild, although nerve function does not seem to improve as a result. Segmental demyelination is commonly observed in nerve biopsies, and the process of remyelination also witnessed. An axonal dying back process may also occur in the dorsal columns of the spinal cord.

Autonomic neuropathy

Most information on autonomic nerves comes from postmortem examinations, although major degenerative changes have been described in vagi removed during gastric surgery (Fig. 17.2). Autonomic ganglia show degenerative changes, and fibre loss or degeneration have been described in corpora caver-nosa of the penis and bladder wall. Inflammatory cellular infiltrates in autonomic tissue (ganglia and nerve bundles of viscera) have been seen in some autopsies from severely affected autonomic neuropathy patients, leading to the suggestion that immunological damage might have some role in the development of this disorder.

Mononeuropathies

Multifocal lesions with patchy fibre loss have been seen in the very rare instances where autopsy examination has been possible. Vascular occlusion may be responsible, but observations are few.

Electrophysiology

Electrophysiological abnormalities occur very frequently in patients with long-standing diabetes whether or not symptoms are present and, conversely, those with the most severe symptomatic painful neuropathies may prove to have almost no abnormal electrophysiological changes. The value of these tests in practice is therefore very limited; their chief use is in the diagnosis of mononeuropathies

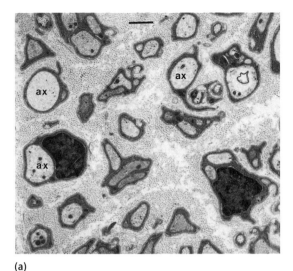

(a)

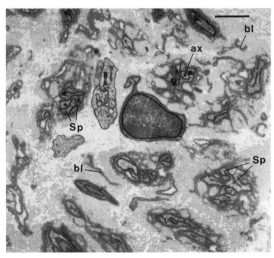

(b)

Figure 17.2 Electron micrographs of transverse section through abdominal vagus nerves: (a) of a normal subject aged 24 years, showing a dense population of unmyelinated axons (ax); and (b) from a severe autonomic neuropathy patient with intractable gastroparesis aged 28 years showing marked reduction of the axons both in density and size (bl, basal lamina; Sp, Schwann cell processes).

and assisting with their distinction from nerve root compressive lesions which require further investigation and treatment.

Electrophysiological abnormalities are numerous. Motor nerve conduction is often moderately re-

duced, although this observation may be the least clinically relevant in diabetic neuropathy, which is predominantly sensory. Sensory conduction and amplitude of evoked responses are helpful tests, showing slowing and reduction, respectively, in disease states, while demonstration of increased F-wave latencies may, in some instances, provide the most sensitive test. Recording from single nerve fibres is now possible and by this technique absence of peripheral sympathetic nerve fibres has been shown to occur more frequently in diabetic neuropathies than in others. This is currently primarily a research tool.

Clinical description of the neuropathies

The diverse clinical neurological syndromes associated with diabetes can be clearly separated into symmetrical sensory and autonomic neuropathy which steadily progresses with duration of diabetes, and is associated with other diabetic complications; and those which are abrupt in onset, often occurring at the presentation of diabetes itself, and not associated with duration or other complications: the latter are expected to recover completely. These clinical observations lead to a suggested classification of the neuropathies shown in Box 17.1.

Distal symmetrical sensory and autonomic neuropathy

This is the most common form of diabetic neuropathy and is associated with autonomic dysfunction. Detectable neuropathy increases as duration of

---

Box 17.1 **Clinical features of sensory neuropathy**

Symptomless
Paraesthesiae
Painful syndrome
Numbness
Sensation of coldness
Neuropathic ulceration
Charcot joints

diabetes lengthens; in long-standing diabetes it often occurs in association with other diabetic complications, although it can develop independently of them. It is permanent and irreversible. Its severity varies greatly from one patient to another, and as with other complications some are spared altogether.

The neuropathy is symmetrical, affecting the feet in a stocking distribution, with rare symptomatic involvement of the hands, possibly because the nerves supplying the hands are shorter. It follows that neurological symptoms in the hands are more commonly caused by carpal tunnel syndrome or ulnar nerve compression. Distal symmetrical sensory and autonomic neuropathy is predominantly a sensory neuropathy in which small nerve fibres carrying pain, temperature and autonomic modalities are affected first. As the disease advances, all fibre types may be affected. Early motor loss is restricted to the nerves supplying the intrinsic muscles of the feet which can lead to anatomical abnormalities as the flexing action of the extrinsic foot muscles is left unopposed.

The neuropathy is often symptomless and this is the chief hazard to the unwary patient who is then prone to foot injuries and sepsis. Later, patients may be aware of numbness; sensations of coldness and paraesthesiae are common (Box 17.1). The disorder sometimes worsens until, rarely, there is almost complete anaesthesia below the knees; at this stage motor involvement, and foot drop in particular, can develop. Proprioceptive loss is also a feature of the most advanced neuropathies, leading to ataxia and making patients feel unsteady and unsafe. Severe pain of the type described on page 161 is occasionally the predominant feature. The most serious consequences of diabetic neuropathy are pain and the development of diabetic foot problems.

Diagnosis and evaluation

Careful examination is needed to detect diabetic neuropathy. Non-diabetic causes must always be considered and investigated when appropriate. Motor weakness is very uncommon and sensory abnormalities can be difficult to detect at the bedside. Ankle reflexes are usually absent, while knee jerks are retained until an advanced stage. Pain and temperature modalities of sensation are lost first and thus, surprisingly, severe lesions of the feet may be seen while light touch sensation remains grossly intact. Light touch and vibration perception are often affected: the distibution of sensory loss is always in a symmetrical 'stocking' distribution. In time, all sensory modalities may be impaired, although the progression of neuropathy is often imperceptibly slow.

Sophisticated techniques are not normally needed for investigation. Electromyogram (EMG) examination rarely helps in cases of symmetrical neuropathy beyond establishing the presence of neuropathy, but in the mononeuropathies it is of value in localizing the lesion. Evaluation of vibration perception threshold using a biothesiometer and of light touch sensation are helpful and recommended (pages 173 and 179) but other tests of sensory function are complex and not suitable for routine clinical use. Sural nerve biopsy is a research procedure and is only performed if there are strong reasons to suspect the presence of other specific neuropathies not resulting from diabetes.

Neuropathy and the hands

Diabetic neuropathy rarely causes symptoms in the hands and, when it does, the disease is already advanced in the feet and legs. Numbness and clumsiness of the fingers are unusual and generally caused by some other neurological disorder, although impairment of sensation is often sufficient to prevent blind people with diabetes from reading Braille. Some patients cultivate longer nails in order to increase tactile sensitivity.

Paraesthesiae and numbness in the fingers especially at night are usually caused by nerve compression syndromes, most commonly carpal tunnel syndrome, which is easy to diagnose and treat by minor surgery under local anaesthetic.

Interosseous muscle wasting is not uncommon and usually a result of ulnar nerve compression at the elbow; it is accompanied by typical sensory defects in the fourth and fifth fingers. Disability is unusual and there is no satisfactory treatment beyond the advice not to lean on the elbows.

Autonomic neuropathy

Autonomic dysfunction is very common in patients with long-standing diabetes but only rarely causes

Table 17.2 Clinical features of autonomic neuropathy.

	Clinical syndromes	Other abnormalities	
Cardiovascular	Postural hypotension Tachycardia		
Sweating	Gustatory sweating		
Genitourinary	Erectile dysfunction Neurogenic bladder		
Gastrointestinal	Diarrhoea Gastroparesis	Oesophageal mobility Gall bladder emptying	
Respiratory	Arrests ?Sudden death	?Sleep apnoea Cough reflex	
Eye		Pupillary responses Pupillary size decreased	all reduced
Neuroendocrine responses		Catecholamines Glucagon Pancreatic polypeptide	

the unpleasant clinical symptoms described in Table 17.2. Even when they do occur, these symptoms are often curiously intermittent, although they continue over many years and rarely remit completely. Sympathetic damage causes a substantial increase in peripheral blood flow together with major changes of vascular regulation which may be related to some of the foot problems experienced by diabetic patients and these are described on page 167.

We have described a very striking syndrome in which younger predominantly female Type 1 diabetic patients develop iritis accompanied by severe 'small fibre' neuropathy causing severe symptomatic autonomic neuropathy together with a dissociated sensory loss (loss of pain and temperature modalities while retaining relatively normal light touch and vibration perception), Charcot joints and foot ulcers with arterial calcification in the feet (page 169). The mechanisms underlying these characteristic features remain to be elucidated, but an immunological basis has been postulated.

Autonomic neuropathy progresses very slowly; when it is associated with postural hypotension mortality is increased, and sudden unexplained deaths possibly as a result of respiratory arrest have been reported in a few cases. The development of nephropathy in these patients is not uncommon and deaths are usually from renal failure or coronary artery disease.

Diarrhoea

This is often a catastrophic watery diarrhoea with severe nocturnal exacerbations and faecal incontinence, preceded by abdominal rumblings. Steatorrhoea is not normally a feature and should lead to consideration of pancreatic exocrine insufficiency. The symptoms are intermittent with normal bowel action or even constipation between bouts. They continue over many years and complete remissions are unusual. Persistent and intractable diarrhoea is very rare. The presence of demonstrable autonomic dysfunction is required in establishing the diagnosis, but there is no direct test of colonic or rectal innervation. It is absolutely essential to exclude other causes of diarrhoea such as coeliac or pancreatic disease, inflammatory bowel disease, malignancy, etc. The diarrhoea is treated with any antidiarrhoea agent, the best of which is codeine phosphate. Metronidazole or a broad-spectrum antibiotic such as tetracycline can have an impressive effect in about half the cases, even after the first two or three doses, and should be used at the onset of exacerbations. Their mechanism of action is unclear but may be a response to the bacterial overgrowth that may occur in semistagnant bowel. The use of clonidine has been described but its efficacy not confirmed. Octreotide can be effective though side-effects are common.

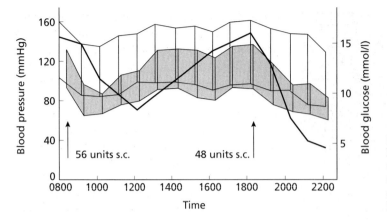

Figure 17.3 Fluctuations in postural hypotension in relation to subcutaneous (sc) insulin injections. Plain area shows recumbent blood pressure and that on standing is shown in the shaded area. Blood glucose is shown by the solid line.

Gastroparesis

Diminished gastric motility and delayed stomach emptying occur sometimes in diabetic patients with autonomic neuropathy but symptoms are rare. Intermittent vomiting may occur and is very rarely intractable. Diagnosis is established by the presence of a gastric splash and screening during barium studies which show food residue, loss of peristalsis and failure to empty. Autonomic dysfunction should be present, while endoscopy is needed to exclude other gastric disorders. Isotopic studies of gastric emptying are helpful but must be performed under near normoglycaemia, as hyperglycaemia delays gastric emptying even in healthy stomachs. Isotopic studies of gastric emptying should be performed and should clearly demonstrate an impairment of emptying times: many patients with advanced disease show no emptying at 90 min (100% retention). Otherwise, the normal values of 54±10% retention at 90 min or 24±13% retention at 140 min should be exceeded usually by a considerable amount.

Any antiemetic can be useful, including metoclopramide or domperidone. Erythromycin given intravenously accelerates gastric emptying by a motilin agonist effect, but the clinical value of small doses of oral erythromycin (50 mg t.d.s.) is very questionable. Cisapride has been helpful to some patients but its use was associated with arrythmias and it is now available only on a 'named patient' basis. Some patients benefit from rotating courses of different agents and some may need H2 blockers to reduce any associated gastritis.

Surgical treatment is occasionally needed for the very rare cases of intractable vomiting from gastroparesis. Percutaneous endoscopic jejunostomy can help and, even more rarely, radical surgery by two-thirds gastrectomy with Roux-en-Y loop may be required and can be successful.

Postural hypotension

This is defined by a postural fall of systolic pressure on standing of more than 20 mmHg; blood pressure may fall progressively for up to 3 or 4 min. The postural fall is very variable and is exacerbated by insulin (Fig. 17.3). Symptoms, which are rare, are also very variable in their severity. Disabling postural hypotension is very uncommon indeed and management is not simple. Patients should stop any medication that aggravates hypotension, notably hypotensive agents, tranquillizers, antidepressants and diuretics; they should sleep with the head of the bed elevated and wear full-length elastic stockings. The most effective measures aim to increase blood volume and include a high salt intake and fludrocortisone, using increasing doses from 0.1 mg/day up to 0.6 mg/day. Failures are common, and the oedema that results from treatment is often unacceptable. Many other agents have been tried, the best of which is the alpha-agonist midodrine. A combination of fludrocortisone, flurbiprofen and ephedrine may help. Erythropoietin injections can increase the systolic pressure both when lying and standing. Variable severity of postural hypotension persists over many years, but

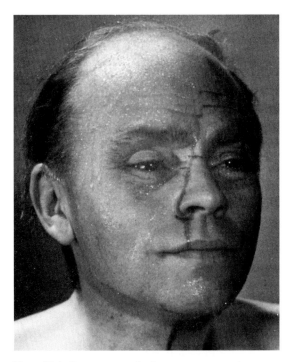

Figure 17.4 Gustatory sweating in a severe autonomic neuropathy patient, shown a few seconds after chewing cheese. The dark line is from application of starch–iodide powder.

only a very small minority of patients become incapacitated.

Respiratory arrests

Transient respiratory arrests occur sometimes if susceptible neuropathic patients are given agents that depress respiration, notably powerful analgesics and anaesthetics. These patients should be monitored carefully even during minor surgery. It is very likely that some sudden unexpected and unexplained deaths amongst these patients are caused by respiratory arrests.

Gustatory and nocturnal sweating

Facial sweating (including scalp, neck and shoulders) which occurs while eating tasty foods, notably cheese, is a common symptom of autonomic neuropathy (Fig. 17.4). In severe cases the sweat pours down the neck and chest, and sufferers feel they are in a Turkish bath and socially embarrassing visible sweating may occur. This symptom provides clinical evidence for the presence of autonomic neuropathy. It tends to persist over many years, although remissions after renal transplantation have been reported. Some patients seek treatment which is effected either by avoiding the offending foodstuffs or by the use of an anticholinergic agent, namely propantheline bromide, although typical anticholinergic side-effects are common. Topical applications of antiperspirants such as glycopyrronium bromide or aluminium chloride can be helpful applied to the areas affected by sweating, avoiding contact with the mouth, nose and eyes. The area should not be washed for 4 h after application and alternate-day or occasional use is recommended. Clonidine is another agent that has been used with reported benefit.

Gustatory sweating is thought to result from disordered innervation of the sweat glands. Nocturnal sweating may be a feature of autonomic neuropathy, although hypoglycaemia is a more common cause and chronic infections and malignant causes must be ruled out.

Neurogenic bladder

Urinary retention is a serious and usually late complication of autonomic neuropathy. It develops following both loss of the normal sensation of bladder distension and failure of detrusor activity. Inadequate micturition and later gross bladder distension occur and may mimic prostatic obstruction; rarely, hydronephrosis develops. Persistent urinary tract infections also occur. Diagnosis is now relatively simple using ultrasound technology before and after micturition, while cystoscopy is needed to exclude other causes of obstruction, notably prostatic. When retention is established, treatment is by self-catheterization two to three times daily.

Erectile dysfunction

Erectile dysfunction is a common symptom especially in diabetic men over 55 years of age. It occurs more often in diabetic men than in non-diabetic men: about half of diabetic men over 55 years of age may be affected, while younger patients in their third and fourth decades sometimes have this problem. While autonomic neuropathy plays an important part, vascular and psychogenic causes

Table 17.3 Normal values for autonomic function tests. These tests decline with age. The figures given here apply generally in those less than 60 years old.

	Normal	Abnormal
Heart rate variation (deep breathing)	>15	<10
Heart rate on standing (at 15 s)	>15	<12
Heart rate on standing 30 : 15 ratio	>1.04	<1.00
Valsalva ratio	>1.21	<1.20
Postural systolic pressure fall at 2 min	<10 mmHg	>20 mmHg

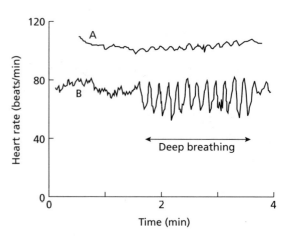

Figure 17.5 Heart rate variation at rest and during deep breathing in a normal subject (B) and in a patient with severe autonomic neuropathy (A). Normally, the heart rate accelerates and decelerates with inspiration and expiration, respectively; these changes are reduced or absent in autonomic neuropathy.

are also relevant. The subject is discussed below (page 163).

Diagnosis of autonomic neuropathy

Autonomic dysfunction is common in long-standing diabetic patients. Its presence is easily confirmed by simple bedside tests described below, although their interpretation in those over 60 years of age is difficult because of their natural decline with age. Symptoms from autonomic neuropathy are relatively uncommon and, before they are attributed to autonomic neuropathy (which must be shown to be present), other disorders must be excluded if serious errors are to be avoided.

Clinical indicators of autonomic neuropathy include the presence of gustatory sweating and, on examination, a resting tachycardia (caused by loss of vagal inhibition), postural hypotension and, rarely, a gastric splash.

The bedside tests of autonomic function are valuable; normal and abnormal values are shown in Table 17.3.

Heart rate variation on deep breathing

The normal acceleration and deceleration of heart rate during respiration (sinus arrythmia) is reduced early in the course of autonomic neuropathy caused by cardiac vagal denervation; diminished heart rate variability provides the basis for the simplest and most sensitive test for the presence of autonomic neuropathy. Heart rate variation is maximal during deep breathing at a rate of 6 breaths/min (5 s in and 5 s out). The average heart rate difference (maximum minus minimum at the end of each breath) over 5 breaths is recorded. While the use of a heart rate monitor is the simplest method of conducting this test (Fig. 17.5), an ordinary electrocardiograph can be used. New methods of spectral analysis of heart rate variability can distinguish sympathetic and parasympathetic defects, and at least for research purposes provide extremely sensitive assessment of the autonomic nervous system.

Heart rate increase on standing

On standing up there is an immediate and rapid increase in heart rate which overshoots the eventual rate on standing, which is higher than that when lying down. Absence of this overshoot is evidence of a cardiac vagal defect (Fig. 17.6). For diagnostic purposes, the heart rate increase is recorded at the peak of the overshoot or, if there is no overshoot, 15 s after standing up. An alternative index is the 30 : 15 ratio which records the ratio of the R : R interval of the 30th in relation to the 15th beat after standing.

Valsalva manoeuvre

This is performed by asking the patient to blow into the empty barrel of a 20-mL syringe attached to a mercury sphygmomanometer; a pressure of 40

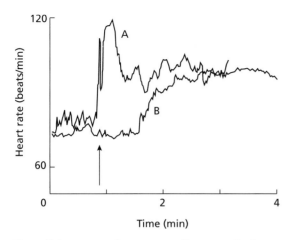

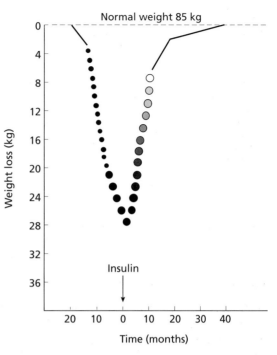

Figure 17.6 Heart rate changes on standing. Normally, the effect of standing (shown by the arrow) from the lying position is to cause an overshoot of heart rate (A), an effect which is lost in autonomic neuropathy (B), together with a progressive reduction in the cardiac acceleration at 15 s.

mmHg should be maintained for 10 s. The ratio of the maximum heart rate during blowing to the minimum heart rate after cessation is recorded. The test should not be performed in patients with proliferative retinopathy.

Blood pressure change on standing
A decrease of more than 20 mmHg systolic pressure is abnormal. Patients should remain standing for at least 3 min during which the systolic pressure may continue to fall.

Loss of sweating from the feet
Bedside sweat tests are not simple and generally used only in research. One test of sweating involves painting the foot with iodine and sprinkling with starch powder. An intradermal injection of acetylcholine is made. In healthy skin, the resultant sweating produces moisture which allows the starch and iodine to interact. Tiny blue spots appear at each sweat gland. In neuropathy, no colour change occurs.

Painful neuropathy

Disabling pain, as opposed to discomfort from paraesthesiae, is an uncommon symptom of diabetic neuropathy. It is to be expected in the thigh of pa-

Figure 17.7 The loss of weight in painful diabetic neuropathy can be profound and has led to the description 'diabetic neuropathic cachexia'. Weight loss increases as pain increases (●) and reduces as pain diminishes (○).

tients with proximal motor (femoral) neuropathy, over the abdomen in cases of truncal radiculopathy, or in the feet and legs if it occurs in symmetrical peripheral neuropathy. The pain causes exceptional distress because it is protracted and unremitting and may last several months or sometimes longer. Constant burning sensations, likened sometimes to walking on burning sand, paraesthesiae and shooting or searing pains are all described. There is a subjective sensation of swollen feet. A highly characteristic feature is that of exquisite sensitivity and discomfort to contact with clothes and bed clothes (allodynia). The symptoms are worse at night causing insomnia and depression, and profound weight loss is usual (Fig. 17.7), often leading to a fruitless search for malignant conditions. Sensory loss is distal, usually less extensive than the pains, and sometimes negligible. Painful symmetrical neuropathy can occur in the initial absence of sensory signs or electrophysiological changes, and patients therefore suspected by some physicians to be malingering; or alternatively it may accompany severe neuropathic loss in which the numb foot is exquisitely painful (the 'painless painful foot'). Patients are so distressed that they may seek several opinions on their condition.

Treatment

Reassurances that painful neuropathy will neither cripple the patient nor result in amputations, and that the most severe symptoms will eventually remit, help to sustain morale. Treatment of painful neuropathy is always difficult. Diabetic control should be optimized, using insulin if necessary. Initially, simple analgesics such as paracetamol taken regularly should be tried. Tricyclic antidepressants have a specific effect in the management of neuropathic pain and are valuable in this condition: a useful combination is a preparation containing a phenothiazine (fluphenazine) with nortriptyline (Motival). Gabapentin is effective, while carbamazepine may help. Capsaicin cream helps sometimes, although it has some side-effects of its own. Topiramate may be used for limited periods in those with severe and protracted pain. Drugs of addiction should be avoided, although just occasionally and for a short period an opioid derivative can be used at bedtime to help distressed patients to sleep.

Application of OpSite (a thin adhesive film) can help alleviate contact discomfort. Electrical nerve stimulators applied to the site of pain may help which enables patients to take an active part in their treatment.

The most severe and unpleasant symptoms of painful neuropathy resolve in 6–8 months, occasionally up to 1 or even 2 years. The symptoms may disappear completely and may leave no residual signs. When the features are less dramatic, some discomfort and paraesthesiae may persist for years although normal body weight is always restored. Relapses are very uncommon indeed.

Mononeuropathies

Single nerves, or groups of nerve roots, are affected. The rapid onset, severity and eventual recovery of these lesions are in striking contrast to the gradually progressive development of diffuse sensory and autonomic neuropathy. The lesions can occur at any age or duration of diabetes, although they are more common in older male Type 2 diabetic patients, and are unrelated to other diabetic complications. It is always important to exclude other causes of nerve or nerve root compression in these cases.

Cranial nerve palsies

Ocular palsies are more common in diabetic than non-diabetic people. Patients tend to be older and the aetiology is thought to be vascular. The cranial nerves most affected are III and VI. The evidence for an association of nerve VII palsy with diabetes is very weak.

The onset of diplopia is abrupt and, in IIIrd nerve palsy, it is often preceded by some pain behind or just above the eye. The pupil is usually spared, and ptosis is very uncommon. Recovery takes place in about 3 months and relapse is very unusual. Extensive investigation is not normally needed unless atypical features are present.

Proximal motor neuropathy (femoral neuropathy; diabetic amyotrophy)

Pain with or without wasting of the thigh is the cardinal feature of this condition. Sometimes the opposite thigh is also affected, usually developing within a few weeks of the first. The quality of the continuous pain that affects the thigh and may extend medially below the knee is identical to that described on page 161. It may cause insomnia and sometimes profound weight loss. The weakness is sometimes sufficiently severe to cause the knee to give way and patients may fall. Examination always shows wasting and weakness of the quadriceps, and usually of the iliopsoas and thigh adductors (innervated by the obturator nerve). The knee jerk is absent, while the ankle jerk may be intact. Diagnosis must be confirmed by careful clinical examination and usually needs electrophysiological confirmation. It is essential to exclude nerve root compression. Magnetic resonance imaging is needed to exclude nerve compression. Cerebrospinal fluid (CSF) proteins are often raised in this condition and may be 1000 mg/L or more but testing the CSF is not a necessary part of diagnosis.

Recovery is the rule, between 6 and 12 months after the onset. The knee reflex is restored in approxi-

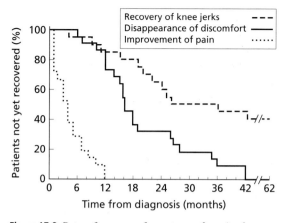

Figure 17.8 Rates of recovery of symptoms of proximal motor neuropathy in 27 patients. The 'improvement of pain' line is the time until the first report of improvement in sensory symptoms, from 22 patients. The 'disappearance of discomfort' line is the time until complete resolution of sensory symptoms in 23 patients. The 'recovery of knee-jerk' represents the time course of return to normal of patella tendon reflexes in 20 patients. No recovery was observed later than 42 months after diagnosis; follow-up was for a median of 62 months. (From Coppack, S. & Watkins, P.J. The natural history of diabetic femoral neuropathy. *Quarterly Journal of Medicine* 1991; **79**: 307–313, with permission.)

mately half of the patients within 3 years (Fig. 17.8). Patients may need a great deal of support especially in the earlier stages of this disorder. Pain management has already been described on page 162; physiotherapy to strengthen the thigh muscles is also valuable and helps to rehabilitate the patient. Recurrence of this condition is extremely rare; occasionally, the opposite thigh develops the same syndrome years later, while relapse in the same leg practically never occurs.

Truncal radiculopathies
Characteristic pain affects areas of the trunk, usually abdominal, in the distribution of groups of nerve roots either unilaterally or bilaterally. It must be distinguished from nerve root compression, and appropriate investigations may be needed. Diabetic radiculopathy does not appear to affect the upper chest or arms. The character of the pain associated with exquisite skin hypersensitivity is as described above. On very rare occasions, motor weakness of abdominal wall muscles causes a striking bulging to

occur. Recovery is expected in 6–12 months or less, severe symptoms rarely persisting for as long as 2 years.

Pressure palsies

Carpal tunnel syndrome is more common in diabetic than non-diabetic people and is the most common cause of paraesthesthiae in the fingers, especially at night. It is easily treated by surgical decompression. Ulnar nerve compression at the elbow probably occurs more often in people with diabetes than others, causing numbness of the fourth and fifth fingers and wasting of the interossei. No disability usually results and there is no effective treatment.

Foot drop results either from pressure on the lateral popliteal nerve at the knee, or from L5/S1 nerve root lesions; it is uncertain whether these problems are causally related to diabetes or merely coincidental. Nerve root lesions require correct diagnosis and treatment in their own right, while patients with lateral popliteal lesions sometimes, but not always, recover spontaneously. Most cases of foot drop in diabetes develop in those with overwhelming sensory and motor neuropathy, in patients who are virtually anaesthetic below the knees (page 156). Foot drop is then usually bilateral and can be disabling.

Erectile dysfunction

The development of erectile dysfunction has three major causes, apart from the reversible form which may develop in almost any state of ill-health. It may be psychogenic, which is probably the most common single cause; neurogenic; occasionally as a result of vascular disease (poor arterial inflow or increased venous leak from the penis); or endocrine. Only neurogenic erectile dysfunction is specific to diabetes; it does not have an endocrine basis and gonadotrophins and testosterone levels are normal.

Neuropathic erectile dysfunction develops in relation to other diabetic complications and it is more likely to be present when there is evidence of both somatic and autonomic neuropathy. It is by no means always present even in patients with severe neuropathy and, conversely, it is sometimes the earliest symptom of neuropathy when there are few other features.

Once present, neuropathic erectile dysfunction is permanent and irreversible. Its onset is always gradual and slowly progressive over months or years. Erectile ability fails first at a time when ejaculation is retained. Retrograde ejaculation sometimes occurs. Nocturnal erections are absent in these patients (they are often retained in psychogenic impotence). Libido is normal. It is important to distinguish neurogenic from psychogenic impotence wherever possible, although this is often difficult. Psychogenic impotence presents in some contrasting ways: it is often abrupt in its onset, sometimes in response to adverse circumstances; nocturnal erections often persist; and the condition is intermittent and potentially reversible.

Diagnosis

A careful history helps to distinguish organic from psychogenic erectile dysfunction. Drug-induced problems, especially from hypotensive agents, should be excluded.

Physical assessment should include examination of the genitalia; endocrine referral is required if there is evidence of hypogonadism. Neurological examination is needed to determine the presence of somatic and autonomic neuropathy. Abnormal autonomic function tests provide some guidance in diagnosis but do not alone establish the presence of neuropathic erectile dysfunction.

The rare endocrine causes of erectile dysfunction are excluded by measurement of testosterone, prolactin and gonadotrophins. Vascular pathology can be established only by complex assessments undertaken in specialist centres: the investigations include assessment of penile blood pressure by Doppler probes, or the use of penile perfusion cavernometry to identify the exact vascular cause for erectile dysfunction.

Treatment

Psychosexual counselling of the couple is sometimes needed, especially if the erectile dysfunction is psy-

chogenic in origin. It can be beneficial in motivated patients and is also of value in conjunction with specific treatments. Neuropathic erectile dysfunction is permanent, but can be considerably assisted by a range of new treatments described below. Oral sildenafil (Viagra) is generally the first choice. Androgen treatment is contraindicated because it merely serves to increase libido without restoring potency.

Oral sildenafil (Viagra)

This can be successful in almost two-thirds of the diabetic patients treated, which is rather less than in non-diabetic people. It is taken 30 min to 1 hour before sexual activity (initial dose 50 mg; subsequently 50–100 mg according to response; not to be used more than once in 24 h). Sexual stimulation and foreplay are necessary for it to be effective. It is contraindicated in those taking nitrates, those whose blood pressure is less than 90/50 mmHg, after recent stroke or myocardial infarction, or in other situations where sexual activity is inadvisable. There are several other potential side-effects which are rarely troublesome. These are listed in the *British National Formulary* and the drug literature.

Sublingual apomorphine hydrochloride (Uprima)

This is rapidly absorbed and acts as a dopamine agonist. It is effective within 10–20 min, requiring sexual stimulation at the same time. The dose range is 2–3 mg. It is effective in approximately 50% of diabetic patients.

Prostaglandin preparations

These include transurethral alprostadil (MUSE) which can provide erections adequate for intercourse. An applicator for direct urethral application is provided. Intracavernosal prostaglandin injection: alprostadil (Caverject; Viridal Duo) is now less used than previously but can be effective; modern injection systems have made its use acceptable to most. Priapism is a possible result and the agents should not be used in the presence of urethral disease or after penile implants have been inserted. The reader is referred to the *British National Formulary* for a full list of possible side-effects.

Priapism can also occur with sildenafil and, if it does not resolve with leg exercise, it can be treated by aspiration of blood from the engorged penis through a butterfly needle inserted into the corpus cavernosum. Phenylephrine is then administered.

Vacuum devices

An external cylinder is fitted over the penis. The air is pumped out creating a semivacuum, resulting in penile engorgement which is then sustained by application of a ring fitted to the base of the penis. This technique is suitable for a wide range of patients and is successful in most cases of erectile dysfunction, although when the problem is of long-standing several attempts may be necessary before a successful erection is achieved.

Penile prostheses

Semirigid, malleable prostheses can be surgically inserted and are particularly valuable for younger patients with confirmed and permanent neuropathic impotence. Ejaculation in some patients is retained.

The Diabetic Foot

Summary

- Foot ulceration and sepsis are due chiefly to injuries in those with neuropathy and/or ischaemia

- Neuropathic ulcers (associated with a good circulation) occur at pressure points (toes, metatarsal heads, heels) in contrast to ischaemic lesions which usually occur on the lateral margins of the feet

- Appraisal of the feet of diabetic patients for risk of ulceration comprises inspection for deformities and skin changes, assessment of neuropathy and of the circulatory status

- General measures for management of ulceration and sepsis include rest, podiatry, eradication of infection, protection from weight-bearing forces by use of appropriate footwear, and appropriate surgery for wound debridement, severe sepsis, osteomyelitis, necrosis or gangrene

- Arterial reconstruction or angioplasty to restore the circulation need consideration when wound healing is delayed in an ischaemic limb

- Detection of critical ischaemia needing urgent revascularisation procedures is crucial

- Prevention of foot problems represents an essential aspect of diabetes care and comprises education, podiatry, regular foot inspection and assessment, and advice regarding appropriate footwear

The popular perception that people with diabetes lose their limbs is in the minds of many patients. Every visible blemish or slightest symptom raises the ogre of an amputation. Many of these symptoms can be eliminated instantly by an understanding physician who in appropriate circumstances explains that amputation is not forthcoming.

Furthermore, both patients and public should know that with proper education and foot care, both prevention and treatment can have a dramatic impact on prognosis; for a relatively low cost these foot problems could be reduced even further.

Clinical features

The chief factors responsible for foot problems in diabetes are neuropathy, ischaemia (or both) and infection. The ischaemic foot is more serious and carries a worse prognosis. The needs of investigation and treatment of these two pathologies are different. Neuropathy results in a warm, numb, dry and normally painless foot in which pulses are palpable (Table 18.1); it predisposes to ulceration, Charcot joints and oedema. In contrast, pulses are absent in the ischaemic foot which may be complicated by

Table 18.1 Characteristics of neuropathic and ischaemic foot ulcers.

	Neuropathic	Ischaemic
Temperature	Warm	Normal or cool
Pulses	Present	Absent
Pain	None	Sometimes severe
Site	Under toes and metatarsal heads	Lateral borders of feet

Table 18.2 Circulatory changes in the neuropathic foot.

Abnormality	Consequence
Increased foot circulation Arteriovenous shunting	Oedema
Increased bone circulation	Osteopenia Charcot joints
Medial calcification	Rigid arteries; high brachial : ankle systolic ratio (pressure index)

pain, discoloration, ulceration from localized pressure, necrosis and gangrene. Foot deformities predispose to problems from ulceration, and sepsis plays havoc with both neuropathic and ischaemic feet.

Pathophysiology

The neuropathic foot

Peripheral neuropathy leads to somatic sensory and autonomic damage (Chapter 17). Small fibre damage predominates initially, causing loss of pain and temperature sensation and later a numb or even anaesthetic foot with loss of all sensory modalities. Sensory loss persists and abnormal forces that deform the foot occur unnoticed by the patient. Motor weakness is not commonly a feature of diabetic neuropathy although it probably causes weakness of the intrinsic foot muscles and leads to clawing of the toes and increased prominence of the metatarsal heads, both of which increase risk of abrasion by footwear.

Sympathetic damage causes loss of sweating and denervates peripheral blood vessels with profound effects. Absence of sweating results in a dry foot sometimes associated with cracked skin which acts as a portal of entry for sepsis. Vascular denervation increases peripheral blood flow, opens arteriovenous shunts bypassing the capillary beds, and leads to arterial medial degeneration with calcification. A warm foot associated with a blood flow (Fig. 18.1) which may be more than five times that of normal are characteristic features of the neuropathic foot. These major haemodynamic changes are at least in part responsible for oedema in the neuropathic foot, occasionally of considerable severity. Increase in bone blood flow also occurs (Fig. 18.2) and may cause os-

teopenia, and this could underlie the development of the destructive bony changes of Charcot joints (Table 18.2). Sympathetic denervation of the arteries to the foot leads to increased vascular rigidity and medial calcification (Fig. 18.3), which is more common after lumbar sympathectomy. While there is no evidence that reduced blood flow results from this, measurement of pedal blood pressure may give misleading results because of the incompressibility of the arteries (page 173).

The ischaemic limb

The blood supply to the foot is reduced by atherosclerosis of large vessels; the disease is more common in diabetics than in people without diabetes, but the histopathology is the same and only the distribution may be different. It is age-related: older patients and those who smoke are more likely to suffer foot problems from ischaemia.

Atheromatous plaques are usually extensive, bilateral and multisegmental; in people with diabetes they are more likely to involve the distal vessels below the knee, so that tibial and peroneal obliteration are quite common. Disease of distal arterioles and capillaries is less well understood and it is not known whether endothelial proliferation or dysfunction, or basement membrane thickening have any significant effect on distal blood flow. This uncertainty should in no way influence proper investigation and treatment of the ischaemic limb.

Precipitating causes of foot lesions

Foot damage and ulceration in both neuropathic and ischaemic feet always result from some noxious

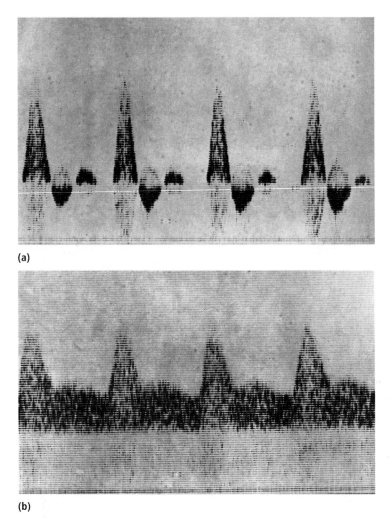

(a)

(b)

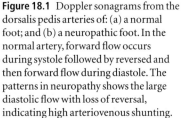

Figure 18.1 Doppler sonagrams from the dorsalis pedis arteries of: (a) a normal foot; and (b) a neuropathic foot. In the normal artery, forward flow occurs during systole followed by reversed and then forward flow during diastole. The patterns in neuropathy shows the large diastolic flow with loss of reversal, indicating high arteriovenous shunting.

stimulus; in the neuropathic foot this may be unperceived by the patient and lesions may progress to an advanced stage before they are detected. Infection is then the final disaster.

Mechanical injuries

The repetitive mechanical forces of normal gait often result in callus formation, especially in neuropathic patients. Callus develops at sites of high pressure and therefore at various points of foot deformity as well as under the metatarsal heads. Tissue necrosis occurs deep to the plaque and eventually breaks to the surface with ulcer formation. The importance of pres-

sure in the development of these lesions has been demonstrated by direct measurement of forces under the foot using pedobarography and vulnerable areas are those where pressure exceeds $10\,kg/cm^2$. Callus removal and alteration of points of high pressure by appropriate footwear are of the greatest importance in both treatment and prevention.

Pressure from tight ill-fitting shoes is a common cause of foot injury, blistering and subsequent sepsis. Shoes which do not accommodate deformities cause a particular hazard and new shoes, which should always be broken in gradually, are frequently the culprits. Oedema poses special problems especially

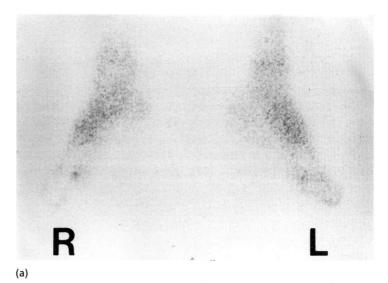

(a)

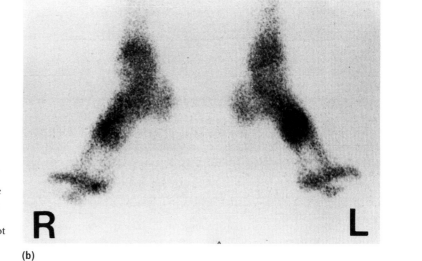

Figure 18.2 Technetium diphosphonate isotope bone scans in: (a) a normal foot; and (b) a neuropathic foot. The huge increase in uptake in the neuropathic foot represents the high bone blood flow. Radiographs were normal.

(b)

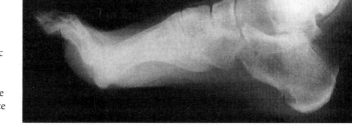

Figure 18.3 Radiograph of a neuropathic foot showing marked arterial medial calcification in both dorsalis pedis and tibialis posterior arteries. It also shows the effect of clawed toes causing protuberance of the metatarsal heads.

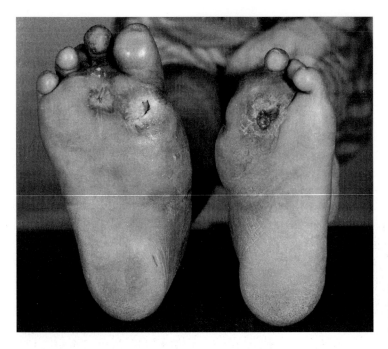

Figure 18.4 Neuropathic ulcers. The surrounding callus, symmetry of the lesions, clawing of the toes and digital amputations are all characteristic.

if it varies a great deal and this needs special consideration.

Heel friction can occur in diabetic patients who for any reason may be confined to bed, even during the relatively short periods needed during, for example, surgical treatments; development of blistering and sepsis can have serious consequences (page 176).

Direct mechanical injuries are common. They occur mainly from stones or protuberant nails inside shoes, or when patients with insensitive feet walk barefoot and encounter sharp objects.

Burns cause blistering with subsequent infection. Hot water bottle burns are the most frequent cause, but unpleasant lesions occur in some neuropathic patients who may fall asleep with their feet too close to an open fire or resting on a radiator. Bathing in excessively hot water or walking barefoot on hot sand during seaside holidays may also cause serious burns.

Chemical injuries occur from the use of keratolytic agents, notably 'corn plasters'; these contain a high concentration of salicylic acid and may cause liquefaction of tissues, sepsis and necrosis which may lead to surgery and amputation. They should never be used by people with diabetes.

Sepsis

Infection gains entry following abrasion of the skin resulting from any of the traumas described above, or just through cracks in hard dry skin that may develop spontaneously. Sometimes, interdigital fungal infection (athlete's foot) serves as the portal of entry. Sepsis is the major cause of the evolution of foot lesions converting simple ulcers into horrendous foot disease.

The organisms are usually *Staphylococcus aureus* or streptococci, but many others are involved including Gram-negative organisms; anaerobes flourish when there is a deep infection and include bacteroides and, more rarely, *Clostridium perfringens*. In recent years the problems arising from infection with methicillin-resistant *Staphylococcus aureus* (MRSA) have grown substantially.

Lesions

Neuropathic lesions
Neuropathic ulcers develop typically at points of high pressure in relation to areas of heavy callus formation (Fig. 18.4; Table 18.3). They most often occur

Table 18.3 Sites of ulceration in neuropathic and ischaemic feet.

Site	Neuropathic (%)	Ischaemic (%)
Toes	68	59
Metatarsal		
plantar	20	3
lateral	3	18
Other	9	20

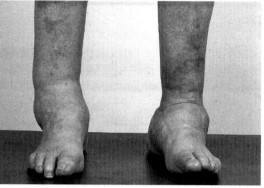

Figure 18.6 Charcot (neuroarthropathic) joints. The feet are grossly deformed from bony destruction and dislocation; the 'rocker' sole is characteristic.

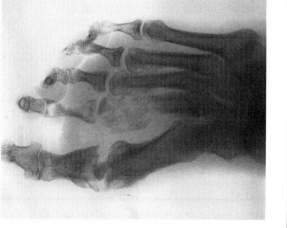

Figure 18.5 Bony destruction from osteomyelitis in a neuropathic foot.

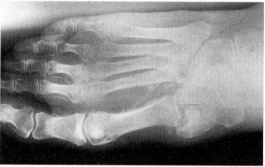

Figure 18.7 Charcot (neuroarthropathic) joints: radiographs showing dislocation of the mid-tarsal joint, bone destruction and new bone formation. Vascular calcification is also visible.

under the tips of the toes, under the metatarsal heads, concealed as interdigital ulcers and occasionally on the heel. Less frequently they are seen on the dorsum of the toes and over bunions. They are frequently circular, punched out in appearance and painless.

Following the entry of sepsis the picture changes, sometimes rapidly. Cellulitis spreads fast, and deep involvement of the foot with abscess formation causes the foot to become dusky, red, swollen and even painful; the development of pain suggests a collection of pus and may indicate the need for urgent surgery. Local arterial thrombosis can cause digital gangrene. Subcutaneous gas formation is a serious development and can occasionally be felt on palpation and seen on radiographs.

The development of osteomyelitis (Fig. 18.5) is always serious because it can rarely be eradicated with-

out surgical excision. Fragments of dead bone are sometimes extruded through open wounds.

In conclusion, neuropathic ulceration and subsequent sepsis develop in a warm insensitive foot with bounding pulses. There is no pain unless deep sepsis and abscess formation occur.

Neuroarthropathy. The Charcot joint (Figs 18.6 and 18.7) is a rare complication which develops in a few patients with neuropathy. Severe bone and joint destruction occurs most frequently in the metatarsal–tarsal region and less commonly at the metatarsophalangeal, ankle or subtalar joints.

The initial presentation is with a hot swollen erythematous yet intact foot, which aches in one-third of cases; it is frequently misdiagnosed as cellulitis or gout. The precipitating cause is commonly minor trauma such as tripping or a mild sprain which may even be ignored at the time. At this early stage, plain X-rays are normal, although isotope bone scans are grossly abnormal showing considerably increased isotope uptake. Distinction from osteomyelitis at this stage can be difficult, but bone biopsy should not be performed and serves only to make matters worse. Magnetic resonance imaging (MRI) of the foot helps in differentiating the conditions. A gallium white cell scan can assist in the detection of infection.

During the following weeks, rapid bony destruction and joint dislocations occur, with grotesque appearance of new bone formation at sites of damage. The foot deforms and classically develops both a rocker bottom deformity because of downward displacement of the tarsus, and medial convexity resulting from displacement of the talonavicular joint or tarsometatarsal dislocation. The evolution of these changes occurs over 2–3 months after which the foot seems to stabilize. Friction within ill-fitting shoes may further aggravate these problems by causing new areas of ulceration. Charcot changes occur bilaterally in about one-third of these patients.

Treatment aims to alleviate early symptoms and attempts to prevent bone destruction leading to major deformity, although there is no certainty that this can be achieved. During the acute stage bed-rest is important and the use of drugs such as non-steroidals can reduce the intensity of the inflammatory response. Novel treatments using biphosphonates aimed at reducing osteoclastic activity are still under investigation. Non-weight-bearing is advisable for some weeks, either by the use of crutches or later a walking plaster cast. When deformities develop it is essential to provide individually made shoes to prevent further friction and ulceration.

Neuropathic oedema can occur in the neuropathic foot and causes problems from friction inside shoes that cannot accommodate the swollen foot; it results from the major haemodynamic changes already described, and is occasionally severe and intractable.

Treatment of neuropathic oedema can be by conventional diuretic treatment, but the use of the sympathomimetic agent ephedrine is specific and effective. Initially, ephedrine 30 mg t.d.s. is used and can be increased to 60 mg t.d.s. Side-effects and tachyphylaxis do not seem to arise.

Ischaemic lesions

The most common manifestation is ulceration presenting as an area of superficial necrosis, surrounded by a rim of erythema which is often painful. The lesions occur chiefly on the great toe or the lateral borders of the feet overlying the first and fifth metatarsal heads. The ulcers are shallow, not associated with callus and quite distinct from those occurring in the neuropathic foot; foot pulses are, of course, absent (Table 18.3).

The development of rest pain in the pink ischaemic foot is always ominous, representing critical ischaemia. Digital gangrene may follow, and spread, and is a much more serious event than in the neuropathic foot with its good circulation. These changes in the ischaemic foot are likely to lead to a major amputation unless urgent revascularization can be achieved.

The introduction of sepsis into the ischaemic foot adds to the severity of the situation and demands urgent attention.

Diabetic patients with peripheral vascular disease describe claudication relatively infrequently; it requires the same attention as in others. It may persist unchanged, regress or progress over months or years. Claudication alone only requires investigation if it causes the patient inconvenience, in which case arteriography with a view to either angioplasty or arterial surgery are required.

Examination and investigation

Inspection

The foot is inspected for deformities, notably clawing of the toes, pes cavus, hallux rigidus, bunions or the more severe abnormalities of Charcot foot changes. The skin should be examined for evidence of dryness, cracking, ulceration and athlete's foot. Examination of footwear is important.

Assessment of neuropathy

Clinical assessment should be undertaken, including knee and ankle reflexes and simple sensory tests, although these may fail to detect pain and temperature sensory deficits. A monofilament sensory test is simple and reliable, and inability to detect 10 g or more indicates risk of foot ulceration (page 179). The use of a biothesiometer is of value to measure vibration perception threshold; a reading of more that 25 V indicates feet at risk of ulceration. The graduated tuning fork is also useful, quick to use and cheap.

Microbiological cultures

Swabs should always be taken from the base of an ulcer, or after débridement of deeper lesions. Blood cultures are taken when cellulitis, fever and systemic illness are present.

Circulation

Palpation of foot pulses is important; if one or both are present, the prognosis is usually good and vascular investigations are not normally necessary. If they are both absent, proximal pulses should also be assessed, and proper vascular investigations performed as follows.

Doppler assessment and measurement of the pressure index

The pressure index is the ratio of the ankle systolic : brachial systolic pressure. Simple Doppler equipment is an essential tool needed in the foot clinic. The pressure index is normally 1.0–1.2; a ratio <0.9 indicates ischaemia and, when it is <0.6, severe ischaemia is present and the prognosis poor. False elevation of this index is unfortunately common because of rigidity and calcification of vessels so that readings may be misleading. Analysis of the wave forms can be helpful.

Angiography

Angiography is needed urgently in all cases of critical ischaemia which includes patients with foot discoloration, and/or pain (the pink painful ischaemic foot) with or without gangrene. It should also be performed if ischaemic foot ulcers do not resolve in 1 month.

Renal protection during arteriography

The intravenous dye used during arteriography can precipitate acute oliguric renal failure in patients with early renal impairment (serum creatinine >130 μmol/L). The following preventive measures should be taken:
- avoid dehydration
- give intravenous fluids starting four hours before the procedure
- intravenous insulin sliding scale should be used
- monitor urine output
- check creatinine before and on the day after the procedure.

Note: metformin should be stopped 48 hours before an angiographic procedure and resumed 48 hours after the procedure has been completed.

Foot pressures

Simple foot pressure pads yield some information regarding sites of excessive pressure. More sophisticated pedobarography may in future identify these areas and also assist in determining appropriate footwear needed to alleviate these high-pressure areas.

Management

General measures for ulcerated and/or infected neuropathic and ischaemic feet

These comprise the following measures.
- *Rest with the foot elevated.*
- *Podiatry.* This is needed to remove callus and permit efficient drainage in the neuropathic foot, and for wound débridement for both neuropathic and ischaemic lesions. Simple ulcers are treated with saline irrigation and non-adhesive dry dressings.
- *Eradication of infection.* Antibiotics are required for treatment of all infected foot lesions and need to be appropriately prescribed according to the severity of the sepsis (Box 18.1).

Treatment is urgent especially if cellulitis develops,

Box 18.1 **Use of antibiotics in the infected foot**

General principles

1 The infecting organisms include Gram-positive (most commonly), Gram-negative and anaerobic organisms, sometimes all together.

2 Take ulcer swabs, and where relevant (especially at débridement) take samples from deeper slough for culture and antibiotic sensitivities.

3 Never delay starting antibiotics.

4 The ischaemic foot is the most vulnerable and added urgency and perseverance are important.

5 If the sepsis is deep and/or extensive, or if the viability of the foot is in any way threatened (bearing in mind that the ischaemic foot represents a particularly high risk), hospital admission for administration of intravenous antibiotics is essential. Multiple antibiotics are used in the first instance until sensitivities are known.

6 Regular monitoring for persistent infection is important. Once the lesions are healing, superficial and sterile, and there is no evidence of cellulitis or local infection, then antibiotics can be stopped, although in the presence of significant ischaemia it may be wise to continue them until healing is complete.

Specific use of antibiotics

Oral antibiotics

1 Superficial ulcers. Amoxicillin and flucloxacillin (or erythromycin or cephadroxyl if penicillin-sensitive).

2 Mild cellulitis ± deep ulcers. Add trimethoprim and metronidazole.

Regularly review activity of infection and modify treatment in the light of antibiotic sensitivities.

Intravenous antibiotics

In the presence of extensive infection or if the viability of the foot is threatened (see 5 above) then intravenous antibiotics are recommended, starting with quadruple therapy and refining this in the light of antibiotic sensitivities. Suitable antibiotics are listed in Table 18.4.

Osteomyelitis

Treat in the same way as described above. Antibiotics with good bone penetration include sodium fusidate, rifampicin, clindamycin and ciprofloxacin. Antibiotics are needed for at least 12 weeks. Fragmented bone requires surgical excision.

Methicillin-resistant Staphylococcus aureus *(MRSA)*

When MRSA is grown in the presence of a locally infected lesion, then appropriate oral antibiotics (Table 18.4) should be given together with topical mupirocin 2% ointment. Even in the absence of clinical signs of infection in an ischaemic foot, MRSA should be treated. When MRSA infection is more extensive, appropriate intravenous antibiotics are required.

Table 18.4 Antibiotics for diabetic foot sepsis.

Symptoms	Antibiotic treatment
Superficial infection No cellulitis Little risk to foot	Amoxycillin and flucloxacillin (or erythromycin in case of penicillin allergy)
Superficial infection Cellulitis Minor risk to foot	Oral amoxycillin, flucloxacillin, ciprofloxacin or metronidazole
Deep infection Major risk to foot	Intravenous amoxycillin, flucloxacillin, ceftazidime, metronidazole
Osteomyelitis	Intravenous as above, then rationalize to according to antibiotic sensitivities (Table 18.5)
Methicillin-resistant *Staphylococcus aureus* (MRSA)	For appropriate antibiotics see Table 18.5

because progression to deep-seated infection and abscess formation can occur with astonishing speed. All patients with recent onset of acute sepsis should be admitted to hospital immediately for administration of intravenous antibiotics. A scheme of antibiotic treatment is shown in Tables 18.4 and 18.5. A combination of at least three antibiotics including metronidazole is required for the first 48 h or perhaps longer if the viability of an ischaemic limb is threatened. Antibiotics are rationalized once sensitivities are known, and changed to oral administration as the infection subsides. Note that it is not sensible to change antibiotic therapy that is associated with clinically obvious improvement in the event that cultures suggest that the organisms may be resistant to the drugs in use. The culture results should be used to select the drugs in a combination that is working best or to indicate rational choices of new agents in the event of no clinical improvement. Treatment with one or two antibiotics is generally continued until the lesion is obviously healing and bacterial cultures from swabs are negative. In those whose foot is at very high risk, notably those with severe ischaemia, antibiotics may be continued until wound healing is complete.

The emergence of MRSA is a very serious problem, first because it can be responsible for the ravages of sepsis and, secondly, because these patients become 'lepers', needing isolation while in hospital and denied access to nursing homes.

Reduction of weight-bearing forces

In the acute stages, bed-rest with the limb elevated is important and both heels must be protected from blistering by elevation on a simple foam wedge under the ankle (Figs 18.8 and 18.9); otherwise non-weight-bearing is achieved by the use of crutches or total-contact walking plaster. In the longer term, specially fitted shoes are needed to ensure redistribution of weight-bearing forces and alleviation of pressure at vulnerable sites.

Various casts that alleviate pressure on the healing ulcer during walking are now available. The Aircast is a prefabricated walking cast lined with inflatable air cells: it can be easily removed for regular foot inspection. The total-contact plaster cast is an efficient method of redistributing plantar pressure, but complications at pressure points can arise and it should only be applied by those with the appropriate experience. The Scotchcast boot is a simple removable boot made from bandages and felt, and held together with fibreglass tape.

Surgical intervention

Surgery is needed to drain pus and to excise necrotic tissue, and when possible in cases of ischaemia to improve the circulation by angioplasty or arterial surgery.

In the neuropathic foot with an intact circulation, swelling, inflammation and pain suggest the development of an abscess needing urgent surgical drainage.

Table 18.5 Useful antibiotics.

Micro-organism	Antibiotic treatment	
	Oral	IV
Streptococcus (inc. Group B, C & G)	Amoxycillin 500 mg t.d.s. Erythromycin 500 mg q.d.s Clindamycin 300 mg t.d.s.	Amoxycillin 500 mg t.d.s.
Staphylococcus aureus	Flucloxacillin 500 mg q.d.s. Sodium fusidate 500 mg t.d.s. Clindamycin 300 mg t.d.s. Rifampicin 300 mg t.d.s.	Flucloxacillin 500 mg q.d.s. Gentamycin 5 mg/kg/day (according to levels)
Anaerobes	Metronidazole 400 mg t.d.s. Clindamycin 300 mg t.d.s.	Metronidazole 500 mg t.d.s. Clindamycin 300 mg t.d.s.
Gram negatives	Ciprofloxacin 500 mg b.d. Cefadroxil 1 g b.d. Trimethoprim 200 mg b.d.	Ceftazidime 1–2 g t.d.s. Ceftriaxone 1–2 g daily Gentamycin 5 mg/kg/day (according to levels) Piperacillin-Tazobactam 4.5 g t.d.s. Meropenem 500 mg t.d.s.
MRSA	Sodium fusidate 500 mg t.d.s. Trimethoprim 200 mg b.d. Rifampicin 300 mg t.d.s. Doxycycline 100 mg daily	Vancomycin 1 g b.d. (according to levels) Teicoplainin 400 mg daily

Intramuscular antibiotics: Ceftriaxone 1 g daily im to treat gram positives and gram negatives . Teicoplainin 400 mg daily im to treat gram positives including MRSA. Imipenem w. cilastatin 500 mg b.d. im to treat gram positives, gram negatives and anaerobes. From Edmonds M. & Foster A. (2000) *Managing the Diabetic Foot*. Blackwell Science, Oxford.

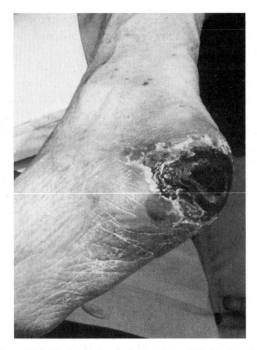

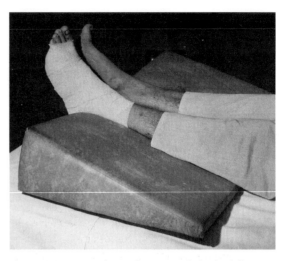

Figure 18.9 Foam wedge used to protect the heels of all diabetics requiring bed-rest.

Figure 18.8 Heel ulcer in an ischaemic foot which developed following a laparotomy because of inadequate heel protection. Below-knee amputation followed.

Digital gangrene obviously requires local amputation although the presence of extensive sepsis in the foot in such cases often demands the more extensive resection of a ray amputation in which the digit and distal metatarsal are removed; this operation is usually highly successful and rapid healing is expected. The presence of osteomyelitis is usually an indication for surgery because infection tends to relapse repeatedly in these patients. Radical amputations are rarely needed in neuropathic limbs with a good circulation, and when they are required it is usually because the patient has come for advice too late.

Surgery for the ischaemic foot is described below.

Additional measures needed in the management of the ischaemic foot

The problems in the ischaemic foot are those of ulceration, gangrene, sepsis and pain. If extensive gangrene is present, major amputation (usually below-knee) should be performed as soon as possible. When digital gangrene occurs, decisions re-

garding treatment are never easy because digital or ray amputations rarely, if ever, succeed and should not normally be attempted unless arterial reconstruction or angioplasty can succeed in restoring peripheral blood flow first. Limited operations in the ischaemic foot (other than wound débridement or drainage of pus) have earned the diabetic foot its bad reputation and may lead to many months of fruitless hospital treatment.

The following plan of investigation and treatment is adopted.

Medical management

Rest, antibiotics, chiropody and elimination of oedema are always needed and have been described in detail above. Drainage of pus or wound débridement may also be required. More than 70% of ischaemic ulcers are expected to heal using conservative measures.

Where limited dry digital gangrene is present, when sepsis has been eradicated and arterial reconstruction is not feasible, it is best not to amputate the digit but to continue conservative treatment with regular attendance for review and continuing chiropody until the necrotic digit auto-amputates. Attempts at surgical amputation usually fail because they do not heal and ultimately result in below-knee amputation. This conservative approach saves many patients from suffering major amputations (Fig. 18.10).

Surgical management

Arterial reconstruction, angioplasty and amputation are the surgical options available for treating the ischaemic foot. The chief urgent indication for attempting arterial reconstruction or angioplasty is the critically ischaemic foot, especially in association with intractable rest-pain and/or pink or mauve discoloration. It is also required in patients with ischaemic ulceration that has not responded to medical treatment. When limited gangrene develops, the need for major amputation may be averted by surgical improvement of the blood supply.

Diabetes is not itself a contraindication to vascular surgery or angioplasty; it is the nature and site of the lesions that determine the procedure to be adopted. Aortoiliac, aortofemoral or femoropopliteal bypass operations are performed as appropriate; distal arterial lesions can be tackled by vascular surgeons performing femorotibial bypass operations, and may be successful.

Balloon angioplasty in which intraluminal balloons are used to dilate stenoses in obstructed arteries (Fig. 18.11) is a major advance and can also be used in patients too frail for major vascular surgery. Lesions that can be treated by angioplasty should be < 10 cm in length. Iliac artery angioplasties are the most successful and those below the trifurcation of the popliteal artery least so. Intractable ischaemic ulcers may heal more quickly after successful angioplasty. As with vascular surgery, the most distal arterial occlusions remain difficult to treat.

Amputation

Surgical sympathectomy is rarely performed now as its usefulness in alleviating ischaemic pain is very limited; it can be tried when other measures have failed but it does not significantly improve blood flow.

The need for below-knee amputations should not necessarily be considered as a failure of treatment; appropriately timed surgery and rehabilitation are often more successful in restoring mobility and good quality of life than prolonged and fruitless attempts at conservative treatment.

Indications for below-knee amputation include extensive gangrene, or more limited gangrene in the presence of gross sepsis. Intractable pain that cannot be relieved by other measures is occasionally an indication for amputation even if the lesions themselves are relatively minor. Limited operations including digital or ray amputations rarely, if ever, succeed in the ischaemic foot unless the blood supply can be improved surgically; the choice then lies between the more radical below-knee amputation or conservative treatment leading to auto-amputation (page 176). Major amputations can be performed readily and rapidly even in very sick elderly patients. There is often a spectacular improvement in the general condition and well-being of patients, especially when sepsis has been present, and these operations should not be delayed. Fortunately, above-knee amputations are rarely needed.

Prevention

Prevention of foot ulcers and sepsis, and in particular

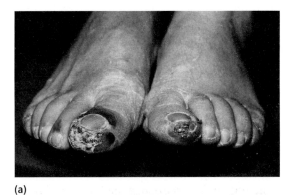

(a)

(b)

Figure 18.10 Terminal necrosis of: (a) the great toes; and (b) recovery with conservative treatment.

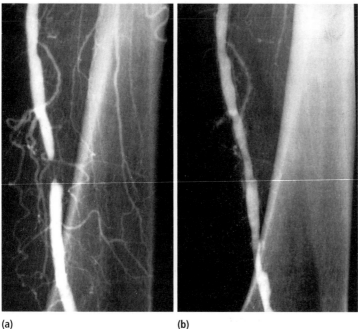

Figure 18.11 Atheromatous narrowing of the superficial femoral artery: (a) before; and (b) after balloon angioplasty.

(a)   (b)

preventing their recurrence, is an exceptionally important aspect of diabetes care; of all the complications of diabetes, foot problems can be the most successfully averted.

1 *Education.* Every diabetic patient needs to be made aware of the potential hazards to the feet and the methods by which they can be avoided. This is done first at diagnosis, but the advice needs to be reinforced at intervals and is most easily done at podiatry attendances. All patients should receive clear printed instructions regarding foot care, an example of which is shown in Fig. 18.12.

2 *Podiatry.* Neuropathic ulcers often begin deep to callus (page 168). Regular attention by a podiatrist is the single most important measure needed to prevent foot ulceration. Furthermore, the spread of sepsis can also be prevented by immediate (same day) treatment which should now be available to all diabetic patients who need it; patients should be seen and treated at the earliest sign of a lesion. Relief of pressure points either by specially fitted shoes or insoles can also be provided by podiatrists. A proper podiatry service is an essential part of diabetic care which should not be neglected.

3 *Foot inspection.* This is routinely undertaken at diagnosis and regular intervals when the diabetes and its complications are brought under annual review. Structural deformities are sought, and examination for the presence of vascular disease and neuropathy is important.

4 *Shoes and insoles.* Correctly fitting shoes are vital in ulcer prevention. They must accommodate any deformities and reduce pressure at major pressure points to eliminate recurring callus formation. Sometimes shoes must be specially made for an individual patient, which is expensive, but there is an increasing range of standard shoes providing sufficient depth to accommodate appropriate insoles. The provision of insoles alone will sometimes suffice. While podiatrists can provide a part of the shoe-fitting service, and often make the insoles themselves, attendance at the foot clinic by an orthotist or shoe-fitter is also extremely important, so that patients can be measured and fitted with proper shoes on the spot.

Examination of the foot: screening

The foot must be examined routinely at the onset of diabetes and at every annual review thereafter.

CARE OF YOUR FEET

To help prevent complications:–

DO

Wash daily with soap and water.
Dry well, especially between toes.
Change socks/stockings daily.
See that your shoes are not too tight.
See a Chiropodist.

DON'T

Walk barefoot.
Sit too close to a fire or radiator.
Put your feet on hot water bottles.
Neglect even slight injuries—see your Doctor.
Attempt your own chiropody—see your Chiropodist.

Figure 18.12 Simple printed instructions regarding foot care.

Essential

1 Each patient should be aware of the need for foot care.

2 Active lesions should be sought (e.g. hidden lesions between the toes) and treated immediately.

3 Deformities, callus, skin cracks and discoloration need to be detected and managed.

4 Critical ischaemia should be identified and treated urgently.

5 A simple sensory test should be performed, e.g. a monofilament sensory test under the great toe (inability to detect 10 g or more indicates risk of foot ulceration) The 10 g monofilament should be pressed against several sites including the plantar aspects of the first toe, first, third and fifth metatarsal heads, the plantar surface of the heel, and the dorsum of the foot. If the patient cannot feel the filament at any of the tested areas, significant neuropathy is present. The presence of callus impairs sensation, and it is not useful to apply a monofilament over such an area.

6 Examination of pulses (dorsalis pedis and posterior tibial).

Desirable

1 Assess ankle reflex.

2 Assess other sensory modalities; e.g. pinprick, vibration perception, temperature and joint position sense (the latter only abnormal in very advanced neuropathy) .

Advice and education must follow the examination.

Care and preventive measures

1 Active lesions should be treated immediately.

2 Written advice and education of foot care should be provided.

3 Advice is needed on appropriate shoes to accommodate foot deformities.

Regular podiatry to remove excess callus and provide nail care is *absolutely essential.*

Guidelines for foot care

Low current risk foot

Normal sensation, palpable pulses.

1 Foot care education.

2 Annual review.

At-risk foot

Neuropathy (inability to detect 10 g monofilament), absent pulses or other risk factors.

1 Enhance foot care education.

2 Podiatrist to inspect feet every 3–6 months.

3 Advice on appropriate footwear.

4 Review need for vascular assessment.

5 If previous ulcer, deformity or skin changes, manage as high risk.

High-risk foot

Risk factors as above, deformity or skin changes or previous ulcer.

1 Arrange frequent review (1–3 monthly) from podiatrist.

2 At each review, evaluate:
   • intensified foot care education;
   • specialist footwear and insoles; and
   • skin and nail care according to need.

3 Review education/footwear/vascular status as for the at-risk foot.

4 Ensure special arrangements for people with disabilities or immobility.

Ulcerated foot

1 Arrange urgent foot ulcer care from the specialist foot care team.

2 Expect the team to ensure as a minimum:
- local wound management, appropriate dressings and débridement as indicated;
- antibiotic treatment as appropriate;
- investigate and manage vascular insufficiency;
- specialist footwear to distribute foot pressures appropriately; and
- good blood glucose control.

Conclusions

It is now possible both to prevent diabetic foot problems and to treat them successfully. More than 90% of neuropathic ulcers and 70% of ischaemic ulcers are expected to heal. The organization of diabetic foot care is extremely important and one of the most optimistic aspects of diabetes management.

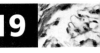

Cardiovascular Disease

Summary

- Morbidity and mortality from cardiovascular disease are substantially increased in both Type 1 and Type 2 diabetes, especially the latter

- Cardiovascular disease is frequently already present at diagnosis of Type 2 diabetes

- Risk factors for cardiovascular disease include smoking, obesity, insulin resistant states, hypertension, hyperglycaemia, hyperlipidaemia

- Patients with either microalbuminuria or established proteinuria have a particularly high risk of cardiovascular disease, and their mortality is increased many fold

- Mortality and morbidity following myocardial infarction are substantially increased in diabetic subjects

- Treatment of myocardial infarction should include the appropriate use of thrombolysis (retinopathy is not a contraindication), aspirin and insulin

- Cerebrovascular disease is also increased in those with diabetes and particular attention needs to be given to control of diabetes (often with insulin) in those suffering acute strokes

Morbidity and mortality from cardiovascular disease are substantially increased in both Type 1 diabetes and Type 2 diabetes, but especially the latter. Indeed, the most serious consequences of Type 2 diabetes arise from cardiovascular problems, so much so that reducing risks of developing coronary artery disease and strokes is now a major aspect of management with a view to preserving health and to some extent prolonging survival.

Diabetes more than doubles the risk of cardiovascular disease (Table 19.1). In the UK, 35% of total population deaths are attributable to cardiovascular causes; this rises to about 60% in those with Type 2 diabetes, and 67% in Type 1 diabetic patients over 40 years of age. The relative risk is greater for women than for men, with total loss of the usual male preponderance in younger age groups—the sex ratio is equal in those with diabetes. The development of myocardial infarction (MI) over a period of 7 years in middle-aged diabetic patients without known pre-existing coronary heart disease (CHD) is the same as that in non-diabetic individuals with existing CHD. Heart failure also occurs more frequently after MI in diabetes, resulting in a poorer outlook for these patients. Even in the absence of MI, the risk of heart failure is substantially increased in diabetes—approximately twofold in men and fivefold in women. Left ventricular mass is increased in about one-third of Type 2 diabetic patients and probably predisposes to left ventricular fibrosis. As a further

Table 19.1 Cardiovascular disease occurring in excess in diabetes.

Coronary artery disease
Frequency increased by two- to threefold (men)
Frequency increased by four- to fivefold (women)

Myocardial infarction mortality
Increased by twofold

Silent ischaemia
Worse prognosis

Stroke
Frequency increased by two- to threefold (men and women)
Mortality and morbidity worse

Heart failure
Increased by two- to fivefold

complication, cardiac denervation is a well-established feature of diabetic autonomic neuropathy, although its functional consequences are uncertain, and whether or not some sudden deaths are related to denervation remains controversial.

Epidemiology of cardiovascular disease in diabetes

Diabetes is an independent risk factor for mortality and morbidity from cardiovascular disease, and the excess is not simply a result of increases in other known risk factors. Estimates of the additional risk are in the range of two- to fivefold and are shown in Table 19.1. Most of the available information includes both Type 1 and Type 2 patients together, with more limited data on Type 1 diabetes alone. It should be noted that the risk of MI is almost as high in people with impaired glucose tolerance as with frank Type 2 diabetes, leading to questions about the role of insulin resistance and postprandial blood glucose peaks in the aetiology of the cardiac disease.

Coronary artery disease is four- to fivefold more common in premenopausal women with diabetes than in non-diabetic women. Young Asian and Polynesian groups have an especially high prevalence of coronary artery disease, and there is an excess of cerebrovascular disease in Africans and Caribbeans. However, the excess cardiovascular risk is not univer-

sal, as in Japan only 7% of deaths in diabetics are brought about by coronary artery disease. This protection is lost by Japanese migrants to Hawaii, suggesting that environmental rather than genetic factors are responsible. Differing cholesterol levels provide one possible explanation. In all groups, patients of low socioeconomic status have both a higher prevalence of and a higher mortality from cardiovascular disease.

Risk factors for cardiovascular disease

1 Smoking.
2 Obesity (especially android obesity with a high waist : hip ratio).
3 Insulin-resistant states.
4 Asian origin.
5 Hypertension.
6 Proteinuria (microalbuminuria and macroalbuminuria of nephropathy).
7 Hyperglycaemia.
8 Hyperlipidaemia.

Hyperglycaemia

Hyperglycaemia represents an independent risk factor for developing coronary artery disease. The UK Prospective Diabetes Survey (UK PDS) study has shown that the hazard ratio increases significantly in relation to the increasing HbA_{1c}, so that for every 1% increase in HbA_{1c} there is a 14% increase in fatal and non-fatal MI (Fig. 14.2). Subjects with impaired glucose tolerance have also been shown by the Bedford and Whitehall studies (West 1978) to have an increased risk of cardiovascular and cerebrovascular disease and this has recently been confirmed still to be true. Associated with this is the growing epidemiological evidence that postprandial spikes of hyperglycaemia may contribute to the development of coronary artery disease, although whether that is secondary to diurnal fluctuations of triglyceride in relation to glycaemic swings is unclear. The relative risks of CHD in impaired fasting glucose states remains to be determined but early evidence suggests that this too is a risk indicator.

The increasing risks of cardiovascular disease from both hyperglycaemia and hypertension are continuous and without threshold levels, and the two taken together have an additive effect.

Hyperglycaemia is a clear risk indicator for CHD but is also likely to be a contributory causative factor. A 16% reduction in rates of MI (non-fatal and fatal) was also demonstrated in the intensively treated arm of UK PDS, although—perhaps as the event rate in this newly diagnosed population was not very high—this did not achieve statistical significance. There may be additional benefits in this regard following the use of metformin.

Hypertension

Hypertension in all populations, including those with diabetes, is one of the strongest risk factors for cardiovascular disease, cerebrovascular disease and mortality, and increases the risk of heart failure. The consequences of hypertension on both microvascular and macrovascular disease together with the benefits of appropriate treatment are described in more detail in Chapters 14 and 20.

Diabetic nephropathy

Cardiovascular mortality in diabetes is very strongly linked to the presence of diabetic nephropathy, even from its early stages. Patients with established proteinuria have a cardiovascular mortality more than 40-fold that of the general population; it is increased in those with microalbuminuria but by less than twofold in those without any albuminuria or proteinuria (Fig. 19.1).

The underlying mechanisms that associate urinary protein loss with development of atheromatous arterial disease are the subject of much investigation. Both may be elements of the metabolic syndrome, and may be linked through abnormalities of endothelial function. The relationship applies both to those with and without diabetes. The excess mortality may be decreased with energetic treatment of any degree of nephropathy with antihypertensive agents, particularly angiotensin-converting enzyme (ACE) inhibitors. Recently, treatment of Type 2 diabetic patients without other risk factors for CHD and cholesterol levels < 5 mmol/L with the lipid-lowering agent simvastatin was demonstrated to reduce risk of

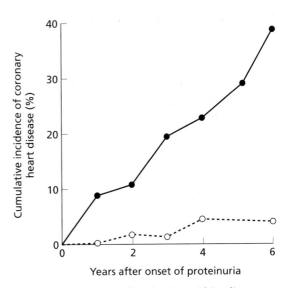

Figure 19.1 Relative mortality of patients with insulin-dependent diabetes mellitus with (●) and without (○) persistent proteinuria, compared with non-diabetic population. (From Jensen, T. *et al.* Coronary heart disease in Type 1 diabetes. *Diabetologia* 1987; **30**: 144–148.)

cardiovascular disease. None the less, the most common cause of death even in those on dialysis or following renal transplantation is still coronary artery disease.

Cardiovascular disease at diagnosis of diabetes

Evidence of cardiovascular and peripheral vascular disease is frequently discovered at the time of diagnosis of Type 2 diabetes, and in the UKPDS study ECG changes indicative of myocardial ischaemia were already present in 16% of men and 20% of women at baseline. It is always important to detect any such complications and reduce the many risk factors as far as possible. Conversely, previously undiagnosed diabetes is quite commonly found at the time of presentation of MI, stroke or peripheral vascular disease; the 'yield' is dependent upon the ethnic and age mix of the population, being highest in non-Europeans and in the elderly. Screening for diabetes should form part of the total risk factor assessment of all such patients.

Metabolic syndrome, 'Syndrome X'
or Reaven's syndrome

The frequent coexistence of obesity, diabetes or impaired glucose tolerance, hypertension and dyslipidaemia has been described variously as Syndrome X or Reaven's syndrome. Microalbuminuria is common. This constellation of factors is associated with insulin resistance and hyperinsulinaemia and there is evidence of endothelial dysfunction. As yet, we do not routinely treat the syndrome but the impetus for active management, at least with lifestyle interventions and possibly with insulin sensitizers, is growing. The diagnosis of the metabolic syndrome is discussed on page 8.

Pathology and pathogenesis

The pathology of atheromatous large vessel disease is probably no different in diabetic patients than in people without diabetes, although it tends to be more widespread and, in particular, more distal in distribution. This applies to coronary vessels, peripheral vessels in the legs and probably cerebral arteries as well. In the cerebral circulation small vessels >0.5 mm diameter may be affected most, leading to lacunar infarcts. There is relatively little evidence for an intrinsic 'small vessel disease' in the brain.

Increased rigidity of both major and minor arteries is a feature of long-standing diabetes. The underlying pathological process determining rigidity is not well understood although some vessels, including coronary arteries, may become calcified. Calcification of the intima and media of the distal arteries in the legs is commonly seen and related to the presence of neuropathy (page 157), although it also occurs in older age groups and those with nephropathy. Mortality appears to be increased in those with coronary artery calcification.

Observations suggest that a specific diabetic cardiomyopathy may exist as a distinct entity. Echocardiographic and various functional studies together with pathological observations, including the development of myocardial fibrosis, are probably responsible for the development of heart failure without any other defined cause. The precise cause of defects in the myocytes is not known.

Among the many candidates for the mechanisms that mediate arterial damage caused by diabetes are increased vascular permeability, increased lipoprotein Lp(a), increased platelet size and/or stickiness, fibrinogen, plasminogen activator inhibitor, reduced nitric oxide generation and other antioxidants and proinsulin.

Clinical presentations of coronary artery disease

Angina, MI and heart failure present in the same way as in the non-diabetic, although the frequency of 'silent' ischaemic heart disease is greater.

Angina

Diagnosis and treatment are conducted in the same way as in non-diabetic patients, while observing that ECG abnormalities occur without symptoms more frequently. The resting ECG does not exclude ischaemia and exercise ECG and thallium scans are needed to diagnose or rule out reversible ischaemia.

Aspirin, nitrates, calcium-channel blockers and beta-blockers are used in the normal way. Negative inotropes should be avoided if there is evidence of heart failure; ACE inhibitors should be used early (with a careful watch on renal function). Cardioselective beta-blockers should be used, although in well-controlled and educated insulin-treated patients there is a small but real risk of loss of hypoglycaemic warning symptoms and delayed recovery from hypoglycaemia, so care should be taken to advise patients to use home blood glucose monitoring to minimize risk of exposure to plasma glucose readings of <4 mmol/L.

Coronary artery arteriography is indicated if medical therapy fails or postinfarction, and may lead to treatment by either angioplasty or coronary artery bypass grafting (CABG). Decisions on the need for invasive coronary artery treatments are made as for people without diabetes. Angioplasty itself can be very effective although restenosis may occur more commonly in diabetic patients. Limited information on heart transplantation suggests that diabetic patients are not disadvantaged.

Myocardial infarction

Mortality and morbidity from MI in diabetic patients is substantially increased. Inpatient and 30-day mortality are approximately doubled from the expected 15–20% to 25–40% in those with diabetes, with a continuing adverse trend for the next 2 years. Infarct size is similar and the increased mortality is mainly caused by heart failure.

'Silent infarcts' without chest pain occur, and any presentation with heart failure, collapse, confusion, vomiting or unexplained uncontrolled diabetes should prompt a 12-lead ECG and cardiac enzyme estimation.

Treatment
Thrombolysis should be used in diabetic patients for precisely the same indications as for those without diabetes. The risk of vitreous haemorrhage in those with proliferative retinopathy is negligible and thrombolysis must not be withheld from diabetic patients because of concerns about their eyes. The benefits to diabetic patients with MI appears even greater than to those without diabetes, yet there is good evidence that some doctors wrongly withhold thrombolysis from diabetic patients.

Aspirin 300 mg is given at the onset of an MI and enteric coated aspirin 75–150 mg/day should be continued indefinitely thereafter.

Insulin treatment leading to optimal glycaemic control and started as soon as possible after the onset of an MI is associated with reduced mortality after discharge from hospital. The admission blood glucose is a predictor of outcome, levels > 20 mmol/L being associated with a high mortality, although whether this reflects the size of the infarct and the initial stress response rather than representing the consequence of glycaemic control is uncertain.

The DIGAMI (diabetes, insulin, glucose infusion in acute myocardial infarction) study examined 620 patients with established or newly diagnosed diabetes (plasma glucose exceeding 11.1 mmol/L). An insulin, glucose and potassium infusion was started at presentation, followed by a multiple insulin injection regimen for at least 3 months. Twelve-month mortality was reduced by 30%. Confirmation of these results is required, but at present this study presents the best evidence available for the management of diabetes after MI.

Thus, strict glycaemic control should be established using an insulin, glucose and potassium infusion at the time of the infarct for about 24 h and all diabetic patients, newly diagnosed and established, should be treated with insulin therafter. In many cases, insulin may wisely be continued indefinitely. Some discretion needs to be used among the elderly or others who cannot easily or comfortably use insulin, in whom other simple measures can achieve very good diabetic control, but, on the present evidence, insulin should be considered the first line of therapy.

After myocardial infarction
Half the patients after their first MI die during the following 12 months, and half of those die before they reach hospital. Continuing optimal management of all risk factors is strongly recommended, and these include:

- cessation of smoking;
- optimal blood pressure management;
- optimal diabetic control, normally with insulin; and
- optimal lipid control use of aspirin, ACE inhibitors and/or beta-blockers, unless contraindicated.

Postinfarction use of beta-blockers is often limited by actual or incipient heart failure. ACE inhibitors should be used wherever possible, with the usual precautions, as these patients are at high risk of heart failure and recent studies suggest particular benefit for diabetic patients.

CABG may offer an improved prognosis to those with diabetes after spontaneous Q-wave infarction compared to angioplasty, and further investigations of this apparent benefit are in progress.

Other cardiac disorders

Cardiac denervation and conduction disorders

Patients with autonomic neuropathy affecting vagal tone to the heart show increased resting and nocturnal heart rates. Q–Tc intervals are sometimes increased leading to a theoretical potential hazard of ventricular arrythmias and sudden death, although there is no evidence that this actually occurs. There are data showing that the Q–Tc interval increases during hypoglycaemia and this has been suggested to indicate that arrythmias may occur in hypoglycaemia. This remains at present only a hypothesis but diabetic patients should have an electrolyte check before invasive procedures and anaesthetics, and continuous cardiac monitoring during them.

Prevalence of conduction disorders among younger healthy diabetic patients is not increased, while the probable increase in first-degree and right bundle branch block presumably reflects the existence of ischaemic heart disease. Diabetes is over-represented among recipients of pacemakers for complete heart block and sick sinus syndrome.

Heart failure

Heart failure is up to five times more common in diabetes, more so among women than men, sometimes without evidence of pre-existing coronary artery disease. Evidence of improved longevity and quality of life from use of ACE inhibitors is encouraging.

Cerebrovascular disease

Stroke occurs more often in both those with diagnosed and previously undiagnosed diabetes, and also in those with impaired glucose tolerance; overall the excess risk is two- to threefold and equal between the sexes. Mortality and residual morbidity is probably higher among diabetic patients, with an increased proportion of cerebral infarcts and fewer cerebral haemorrhages. Good glucose control is important during the management of strokes and a 'DIGAMI' style trial of insulin, glucose and potassium infusion during the acute stroke is in progress.

Hypoglycaemia can cause a reversible hemiplegia, which may recover immediately or persist for several hours after the glucose has been restored. The hyperosmolar state can cause a variety of transient central nervous system abnormalities.

Treatment and prevention of risk factors

An assessment of vascular risk, with appropriate advice and treatment, should form part of the ongoing management of all diabetic patients.

Hypertension

Detection and management of hypertension is now a crucial aspect of diabetes care, leading to substantial benefits in ameliorating both macrovascular and microvascular complications (described in detail in Chapters 14 and 20).

Smoking in diabetes

Smoking reduces life expectancy and its effects are potentially reversible. The extent of the attributable risk in coronary heart disease is shown in Table 19.2. Cerebrovascular disease and especially peripheral vascular disease are also increased in smokers. Smoking may also accelerate the progression of diabetic nephropathy and retinopathy.

Table 19.2 Relative and attributable risk in the Multiple Risk Factor International Trial (MRFIT) study. Risks are 10 year coronary heart disease mortality per 1000 subjects screened. (Data from Stamler, J. *et al. Diabetes Care* 1993; 16: 434–444.)

	Smokers (A)	Non-smokers (B)	Relative risk (B/A)	Attributable risk (B/A)
Diabetic subjects	69	45	1.6	24
Non-diabetic subjects	24	10	2.4	14

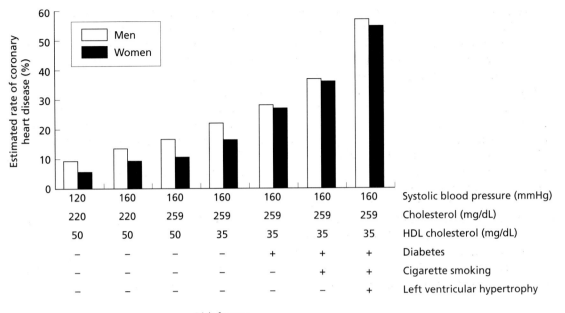

120	160	160	160	160	160	160	Systolic blood pressure (mmHg)
220	220	259	259	259	259	259	Cholesterol (mg/dL)
50	50	50	35	35	35	35	HDL cholesterol (mg/dL)
–	–	–	–	+	+	+	Diabetes
–	–	–	–	–	+	+	Cigarette smoking
–	–	–	–	–	–	+	Left ventricular hypertrophy

Risk factors

Figure 19.2 Estimated coronary heart disease rates according to various combinations of risk factors over 10 years. (From Kannel, W.B. Blood pressure as a cardiovascular risk factor. *Journal of the American Medical Association* 1996; **275**: 1571–1576.)

Lipids and cardiovascular disease in diabetes

Cardiovascular mortality rises with increasing total cholesterol or low-density lipoprotein (LDL) levels. The evidence is stronger for men than women (Fig. 19.2), but also suggests that low high-density lipid (HDL) concentrations and high triglycerides are risk factors.

Lipids in Type 1 and Type 2 diabetes

Some lipid abnormalities are shown in Box 19.1. Hypercholesterolaemia is no more (and no less) common in Type 1 diabetes than in the background population and well-controlled patients with Type 1 diabetes have minimal, if any, lipid abnormalities unless nephropathy is present, when a high-risk pattern (high total : LDL cholesterol ratio, low HDL, high triglyceride) is seen, increasing in severity with worsening renal function. In Type 2 diabetes, lipid abnormalities are common. Lipid profiles improve with

---

Box 19.1 Lipid abnormalities

Primary hyperlipidaemias
Polygenic hypercholesterolaemia
Familial hypercholesterolaemia
Familial combined hyperlipidaemia
Familial hypertriglyceridaemia

Secondary causes
Renal impairment, including nephropathy
Primary hypothyroidism
Alcohol excess
Thiazide diuretics
Beta-blockers

---

better control but do not generally return to normal, the high-risk pattern still remaining. Indeed, even when LDL cholesterol is normal or even slightly raised in Type 2 diabetes (the major abnormalities being low HDL cholesterol and high triglyceride), the LDL particles may be qualitatively different and more atherogenic. Glycosylation of lipids and/or oxidation by increased free radicals may alter their handling and render them more atherogenic than natural lipids.

Patients may have lipid disorders independent of their diabetes and a family history, including ages and causes of death, can be important.

Investigations

Except in special circumstances (e.g. eruptive xanthomas), measurement of lipids is most appropriately undertaken when diabetic control has become stable for some months. Cholesterol measurements are reliably made on blood samples from non-fasting patients; these are also suitable for triglyceride screening. Elevation of triglycerides needs to be confirmed in the fasting state prior to instituting treatment. Although there is increasing concern that postprandial triglyceride excursions may be important in the pathogenesis of cardiovascular disease, today's treatment guidelines are based on fasting levels.

Routine screening for lipid abnormalities is an essential aspect of the annual review. If the lipid profile is entirely normal, further screening could be postponed for 3–5 years unless circumstances change.

Lipid levels change only slowly after dietary or therapeutic changes, and at least 3 months should be allowed before such changes are reassessed.

Treatment of hyperlipidaemia

Lifestyle measures
Weight reduction. The importance of weight loss cannot be overemphasized. LDL cholesterol and triglycerides decrease and HDL levels rise proportionately; each kilogram of weight loss produces approximately 1% fall in the elevated levels. There are additional benefits from weight loss on diabetes control and blood pressure.

Dietary advice. The general principles of a healthy diet for diabetes apply. Specific recommendations beyond weight loss and reduced alcohol consumption include:
* replacement of fat with complex carbohydrate;

* substitution of saturated fat with monounsaturated and polyunsaturated fatty acids; and
* increase in dietary fibre content, especially leguminous, soluble and gel-forming types.

The effects of changes in diet may take several months to yield changes in lipid levels (and in glycaemic control). Many patients are unable to achieve full compliance with dietary targets, or indeed with the multiple lifestyle changes advised.

Drug therapy
Statins are the first line of drugs for treating hypercholesterolaemia; and fibrates for treating hypertriglyceridaemia. Statins and fibrates can be used alone or together for treating mixed hyperlipidaemia, although care must be taken to warn patients of the potential risk of muscle pain with statins, especially when mixed with fibrates. Fibrates are particularly effective in reducing triglycerides, with smaller improvements in LDL and HDL, while statins produce a 30–40% decrease in LDL with small improvements in triglycerides and HDL. Apart from cholestyramine, the other agents are little used.

Specialist advice should be sought on resistant or complex hyperlipidaemic states.

Targets for treatment (Box 19.2). The current targets for cholesterol and other lipid fractions are the same for primary prevention in diabetes as for secondary prevention in people without diabetes. They are as follows.
* Total cholesterol < 5.0 mmol/L.
* Fasting triglyceride < 2.0 mmol/L.
* LDL cholesterol < 3.0 mmol/L.
* HDL cholesterol > 1.1 mmol/L.

It is desirable that the (HDL cholesterol)/ (total cholesterol − HDL cholesterol) ratio should be

---

Box 19.2 Targets for plasma lipids and lipoprotein levels

Lipid/lipoprotein	Recommended level
Total cholesterol	< 5.0 mmol/L
Fasting triglyceride	< 2.0 mmol/L
LDL cholesterol	< 3.0 mmol/L
HDL cholesterol	> 1.1 mmol/L

> 0.25 mmol/L or total cholesterol/HDL cholesterol should be < 3.0.

Heart Protection Study

This huge double blind trial of 20 000 people at increased risk of vascular disease examined the benefits of treatment with simvastatin 40 mg/day, and reported its results in March 2002. The vascular event rate curves began to separate by the end of the first year, and the absolute benefits of treatment were seen to increase over time, becoming very obvious after 5–6 years. The major results were as follows.

- 17% reduction in vascular deaths.
- 24% reduction in major vascular events.
- 27% reduction in strokes.

Treatment benefits were not only obvious among patients who had previously had an MI but also in those with prior cerebrovascular or peripheral vascular disease. Benefits were also demonstrated for diabetic patients without prior CHD. Both sexes benefited equally, and elderly patients over 75 years of age were seen to benefit to the same extent as younger patients. Whether all Type 2 diabetic patients should automatically be given statin therapy (as opposed to only those with a calculated risk of 15% or more of a cardiac event within 10 years) is not yet clear but the threshold for starting therapy in this group of patients should be very low.

Strategies for prevention of cardiovascular mortality

All diabetic patients are at increased risk of cardiovascular mortality, and this risk increases substan-

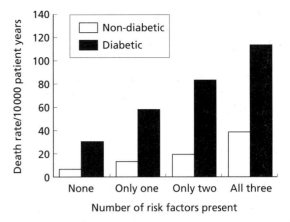

Figure 19.3 Age-adjusted cardiovascular death rates by number of risk factors for diabetic and non-diabetic men. (From Stamler, J. *et al. Diabetes Care* 1993; **16**: 434–444.)

tially in the presence of other factors (Fig. 19.3), notably nephropathy and hypertension. Reduction of morbidity and mortality by attention to the many risk factors represents a key facet of management of diabetic patients. It can be difficult to achieve in practice, and much emphasis needs to be given to lifestyle changes which may be more effectively conducted in groups than by individuals alone. Motivation needs to be assessed and understood when giving patients choices of treatment. Skilful clinical judgements are required throughout.

20

Hypertension

Summary

- Hypertension has adverse effects, accelerating macrovascular disease (cardiovascular and cerebrovascular disorders) and increasing both morbidity and mortality of patients

- Hypertension also accelerates decline of renal function in patients with diabetic nephropathy, and worsens some aspects of retinopathy notably the development of maculopathy

- Effective treatment of hypertension can ameliorate all of the above problems

- Targets for control of blood pressure are presented

- The key objective is to lower blood pressure by any means since most of the benefits relate to the blood pressure achieved rather than the agent used

- Angiotensin-converting enzyme inhibitors or angiotensin 2 receptor blockers have additional advantages and are the agents of first choice

- Other hypotensive agents need to be added as required

The numerous hazards of hypertension lead to disability and death. Coronary artery disease, strokes and heart failure represent some of the very damaging consequences of raised blood pressure. More recently, it has also been shown that in those with diabetes, renal damage is promoted and renal failure from diabetic nephropathy accelerated, while changes in retinopathy—particularly those predisposing to maculopathy—are also made worse. One of the major developments of the last quarter of the 20th century was the demonstration that by rigorous treatment of hypertension, all of the risks described are reduced. At the same time the introduction of effective medication with minimal side-effects transformed the potential benefits into clinical reality. Amongst diabetic patients in particular, microvascular hazards especially affecting the eye and kidney, as well as the dire consequences of macrovascular

disease, are substantially ameliorated by successful blood pressure management and it is obvious that health and longevity benefit greatly. Treatment of hypertension has become a major aspect of diabetes management.

Hypertension in diabetes (Table 20.1)

Hypertension in all populations, including those with diabetes, is one of the strongest risk factors for cardiovascular disease. This has been confirmed in the Framingham, Bedford, Whitehall and Multiple Risk Factor International Trial (MRFIT) studies. Type 2 diabetes and hypertension are commonly associated: the prevalence of hypertension among this population is approximately 40% at 45 years of age increasing to 60% in those aged 75 years. As well as

Table 20.1 Causes of hypertension in diabetes.

Type 1 diabetes
Diabetic nephropathy (including microalbuminuria)
Coincidental essential hypertension
Isolated systolic hypertension, usually associated with arterial
    disease
Diabetic nephropathy

Type 2 diabetes
Hypertension of obesity
Coincidental essential hypertension
Isolated systolic hypertension, usually in the elderly

Secondary diabetes with hypertension
Acromegaly
Cushing's syndrome
Phaeochromocytoma
Drug-induced (e.g. steroids, oral contraceptive)

Coincidental secondary hypertension with unrelated diabetes

increasing the risks of cardiovascular disease, hypertension also accelerates evolution of retinopathy and proteinuria.

The UK Prospective Diabetes Survey (UKPDS) of Type 2 diabetes (page 129) has shown that for every 10 mmHg increase in systolic blood pressure:
• any complication related to diabetes is increased by 12%;
• deaths related to diabetes are increased by 15%;
• myocardial infarction (MI) is increased by 11%; and
• microvascular complications are increased by 13%.

Benefits of tight blood pressure control

Microvascular disease

UKPDS shows the considerable benefits of tight blood pressure control (see Fig. 14.4, p.130). By achieving a mean blood pressure of 144/82 mmHg, representing a reduction of systolic blood pressure of 10 mmHg compared to the less intensively treated group. Microvascular endpoints (chiefly the need for photocoagulation) were reduced by 37%; and risk of vision declining by three lines on the Snellen chart was reduced by 47%, chiefly by protection from the development of macular disease.

The benefits of intensively managed blood pressure control in reducing the proteinuria of nephropathy and retarding the decline of renal function are described in detail in Chapter 15.

Macrovascular disease

Those with a high risk of cardiovascular disease stand to gain proportionately greater benefit by reduction of risk factors. The following recently published major trials demonstrate exactly what can be achieved.

UK Prospective Diabetes Study (see Fig. 14.4)
Tight vs. less tight blood pressure control (mean 144/82 vs. 154/87 mmHg).
    Benefits:
• heart failure reduced by 56%;
• strokes reduced by 44%; and
• combined MI, sudden death, stroke, peripheral vascular disease (PVD) reduced by 34% (MI alone was reduced non-significantly by 16%).

HOPE and MICROHOPE studies
These studies over 4.5 years comprised 9297 patients overall and included 3577 diabetic patients (98% with Type 2 diabetes). Patients with diabetes and one other risk factor for cardiovascular disease were randomly treated with the angiotensin-converting enzyme (ACE) inhibitor ramipril 10 mg/day. Systolic blood pressure decreased by approximately 2–3 mm and yielded a reduction of combined MI, strokes and deaths from cardiovascular diseases of 25%. The demonstrated benefits included:
• MI relative risk reduced by 22%;
• stroke relative risk reduced by 33%; and
• cardiovascular death relative risk reduced by 37%.

Questions have been raised regarding matching of the baseline characteristics of the two study groups, but the conclusions from this trial strongly support the view that ACE inhibitors are the first-line treatment for blood pressure control in diabetes.

A good critique of recent multicentre trials is to be found in Bilous, R. *Horizons in Medicine* (ed. S. Amiel), Vol. 13, pp. 195–206. Royal College of Physicians of London, 2002.

Management of hypertension

Hypertension normally causes no symptoms and most cases are detected either during routine screening, or when complications develop. All diabetic patients should have blood pressure carefully recorded at least annually. Those with borderline or abnormal levels, especially in the presence of vascular complications or early nephropathy, should be checked more frequently. Except in emergency, at least three separate blood pressure readings should be recorded; large cuffs must be used for obese patients, otherwise artificially high readings will be obtained.

Indications for treatment, according to the National Institute for Clinical Excellence guidelines

Blood pressure >160/100 mmHg should always be treated, aiming for a level of <140/80 mmHg (audit standard <140/90 mmHg).

Blood pressure ≥140/90 mmHg should be treated in diabetic patients at risk of cardiovascular events >15% in 10 years, with a target of <140/80 mmHg. Blood pressure >140/80 mmHg should also be treated if there is evidence of target organ damage (microalbuminuria or proteinuria), aiming for a level of 135/75 mmHg. It is our opinion that in the presence of nephropathy the lowest blood pressure that can be achieved without side-effects is ideal. (Note that microalbuminuria or proteinuria in the absence of hypertension may also require treatment; Chapter 15).

Blood pressure > 130/80 mmHg should be treated in those with microalbuminuria or macroalbuminuria (page 138), and the aim of therapy should be to achieve the lowest blood pressure the patient can easily tolerate.

Treatment of hypertension

When nephropathy is present a high priority is given to lowering blood pressure (discussed in more detail on page 139).

Unless hypertension is severe, initial treatment should be by lifestyle and non-pharmacological measures (see Box 20.1). These include weight reduc-

---

Box 20.1 Lifestyle and non-pharmacological therapy for hypertension

Weight reduction
Dietary sodium reduction, even to 80–120 mmol/day is beneficial
Reduced alcohol consumption where excessive
Increase in physical exercise

---

tion achieved by healthy eating and exercise (which also assist diabetic and lipid control) salt restriction and reduced alcohol consumption.

Drug therapy

Once lifestyle changes have proved inadequate, pharmacological treatment is needed. Where there is continuing doubt about blood pressure levels, 24-h monitoring may be of value, as is echocardiography. Left ventricular hypertrophy is both a good measure of sustained hypertension and an independent risk factor for cardiovascular death. Some antihypertensive agents have limitations when used in diabetic patients, either because of metabolic changes they induce (worsened glucose tolerance or lipid patterns) or because their side-effects may be particularly relevant to the diabetic patient (e.g. erectile dysfunction, worsening of claudication, diminished warning of hypoglycaemia).

Drug therapy needs to be tailored for the individual patient. The choice needs to take into account age, sex, ethnicity, diabetic complications as well as cardiac and renal function.

Choice of antihypertensive drugs (Table 20.2)

The key objective is to lower blood pressure by any means because most of the benefits relate to the blood pressure achieved rather than the agent used. However, there are additional advantages of using ACE inhibitors or angiotensin 2 (AT2) receptor antagonists. Several trials have indicated specific benefits of various ACE inhibitors; the losartan intervention for end-point reduction (LIFE) study demonstrated additional benefits resulting from the use of the AT2 receptor antagonist losartan when compared to

Table 20.2 Problems in the use of antihypertensive drugs in diabetes.

Group of drugs	Some side-effects or limitations
Angiotensin-converting enzyme inhibitors	
Ramipril, lisinopril, enalapril, etc.	Renal impairment Hyperkalaemia
Angiotensin 2 receptor blockers	
Losartan, irbesartan, etc.	
Calcium antagonists	
Amlodipine, verapamil	Negative inotropes to variable degree Headaches, flushing, oedema Short-acting dyhydropyridine calcium-channel antagonists may worsen microalbuminuria
Cardioselective beta-blockers	
Atenolol, etc.	Impairment of glucose tolerance Worsened lipid profile Poor recovery from hypoglycaemia Sexual dysfunction Worsen claudication symptoms
Thiazide diuretics	
Bendrofluazide (2.5 mg dose is free from most problems)	Impairment of glucose tolerance Worsened lipid profile Sexual dysfunction Hypokalaemia
Alpha-blockers	
Doxazosin, prazosin, etc.	Adjuncts to treatment
Vasodilators	
Hydralazine, minoxidil	

the beta-blocker atenolol, despite comparable blood pressure reduction. Many, and probably most patients will need more than one drug to achieve the intended goal. A pragmatic approach to treatment is often required.

ACE inhibitors or, if these provoke cough, AT2 antagonists are the first choice in those with microalbuminuria. There is evidence that adding an AT2 antagonist to an ACE inhibitor may have extra benefit on the blood pressure but no additional benefit for renal disease.

ACE inhibitors, AT2 antagonists, cardioselective beta-blockers or thiazide diuretics are reasonable first-line treatment in those without microalbuminuria. Both thiazide diuretics and, more recently, indapamide have been shown to reduce the risk of stroke in non-diabetic populations.

Long-acting dihydropyridine calcium-channel antagonists (e.g. amlopidine) are effective at lowering blood pressure and are second-line agents. There are unresolved issues about their ability as first-line agents to reduce ischaemic heart disease as effectively as other agents, although paradoxically they may reduce risk of stroke. The use of nifedipine has been associated with oedema and there are concerns about its effects on albuminuria, but other calcium-channel blockers can be useful as second-line agents where the ACE inhibitor fails to achieve adequate blood pressure reduction. Aspirin 75 mg/day should be recommended in addition to people with manifest evidence of cardiovascular disease and for those with a 10-year coronary heart disease risk > 30%, bearing in mind the contraindications for using aspirin.

Further useful guidelines are as follows.

•   Those with overt or incipient heart failure should have an ACE inhibitor wherever possible, which can be combined with a diuretic.

•   Conversion to an AT2 antagonist is helpful if the patient develops cough on the ACE inhibitor. It is likely to have similar benefit. Addition of an AT2 antagonist to an ACE inhibitor will have additive benefit on blood pressure but not on microalbuminuria.

•   Negatively inotropic agents should be avoided.

•   Blood pressure in African and Caribbean patients may respond better to diuretics and calcium antagonists than to beta-blockers and ACE inhibitors, although there is no evidence to show whether they benefit less from the other actions of the ACE inhbitors. It may therefore be reasonable to use such agents as first line in cases of very severe hypertension, with the intention of introducing ACE inhibitors later. There is no real evidence base for this.

•   Beta-blockers should be avoided in those with claudication.

•   The combination of beta-blockers and diuretics should be avoided, as it substantially worsens glucose tolerance and, frequently, lipid profiles.

•   The aim should be to reduce blood pressure gradually not abruptly, as the latter may worsen renal function, especially in those with nephropathy.

•   Where there is doubt about response, an echocardiogram is of value but progressive reduction in left ventricular mass goes on for months and even years.

When one agent alone (in full dosage) is insufficient, a second should be added; choice of the second agent should follow the guidelines.

Regular assessment is needed to ensure that the drugs are well tolerated, including a specific enquiry about potency in men. Renal function and potassium should be monitored in those taking ACE inhibitors and diuretics.

Diabetic Care

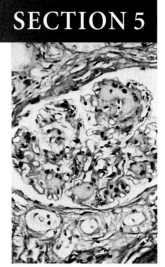

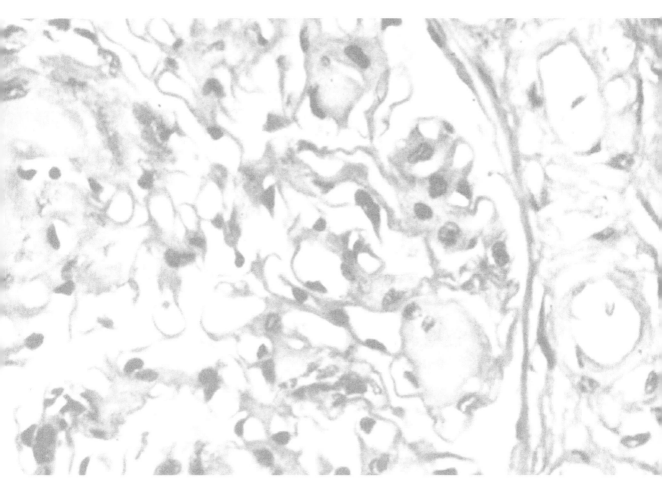

Living with Diabetes

Summary

- Understanding diabetes should of necessity include an understanding of the concerns of those who live with it

- Effective diabetes care should address individual psychological, social and cultural needs as well as the biomedical needs

- Depressive illness is three times more likely in people with diabetes

- Two-thirds of cases of depression in people with diabetes go undetected by healthcare professionals

- Professionals need to be able to give specific, realistic and relevant advice, e.g. travel, employment, to those living with diabetes

- Some medico-legal pitfalls are discussed

Psychosocial consequences of diabetes and legal issues

It is becoming increasingly accepted that for diabetes care to be effective it is necessary to focus on the psychosocial needs of the person with diabetes as well as the pathophysiology of the condition.

The transition in health status from a relatively healthy person to a person with a chronic illness can cause a wide range of emotional reactions. Feelings of anger, denial, sadness and distress may be evoked. These feelings may, or may not, result in a process of adjustment and acceptance of the condition. However, even those who appear to have adjusted well to diabetes will at times experience changes in their physical, emotional or social status that may disrupt their equilibrium and their ability to cope.

Principles for a holistic approach to management

A holistic management plan should encompass psychological, social and cultural factors as well as physical status. Discussion and exploration of the following can help identify psychosocial issues that need to be addressed before knowledge, understanding and self-management of the condition can be achieved, and appropriate lifestyle changes considered.

What are the person's beliefs about their diabetes and diabetes in general?
- What or who do they think caused their diabetes?
- What is their experience of the condition?
- Where are they in the adjustment process?
- What are the social circumstances of their lives?
- What are their fears and uncertainties surrounding their condition?
- What do they need/want to know to enable them manage their condition on a day-to-day basis?

The lived experience of diabetes

Understanding diabetes should, of necessity, include an understanding of the concerns of those who live with it. Qualitative research has provided health care professionals with valuable insight into issues that people living with diabetes face in their daily lives. These include uncertainty surrounding symptoms and prognosis, societal and personal stigma, the management of treatment regimens and professional–patient relationships. The ability and skills of professionals to acknowledge and understand these issues greatly influence clinical outcomes such as self-care skills, concordance with treatment regimens, appointment attendance and the level of patient satisfaction with service provision.

Depression and diabetes

It is generally accepted that people with a chronic physical illness such as diabetes have an increased risk of psychological disturbance and psychiatric illness. All diabetes care teams should have easy and immediate access to a clinical psychologist and/or a liaison psychiatrist who has specialist knowledge of diabetes and its management.

The most common psychiatric disorder in people with diabetes is depressive illness, with or without anxiety. The prevalence of depression in those with diabetes is at least three times more common than in the general adult population. The incidence is similar for both those with Type 1 and Type 2 diabetes, but as in the background population the risk of depression is higher among women.

The increased prevalence of depression is strongly associated with the psychosocial difficulties that arise from living with diabetes. However, it has also been suggested that physiological factors may be important.

Additionally, depression may be a risk factor for diabetes, especially Type 2, because of its effects on health behaviours influencing diet, activity levels, smoking and alcohol consumption. The evidence that poor glycaemic control is associated with depression is well established. Further studies are required to clarify this relationship, but it is clear that in many cases one exacerbates the other.

Those suffering with depression are more likely to:
• be less active;

• have an increased risk of obesity;
• find it more difficult to concord with agreed treatment regimens;
• indulge in high-risk health behaviours;
• be less effective in their social roles; and
• have an increased risk of micro- and macrovascular complications.

Identifying those at risk of depression

It is reported that in as many as two-thirds of cases the presence of depression in those with diabetes goes undetected by health care professionals.

Warning signs related to depression are the following.
• Previous history of depression, anxiety or substance abuse.
• Previous history of mental health treatment.
• Family history of depression.
• Reported sexual dysfunction.
• Chronic pain as a primary complaint.
• Symptoms that are out of proportion to the objective findings.
• Poor glycaemic control and/or poor self-care actions.
• Diabetes-related emotional distress.

Diagnosing depression

Clinical depression is diagnosed when five or more of the specific symptoms are present for a period of at least 2 weeks. The essential features of depression are first a persistent lowering of mood and second a loss of pleasure in usual activities for most of the time (anhedonia).

Other characteristic features of depression include the following.
• Fatigue or anergia (reduction of energy).
• Sleep disturbances.
• Diurnal variation of mood (a particular pattern of mood that is worst first thing in the morning and tends to improve as the day goes on).
• Reduced appetite with weight loss/increased appetite with weight gain.
• Impaired attention and concentration (slow thinking/speech/movement).
• Agitation or psychomotor retardation.

- Negative cognitions of self (guilt, low self-esteem).
- Feelings and expressions of hopelessness.
- Suicidal ideas or thoughts.

Management

Apart from an awareness of the signs and symptoms of depression, health care professionals need to create a clinical environment that encourages people to talk about and reflect upon their emotional state.

The initial treatment plan for mild forms of depression should incorporate supportive strategies that encourage a problem-solving approach to distress. This approach can enhance feelings of control and increase levels of self-esteem. Specific causes of depression and/or anxiety that are related to issues such as fear of complications, infertility or premature death should be identified and discussed sympathetically but realistically.

Moderate or severe depression requires treatment with antidepressants of which tricyclic agents such as amitriptyline are the first choice, but selective serotonin inhibitors and newer antidepressants are becoming increasingly popular because of their lower side effect profile.

The source of the depression and/or distress should also be identified, acknowledged and resolution sought through specific psychological interventions such as psychodynamic psychotherapy or cognitive–behavioural therapy. Individuals expressing suicidal ideas or thoughts need urgent psychiatric referral.

Problems arising from employment difficulties, domestic violence, housing, finances and child care may perpetuate depression and need help from social services or community mental health teams.

Conclusions

Living with diabetes requires a conscious effort to take over what is normally an unseen physiological process. To allow people with diabetes to achieve this, health care professionals need to be able to give specific, realistic and relevant advice regarding employment, travel, insurance, leisure activities and the management of concurrent illness.

Employment and leisure activities

Diabetic patients who are treated by diet alone or with oral hypoglycaemic agents and who are otherwise fit should normally be permitted to undertake any occupation or hobby. When correctly treated their risk of hypoglycaemia is negligible. For those treated with insulin, the guiding principle in making difficult assessments for employment or leisure activities is whether or not the individual concerned is prone to impaired warning of hypoglycaemia leading to diminished cognitive function and confusion during hypoglycaemia, and whether any risks from hypoglycaemia affect the individual only or in addition place the safety of others at risk. Individual organizations generally have their own guidelines regarding the suitability of diabetic patients for particular activities. If candidates are rejected unreasonably they may appeal. Insulin-treated patients are not normally accepted *de novo* by the armed forces, the police, the merchant navy or the fire brigade; they may not serve as pilots and cannot hold driving licences for passenger-carrying vehicles or large heavy goods vehicles. Shift work, especially night-shift work, should be avoided if possible by those on insulin, but sensible diabetic patients can make appropriate adjustments and may successfully cope with such work. Some leisure activities are obviously risky, including mountaineering and scuba diving (the latter is not usually allowed) where the hazards to others can be very great.

Driving

All diabetic patients who are otherwise physically fit and not suffering from blackouts, or other prescribed or relevant medical conditions, are normally allowed to hold ordinary Group 1 (category B) driving licences, i.e. vehicles up to 3500 kg with up to nine seats and with a trailer up to 750 kg. The law demands that diabetic patients treated by tablets or insulin (but not those on diet alone) should inform the Driver and Vehicle Licensing Agency (DVLA) in Swansea. If applying for a licence for the first time the appropriate declaration must be made on the application form. It is helpful to indicate whether or not insulin is being used. Driving licences are granted for 3 years and are reissued (at no extra fee) subject to a satisfactory medical report for those on insulin, and up to 70 years of age for those on diet or tablets subject to any change of their health or treatment.

Healthy people with diabetes who are treated with diet or tablets are normally allowed to drive vehicles larger than those defined above (i.e. Group 2), provided they pass a separate test to meet the higher Group 2 standards. Group 2 or vocational licences include those for Large Group Vehicles (LGV) and Passenger Carrying Vehicles (PCV). Those taking insulin are not permitted to hold Group 2 licences, unless these were granted before 1991 and subject to satisfactory medical reports, because of the serious potential consequences of hypoglycaemia, no matter how small the risk may be for any individual patient. However, exceptional cases based on individual assessment of the risk of experiencing diminished awareness of hypoglycaemia can be identified and enable some people to hold C1 licences, i.e. vehicles between 3500 and 7500 kg, although D1 vehicles (minibuses) do not fall into this category.

Visual acuity must be better than 6/12 in the best eye, and the visual field should exceed 120° horizontally and 20° above and below throughout 120°.

Accidents, sometimes fatal, still occur in people with diabetes who become hypoglycaemic while driving. Alcohol, apart from its own inherent risks, can exacerbate hypoglycaemia especially in those taking sulphonylureas or insulin. It is essential that guidelines should be followed in order to make driving safe and to maintain a good reputation for the diabetic driver. Thus, patients on insulin and insulin secretagogues should never drive if they are late for a meal, when the danger of hypoglycaemia is particularly great; the latter half of the morning may be a dangerous time for this. Patients should normally measure their blood glucose before driving; failure to do so will become increasingly difficult to defend. They should always keep a supply of sugar within immediate reach in their cars. If they do experience warning symptoms of hypoglycaemia they should stop, switch off the ignition and leave the car, because they are otherwise open to a charge of driving under the influence of drugs (insulin). They should treat the hypoglycaemia and then wait at least 15–20 min, or

until the symptoms have completely disappeared; indeed there is now evidence that impaired cognitive function following hypoglycaemia may last even longer. Patients who have experienced a severe hypoglycaemic attack with loss of consciousnesss during the day must inform the DVLA, as would any person experiencing a seizure. This will normally result in the withdrawing of the licence for a period of no less than 3 months, after which the position will be reassessed. Diabetic patients who are prone to disabling hypoglycaemic attacks without warning *must not drive* and their doctors or nurses should make this advice very clear. However, this warning should be followed by attempts to restore hypoglycaemia awareness (Chapter 9).

Insurance and pensions

Driving insurance with a normal premium should be issued subject to a satisfactory medical report; diabetes must be declared. Life assurance premiums are often raised by amounts that depend on the result of a medical examination. Sickness and holiday insurance premiums are also likely to be higher than normal. Diabetes UK offers helpful advice.

Travel

Diabetes control is easily upset by the rigours of travelling. Regular monitoring needs to be undertaken and appropriate adjustments made to the insulin dose. Dieting easily goes astray and changes of activity, which may be more or less than normal, can lead to hypoglycaemia or hyperglycaemia respectively. Foot care remains important; burning feet on hot sand or stones easily occurs, making foot protection with sandals or trainers extremely important. Ample equipment and insulin should be taken, preferably kept in two separate places. When flying insulin should be kept with the hand baggage and not in an aircraft hold where it may freeze. Insulin will keep for some months at room temperature in temperate climates, but should preferably be kept in a refrigerator in tropical climates, although even then decline in potency is very small; it should never be deep-frozen. If insulin supplies are lost, patients should remember that almost any type of insulin that can be purchased locally is suitable for temporary use for survival. Inoculations should be given as for non-diabetic people.

Some form of identification is essential, especially for those travelling alone. All diabetic patients should carry with them a statement that they have diabetes together with details of their treatment and their usual physician or clinic. Identification also helps if customs officials query the possession of syringes and needles. Medic-Alert Foundation International offers a valuable service and their ID products are widely known. Ideally, people with diabetes travelling to remote parts of the world should be accompanied, especially if they are insulin-treated and prone to hypoglycaemia.

Measures described in Chapter 11 should be adopted in the event of illness, especially if vomiting occurs, and insulin treatment maintained throughout. The usual antiemetics can be used, including those used for motion sickness; apart from causing some drowsiness they do not interfere with diabetes control.

Time changes on long distance air travel inevitably cause some disturbance of diabetic control for a few days.

Flying west. The time between injections can, with little problem, be lengthened by 2–3 h twice daily. Regular blood tests should be performed and if they are excessively high (around 15 mmol/L or more) extra soluble insulin (4–8 units) can be given. If the time gap between injections is lengthened still further, a small supplementary injection of soluble insulin (4–8 units) is given between the usual injections.

Flying east. The time between injections will need to be shortened by 2–3 h each time, which could result in rather low blood glucose readings. Careful testing should be performed and, if required, each dose can be reduced by a small amount (4–8 units on average). Regular meals should be taken as normal. Many airlines will make special provision for those with diabetes if notified in advance; it is nevertheless strongly advisable to carry a food pack in case of delays or other emergencies.

Dental treatment

Dental treatment should not be affected by diabetes, nor is there any good evidence that dental or gum disease is exacerbated by diabetes, although risks of periodontal disease may be increased in very poorly controlled diabetes associated with poor dental hygiene. Dental sepsis, if it occurs, can upset diabetic control just as is the case in the presence of any other infection. Treatment under local anaesthetic is carried out as normal, but when general anaesthesia is needed, a brief hospital admission is wise for insulin-treated diabetic patients, and measures are taken as described on page 97.

Legal aspects

Litigation, when standards fall below those expected in the delivery of care, occur especially in relation to failures in the management of retinopathy resulting in decline of vision, or foot care leading to amputation. Such deficiencies are sometimes related to systems failures where, for example, urgent referrals or consultations are not enacted. Individual incompetence and, above all, failure to see or examine the patient at the appropriate time are very serious indeed. The consequences of prolonged hyperglycaemia frequently lead to legal actions. Potential harm from delayed diagnosis of diabetes or years of inadequate control are other issues often considered by lawyers. Failure to diagnose acute Type 1 diabetes is not rare, and on occasions diagnosis is made so late that presentation is in advanced ketoacidosis, which may have fatal consequences. The implications of accidental injuries on diabetes and its complications represent another area where legal action is often sought.

Foot problems. Failure to recognize the seriousness of, for example, foot sepsis before referral for expert assistance can have devastating consequences and is sometimes the result of a lack of continuity of care resulting in the inability to recognize either vascular insufficiency or deterioration of the lesion requiring urgent attention. Failure by health professionals to seek appropriate medical help may also lead to substandard care. Management of foot infections in diabetes should only be undertaken by those with sufficient experience; general practitioners in general do not have that experience.

Retinopathy. The issues here often relate to inadequate eye screening. While frequency of screening is one concern, adequacy of the technology whether by an individual observer or retinal photography represents another. Furthermore, failure to recognize lesions requiring referral to an ophthalmologist can result in unacceptable delay during which vision deteriorates. Sometimes urgent referrals are made, but appointments not appropriately arranged, again leading to disastrous delays.

Trauma

There is nothing to support the notion that trauma causes diabetes. Difficulties do arise, nevertheless, when diabetes is discovered after an accident. In most cases there is no definite proof that the patient did not have diabetes before the accident. However, there is always the possibility that trauma may precipitate overt diabetes rather than cause it. This is because stress and changes of lifestyle will exaggerate the hyperglycaemia of pre-existing diabetes. Signs of retinopathy or other long-term complications may prove that the diabetes was present long before the injury but their absence does not prove it was not. In established diabetes, trauma frequently causes a temporary deterioration of control, but is unlikely to have long-term consequences.

Hypoglycaemia

Diminished cognitive function during unrecognized hypoglycaemia can result in accidents in the workplace, at home or when driving, or lead to disturbances of behaviour in relation to other people or to uncharacteristic actions such as shoplifting. When assessing cases where hypoglycaemia may have precipitated an untoward event it is obviously essential to make a rigorous ascertainment of whether or not the person was hypoglycaemic at the time. It is also important to determine whether impaired awareness of hypoglycaemia was already known to occur in the individual concerned, whether advice had already been proffered by health professionals, or whether the event in question was a one-off occurrence.

Hypoglycaemia is one of several causes of 'automatism', which is defined as 'the existence in any person of behaviour of which he/she is unaware and over which he/she has no conscious control'. During this state, criminal acts may be performed, especially shoplifting, driving offences and breaches of the peace.

A person can be guilty of a crime only if he/she is engaged in a certain conduct (*acta reus*) with a certain state of mind (*mens rea*), the latter indicating guilty intent and implying that the individual committed the crime of his/her own volition. An automaton-like state relieves the offender of '*mens rea*' (the guilty intent) and can be advanced as a defence to criminal charges. In practice, this means that if the presence of hypoglycaemia at the time of the act can be established, some offenders are acquitted. However, lawyers are cautious in their use of this defence because of the readiness with which it might be abused. Furthermore, if it can be shown that the hypoglycaemic state was the result either of carelessness or even deliberately induced, it can cease to be a valid defence. The law regarding automatism is extremely confused. A defence of automatism strictly means that a state of insanity, albeit temporary, must be pleaded, scarcely sensible in a case of hypoglycaemia.

Prison and custody

Care of diabetic patients in prison can result in serious problems of control and often leads to either hypoglycaemia because of the type of diet and its daily distribution, or to ketoacidosis in those refusing to take insulin. The introduction of a specialist diabetes clinic in a local prison in Liverpool led to great improvements in care. Diabetes UK have made recommendations for improvement of diabetes care in prisons and, at the very least, all prisoners on insulin or sulphonylureas should be given a supply of dextrose tablets, have a late evening snack and, ideally, should not be in solitary confinement so that others can recognize impending hypoglycaemia.

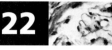

Organization of Care

Summary

- High-quality, comprehensive care is essential in order to prevent acute and long-term complications of diabetes

- National Service Frameworks (NSFs) have been established to enhance quality and eliminate variations in care provision

- Integrated care pathways should be developed between care sectors

- IT systems are important both for the retrieval and dissemination of information

- Up-to-date practice-based registers should be established in all localities

- Screening for diabetes should target those at high risk of developing Type 2

- Structured education is a fundamental component of diabetes care

- Regular clinical audit allows a systematic, critical analysis of clinical outcome and service provision

In order to achieve the stated aims of diabetes care (Box 22.1) it is essential that people with diabetes receive high-quality comprehensive care that is delivered by a variety of providers, in a range of different settings. The patterns of service provision will vary from locality to locality depending upon the needs of the local population, the human and material resources available and the level of skills and expertise of the service providers. In order to achieve these aims, health care providers should:
- establish a diagnosis and initiate treatment;
- provide continuing education programmes for those living with diabetes;
- achieve optimal and appropriate diabetes control;
- offer holistic and effective continuing care;
- screen for and detect complications;
- effectively treat complications;
- provide structures and systems to enable quality

assurance of the processes and outcomes of service provision;
- provide continuing education programmes for professionals to enable them to achieve these aims.

In recent years a number of health policy frameworks have been published that aim to facilitate high-quality equitable services for people with diabetes whatever their geographical location and individual needs.

The New NHS: Modern, Dependable, published by the Department of Health in 1997 first introduced the term 'clinical governance', which was broadly defined as an initiative both to assure and to improve clinical standards of care at local level. The following year *A First Class Service* provided a clinical governance framework (Fig. 22.1) to enable quality standards to be achieved and make organizations accountable for the quality of service they provided. In

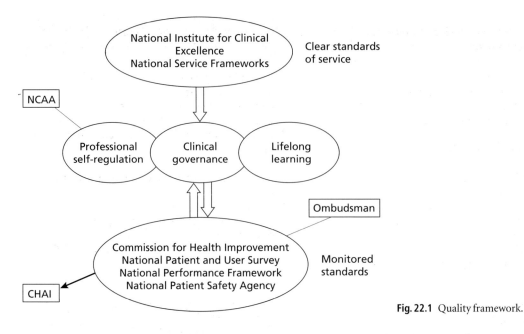

Fig. 22.1 Quality framework.

Box 22.1 **The aims of diabetes care**

Prevention of symptoms of diabetes and prescribed treatment.

Prevention of acute and long-term complications.

Prevention of physical disability.

Prevention of psychological barriers to self-care.

a nutshell, clinical governance is really about doing what we already do, but doing it better and about making changes that result in tangible improvements to services for those living with diabetes as well as the health care professionals working with them.

The following key activities have been shown to have a positive impact on the quality of service provision and clinical outcome.
• Clinical audit and standard setting.
• Clinical effectiveness, incorporating evidence-based practice.
• Clinical risk management (and, as a logical follow on, lessons learned from complaints).

• Continuing professional development (lifelong learning).
• Professional self-regulation.
• Service accreditation.
• Research and development strategies.

On a national level, local clinical governance initiatives are supported by National Institute of Clinical Excellence (NICE) guidelines (Box 22.2), Commission for Health Improvement (CHI) reviews, NHS performance indicators and National Service Frameworks (NSFs).

National Service Framework for Diabetes

The NSF programme was established to improve services and outcomes by setting national standards to enhance the quality of service provision and to tackle variations in care. The NSF for diabetes aims to:
• decrease the incidence of Type 2 diabetes;
• identify people with diabetes earlier;
• allow people with diabetes to have greater control of their condition;
• decrease the rate of complications;

Box 22.2 **NICE appraisals and guidelines (www.nice.org.uk)**

Appraisals date
Rosiglitazone for Type 2 diabetes
August 2000
Pioglitazone for Type 2 diabetes
March 2001
Orilstat for the treatment of obesity
March 2001
Sibutramine for the treatment of obesity
October 2001
Ramipril and other ACE inhibitors
November 2002
Surgery for obesity
June 2002
Insulin pump therapy for people with Type 1 and Type 2 diabetes
April 2003
Long-acting insulin analogues
December 2002
Patient education models for diabetes
March 2003
Clinical guidelines
Management of Type 2 diabetes and its complications
Spring 2002
Management of Type 1 diabetes
December 2003
Management of hypertension in primary care
March 2003
Management of medical emergencies in primary care
To be confirmed

Clinical audit tool
Quality Indicators for Diabetes Services (QUIDS): a project to develop tools for clinical data validation and case mix adjustment for benchmarking services
July 2002

Box 22.3 **NSF standards and cross-cutting issues**

Standards
Prevention of Type 2 diabetes
Identification of people with diabetes
Empowering people with diabetes
Clinical care of adults with diabetes
Clinical care of children and young people with diabetes
Management of diabetic emergencies
Care of people with diabetes during admission to hospital
Diabetes and pregnancy
Detection and management of long-term complications

Cross-cutting issues
User–patient empowerment
Ethnicity
Inequalities and social exclusion
Inpatient management
Primary–secondary care interface
Health–social care interface
Economic analysis

ple with diabetes, whatever their social location, to participate in their care (Box 22.3).

Specialist service provision

To provide a service in keeping with the standards and principles of the NSF adequately staffed and resourced specialist centres as well as adequately developed primary care diabetes services are required.

Diabetes centres have now been established in many parts of the country to provide accommodation and facilities for the provision of education and information to both patient and professional groups as well as the full range of diabetes care.

A core objective of a diabetes centre is to provide rapid access to problem-solving advice for those living with diabetes and for colleagues working in both primary and secondary care. In response to this core function, many centres provide daily 'drop in' sessions for those living and working with diabetes. At

• identify and treat complications earlier;
• provide effective inpatient care; and
• facilitate healthier pregnancies in women with diabetes.

The NSF sets out 12 standards with a number of cross-cutting issues for the prevention and management of diabetes and for strategies to enable all peo-

King's we have established a dedicated advice 'hot line' (*not* an answer phone) for colleagues working in primary care. The diabetes centre may also 'house' and act as an organizational base for the multiprofessional specialist team.

The multiprofessional specialist team

The multiprofessional specialist team needed to provide comprehensive diabetes care should comprise the following.
• Consultant physicians with specialist training in and responsibility for diabetes (at least 28.75 sessions per week per 250 000 population).
• Non-consultant clinical medical staff (associate specialists, hospital practitioners, clinical assistants, specialist registrars).
• Diabetes specialist nurses (at least 4.0 whole time equivalent (WTE) per 250 000 population).
• Diabetes facilitator/coordinator (full-time).
• Specialist dietitians (1.5 WTE per 250 000 population).
• Specialist podiatrists (2 WTE per 250 000 population).
• Clinical psychologist/liaison psychiatrist with an interest in diabetes.
• Consultant paediatrician supported by paediatric diabetes specialist nurses and specialist paediatric dietitians and psychologists.
• Consultant obstetrician supported by specialist midwives.
• Consultant ophthalmologist.
• Consultant nephrologist.
• Consultant neurologist.
• Consultant vascular surgeon.

Joint specialist clinics

One of the most important elements of secondary care provision is the joint specialist clinic. This facility allows the individual to be seen jointly by the diabetes team and the team with specialist expertise, optimizing care provision and saving duplication of clinic appointments. At King's, specialist joint clinics are provided for pregnant women, those transferring from paediatric to adult services, those requiring ophthalmic intervention and those with identified renal and/or neuropathic complications. Local referral guidelines into specialist clinics should be available and should include agreed clinical criteria and the process for referral.

Special groups such as children, young adults, pregnant women, those with complications requiring specialist intervention and those experiencing psychological barriers to self-care generally require specialist care.

To ensure that all people with diabetes receive the right care, at the right time and in the right place, integrated care pathways, shared protocols, agreed roles and responsibilities and collaborative formal systems of audit and evaluation need to be created between care sectors. There is often a misconception that a 'collection' of professionals constitutes a team approach to diabetes care. However, an effective team cannot function without regular meetings, collaborative working and reliable systems of communication.

Integrated care pathways

Integrated care pathways manage clinical and educational processes and measure patient outcomes. Care pathways cross the boundaries of primary and secondary care and predict the course of events (or map the route) for the management of patients with similar problems, e.g. those with newly diagnosed Type 1 diabetes, Type 2 diabetes and women diagnosed with gestational diabetes. The patients' route is specified on a timeline that states the expected patient 'journey', and the predicted interventions/contents of the care package. Any deviation from the route is recorded and used to inform audit and evaluation processes (variance analysis). Evaluation and analysis of the variance data can highlight shortfalls in the level of service provision and demonstrate a commitment to clinical governance (Fig. 22.1).

It has been suggested that the collaborative working needed to develop integrated pathways can create positive team-building dynamics and an environment for the implementation of evidence-based practice. It is also suggested that care pathways are likely to improve documentation and record keeping and have a positive impact on limited resources.

Information technology

Information technology (IT) is increasingly important in the organization of diabetes care and in the retrieval and dissemination of information and knowledge for both patients and professionals. However, it is essential that IT systems are developed to support services with the intention of improving care delivery — service design should not be driven by the requirements of the IT! Nevertheless, IT does have enormous potential to improve service delivery. Electronic records have the ability to prompt the user to perform important functions (e.g. the requirements of an annual review) and should facilitate transfer of clinical information and pathology data between care sectors. Such IT utilization is becoming more common but the standardization and user friendliness of software require further development.

Software packages have the potential to review record systems using built-in data prompts and risk assessment programs. Digital images can be captured, thus enabling retinal photographs, foot lesions and angiography films to be incorporated into electronic patient records and these may be relayed for expert assessment at another site. Programs for automatic assessment and diagnosis are in development. Increasingly, electronic referral and care pathways are becoming available.

The national Primary Care Information Services (PRIMIS) programme is currently working with a number of diabetes specialist teams to develop a minimum data set, computer screen templates and data analysis tools in preparation for the implementation of the NSF.

Local Diabetes Services Advisory Groups Diabetes Steering Groups/NSF Implementation Groups

Such groups should be established in each locality to monitor and advise on the range of services that need to be commissioned in order to reach the NSF standards.

The composition of the group and the methods of working should meet the needs of the local population. The membership of the group should be multiprofessional and include managerial representatives from primary care, secondary care and community health services as well as service users. The major aim of such groups should be to ensure equity of service provision for all users including those that are disadvantaged by social status, ethnicity, age or disability.

Objectives of the group should include the following:
• to agree a strategy for improving the health of local people with diabetes that includes setting specific objectives and key performance indicators;
• to ensure that systems are in place to allow regular audit and evaluation of services;
• to advise on the services required within the locality;
• to monitor the level, range, quality and coordination of services provided locally against agreed local and national standards; and
• to monitor the health status of people with diabetes and progress towards the agreed health improvement targets.

Diabetes registers

Diabetes registers should be established in all localities. They are essential for auditing the quality of the processes and outcomes of care, and for monitoring progress towards agreed local and national standards. Statistical data can be extracted and combined to provide material for large-scale comparative clinical and management audits.

To be effective in achieving their purpose, diabetes registers should meet the following criteria:
• include all known people with diabetes within a given locality;
• be regularly updated (with data on deaths, movement and change of address, etc.); and
• contain data on the process and outcome of care.
Data should conform to the recommended national data set for diabetes and adequate measures should

be put into place to ensure confidentiality of the data held on the register.

Local guidelines for management

Local guidelines for management of people with diabetes should be prepared and agreed by all local providers of diabetes care. They must be based on national and international evidence-based guidelines. They should clearly define specific roles and responsibilities of professionals in local diabetes strategies, taking into account the different levels of interest and skills among primary and secondary health care teams. Most importantly, it is essential that agreed referral pathways between primary and secondary care are appropriate (e.g. pregnant women should have a referral pathway immediately into secondary care), accessible and widely disseminated to all health care professionals via the local diabetes policy document.

Individual management plans should be agreed between each person with diabetes and the key professionals working with them. The responsibility for various elements of the care package should be made clear to all those involved (documented in the individualized integrated care pathway). A patient-held document, containing information such as management targets, first-line advice, impending appointments and useful contact numbers is an effective way to facilitate greater patient involvement and responsibility in their management plan. At King's we have incorporated all of the above into a self-monitoring diary.

Expert patients

The idea of developing a major initiative on expert patients was set out in the 1999 White Paper, *Saving Lives: Our Healthier Nation*, and for the past 3 years modernization policies have consistently emphasized the importance of the patient in the design and delivery of services. In the management of chronic diseases, such as diabetes, arthritis and multiple sclerosis, self-care programmes are being specifically designed to reduce dependence on health care

Box 22.4 **Sharing expertise**	
Patient	Professional
Experience of illness	Diagnosis
Social circumstances	Disease aetiology
Attitudes to risk	Prognosis
Values	Treatment options
Preferences	Outcome probabilities

professionals by improving patient confidence, resourcefulness and self-efficacy. These fundamental changes to service provision are based on the recognition that patients and professional each have their own area of knowledge and expertise (Box 22.4) and that both are necessary if positive biopsychosocial outcomes are to be achieved.

Screening for diabetes

The focus of the continuing debate surrounding screening for Type 2 diabetes has shifted from should we screen, to how and whom should we screen?

We are currently facing an epidemic of Type 2 diabetes. Prevalence rates are quoted as 2–3% of people within the UK population diagnosed as having diabetes and approximately one million people with undiagnosed diabetes. The number of people with diabetes is expected to double by 2010.

Why screen? The UK Diabetes Information Audit and Benchmarking Service (UKDIABS) data show that people with Type 2 diabetes could have had the condition for between 9 and 12 years before diagnosis. Additionally, the UK Prospective Diabetes Survey (UKPDS) found that up to 50% of those newly diagnosed had already developed one or more of the long-term complications of diabetes. We also have evidence to show that active management of specific risk factors can slow the progression towards or even prevent the development of Type 2 diabetes. In the light of this evidence the question of should we screen for Type 2 diabetes is hardly justified. However, the question of whether Type 2 diabetes fulfils national screening criteria (Box 22.5) needs to be explored.

The UK National Screening Committee (NSC) has

reviewed the evidence for introducing population screening for Type 2 diabetes against the screening criteria. This review confirmed that it would not be cost-effective to screen the whole population. However, although currently there is no clear evidence to suggest that screening for Type 2 diabetes in high-risk populations is efficacious, there is an emerging consensus that this should happen. The NSC has now recommended that further analysis of existing evidence as well as further research should be undertaken to identify the methodology for targeted screening (how, who and how often people should be screened for diabetes). The NSC is expected to report its findings in 2005.

A recent position statement from Diabetes UK states that there should be screening programmes for Type 2 diabetes, but that these should be restricted to the adult population with two or more risk factors of Type 2 diabetes (Box 22.6). Diabetes UK currently recommends active case finding of those with increased risk of developing diabetes every 3 years by:
- fasting plasma blood glucose assay (although this will miss 20–30% of cases);
- plasma glucose asssay 2 h after glucose load; and
- postprandial urinalysis for glycosuria is less sensitive and is not recommended but could be used where other methods are not practicable.

The diagnosis of diabetes must be made on an accredited laboratory method. Treatment should not be started on the basis of a screening result. Screening programmes outside of primary care, e.g. in pharmacies or as part of awareness campaigns, should be conducted by adequately trained staff with clear referral guidelines (Box 22.7) to general practice where diagnosis can be confirmed.

Annual review screening for complications

Once diabetes is diagnosed, it must be actively managed to minimize the risk of complications and avoid disability from advanced complications. The annual review sets out to record risk factors for complications and seeks evidence of early, ideally asymptomatic, established complications, with a view to active management to prevent progression. The annual review is thus an integral part of diabetes management. If well organized, as well as providing an effective systematic structure to screening for complications, the process can identify educational needs and provide a forum for people with diabetes to discuss any problems or concerns they may have. The annual review should include the same components whether it is conducted in primary or secondary care (Chapter 14)

Box 22.7 **Response to screening results**
(Diabetes UK 2001)

Screening test positive
Reassure individual (explanation that result of screening test is not diagnostic but suggests the need for further investigation by GP).

Give written details of screening procedure and result of test.

Instruct not to make any changes to diet or medication.

Individual to arrange routine GP appointment 2–4 weeks following screening (sooner if symptomatic).

Screening test negative
Asymptomatic—no action required.
Symptoms of diabetes and/or complications—seek advice from GP who should be informed of negative test result but told that diabetes has not been excluded.

Education

The supplementary information published with the NSF Standards document states that:

'People with diabetes need to be supported to come to terms with having a long-term condition, which needs to be managed on a day-to-day basis. They also need to be able to make choices about the management of their diabetes based on a sound understanding of the condition and its management.' (www.doh.gov.uk/nsf)

This can be best achieved by the effective provision of information, education and psychological support.

However, the Audit Commission Report, *Testing Times*, showed that only one-third of diabetes services offered a structured patient education programme and only two-thirds of those people in the audit sample had had access to an education programme in the previous 12 months. Data from the National Centre for Social Research report, *Listening to Diabetes Service Users*, also identified that people generally have a poor knowledge of care and that there is no consistency in the way information is delivered to people with diabetes.

Diabetes education should be a planned, dynamic, life-long process and a fundamental component of continuing care. The starting point of the educational process has traditionally been at diagnosis of diabetes and delivered by health care professionals. The emerging evidence surrounding the prevention of Type 2 diabetes suggests that the starting point should shift to primary prevention programmes, provided by community health promotion workers working in a variety of settings, such as schools and community projects, but supported by diabetes care specialists. However, whatever their discipline, all those providing and delivering diabetes education require dedicated time, specific training, teaching and communication skills, a supportive attitude and a readiness to listen and negotiate.

Structured education programmes, such as Dose Adjustment For Normal Eating (DAFNE), which train and motivate patients to gain and utilize appropriate self-management skills, are regarded as crucial to both biomedical and quality of life outcome. The aims of such programmes are to optimize knowledge about the condition and its management, to encourage effective patient–professional partnerships and to promote health behaviours that interact positively with individual lifestyle and diabetes management. The content (Box 22.8), focus, timing and method of provision of programmes need to be determined by the stated educational outcome and the specific individual needs.

Continuing education programmes should further expand on the themes in Box 22.8 but also focus on specific issues that are relevant and meaningful to the individual at a particular time. These can include strategies for travelling when going on holiday, family planning and pregnancy for sexually active females, foot care for those identified with foot complications, substance misuse (including alcohol) in adolescent clinics and so on. Additionally, people with diabetes require comprehensive ongoing education that reinforces key messages periodically and incorporates behavioural change strategies to enable and support lifestyle change. Family members, partners and carers should be included in the education process where appropriate.

Education models/approaches that encourage individuals to participate actively in the learning

The nature, symptoms and outcomes of diabetes—'what is diabetes'?

Dietary aspects of management including alcohol.

Self-monitoring diabetes—rationale, techniques and interpreting results.

The importance and effects of exercise/activity.

Treatments—oral therapy, insulin.

Awareness of acute complications—hypoglycaemia, hyperglycaemia.

Life issues such as identification, prescription exemption, driving, insurance, employment/school.

Contacts—who, how and when.

Reducing the risk of developing complications.

Managing concurrent illness.

Box 22.9 **Teaching the management of hypoglycaemia**

Discussion
Establish group's understanding of the term hypoglycaemia.

Experiential learning
Ask the group about their experiences of hypoglycaemia and their individual signs and symptoms.
Ask the group how they treat hypoglycaemia and the consequences of their treatment.

Problem solving
Present the group with scenarios and facilitate discussion of the problem, possible causes and solutions.

Skills-based training
Present the group with management guidelines.

process are more effective than those interventions where learners are passive recipients of information giving (the 'pot filling' model). Participation can be facilitated by using experiential learning methods (using individuals' own experiences to reach stated learning outcomes), problem-based learning processes, 'hands on' skills training and interactive group work. All of these methods can be utilized in many aspects of diabetes education; for example, facilitating a group session on the management of hypoglycaemia (Box 22.9).

In order to optimize the effectiveness of any education intervention, individuals need the opportunity to acknowledge and discuss concerns and anxieties surrounding their condition, social situation and ability to self-manage; anxiety is a powerful barrier to learning! Other barriers to learning include sociocultural barriers such as language and customs, hearing, visual and cognitive impairment, inexperienced facilitators/educators, inappropriate environment and an *ad hoc* approach to the delivery of education programmes. The effectiveness and quality of diabetes education should be evaluated regularly by well-designed audit/research studies assessing both the processes and outcomes of the intervention.

Clinical audit

Clinical audit (Fig. 22.2) is a fundamental part of the quality framework (Fig. 22.1) and can be defined as a systematic and critical analysis of the quality of service provision and its effect on clinical outcome and quality of life for people with diabetes. It helps to determine whether the best practice is, in fact, being delivered to all patients all of the time. There is a very close relationship between research and clinical audit but there is often confusion between the two and how they are connected. Put simply, research tells us what to do and audit explores the extent to which we are doing it. For example, we have an evidence base for the treatment of hypertension in diabetes, the process of clinical audit will reveal the extent to which the evidence is being translated into clinical practice.

Conclusions

The era of people with diabetes as passive recipients of care is changing and being replaced by one where genuine partnerships between health care profes-

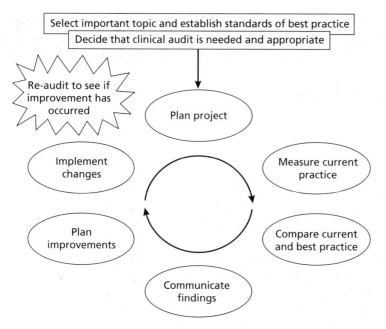

Select important topic and establish standards of best practice

Decide that clinical audit is needed and appropriate

Re-audit to see if improvement has occurred

Plan project

Implement changes

Measure current practice

Plan improvements

Compare current and best practice

Communicate findings

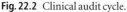

Fig. 22.2 Clinical audit cycle.

sionals and the individuals they care for being developed. There is undisputed evidence that active management of glycaemic control, blood pressure, lipids and obesity substantially reduce the risk of the long-term complications of diabetes and that, once developed, active management of complications can prevent further progression and disability. For some, coping with diabetes on a daily basis can result in psychological morbidity.

It follows then that services must be organized to allow all people with diabetes access to care that facilitates effective self-management, reduces the risk of complications to a minimum and supports individual psychosocial need. In recent years, studies have confirmed variations in service provision and clinical outcome across geographical locations and between clinical teams. Implementation of the quality framework and the NSF standards will go some way in addressing these variations.

Body Mass Index Chart

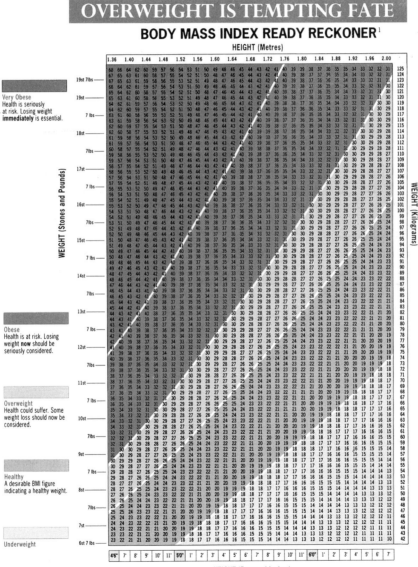

Appendix 2

Cardiovascular Risk Chart

See Plate 6, facing page 148.

Diabetes Associations for Patients and Health Professionals

American Diabetes Association (Patient and Professional), 1660 Duke Street, Alexandria, Virginia VA 22314. Tel: 703-549-1500, Fax: 703-549-6995.

Australian Diabetes Society (Professional), 145 Macquarie Street, Sydney, NSW 2000. Tel: 02-9256-5462, Fax: 02-9241-4083. www.racp.edu.au e-mail: sneylon@racp.edu.au

Canadian Diabetes Association (Patient and Professional), PO Box 12013, Station BRM B, Toronto, Ontario, M7Y 2L3. www.diabetes.ca

Diabetes Australia (Patient), 1st Floor Churchill House, 218 Northbourne Avenue, Braddon ACT 2612. www.diabetesaustralia.com.au

Diabetes New Zealand (Patient), PO Box 54, 1 Conquest Street, Oamaru. Tel: 0800 342 238, Fax: 03-434-5281. www.diabetes.org.nz e-mail: info@diabetes.org.nz

Diabetes UK (Patient and Professional), 10 Parkway, London NW1 7AA. Tel: 0044 20 7424 1000. www.diabetes.org.uk

European Association for Study of Diabetes (Professional), Rheindorfer Weg 3, D-40591, Dusseldorf, Germany. Tel: 0049 211-758469, Fax: 0049 211-7584690. www.easd.org e-mail: easd@uni-dusseldorf.de

Irish Diabetic Association (Patient), 76 Lower Gardiner Street, Dublin 1. Tel & Fax: 00353(0)1-8363022.

Juvenile Diabetes Research Foundation, 19 Angel Gate, London ECIV 2PT. Tel: 0044 20 7713-2030, Fax: 0044 20-7713-2031. www.jdrf.org.uk

Juvenile Diabetes Research Foundation International, 120 Wall Street, New York, NY 10005-4001, USA. Tel: 212-785 9595. www.jdrf.org/index.php

National Diabetes International Clearing House, Box NDIC, Bethesda, MD 20205, USA.

New Zealand Society for the Study of Diabetes (Professional), East Riding, Whiterocks Road, 6-D RD Oamaru. Tel & Fax: 03-434-8188.

Society for Endocrinology, Metabolism and Diabetes of Southern Africa (Professional), PO Box 783155, Sandton 2146, Johannesburg, South Africa. Tel: 27-11/807-0794, Fax: 27-11/807-7989. e-mail: rsh@novonordisk.com

South African Diabetes Association (Patient), PO Box 3943, Cape Town 8000. Tel: 21-461-3715, Fax: 21-462-2008.

USEFUL WEB SITES

Clinical Standards for Diabetes (Scotland) www.clinicalstandards.org

Exeter genetic screening service www.diabetesgenes.org

Heart Protection Study www.hpsinfo.org

National Service Framework for Diabetes www.doh.gov.uk/nsf/diabetes

Scottish Intercollegiate Guidelines Network (SIGN) www.sign.ac.uk

Warwick Centre for Diabetes Education and Research www.diabetescare.warwick.ac.uk

Appendix 4

References and Further Reading

Alberti, K.G.M.M., Defronzo, R.A., Keen, H. & Zimmet, P., eds. (1997) *International Textbook of Diabetes Mellitus*, 2nd edn. John Wiley & Sons, Chichester. [A two-volume comprehensive review.]

Amiel, S. (2002) Is there anything new about insulin therapy? In: *Horizons in Medicine* (ed. S. Amiel), pp. 175–184. Royal College of Physicians, London.

Angel, A., Dhalla, N., Pierce, G. & Singal, P. (2001) *Diabetes and Cardiovascular Disease*. Kluwer Academic Publishers, Netherlands.

Besser, G.M., Bodansky, H.J. & Cudworth, A.G. (1988) *Clinical Diabetes: An Illustrated Text*. J.B. Lippincott, Philadelphia. [An extensively illustrated text.]

Bilous, R. (2002) HOPE and other recent trials of antihypertensive therapy in Type 2 diabetes. In: *Horizons in Medicine*. (ed. S. Amiel), pp. 195–206. Royal College of Physicians, London.

Bliss, M. (1983) *The Discovery of Insulin*. Paul Harris Publishing, Edinburgh. [A masterful account of the events surrounding the discovery of insulin.]

Bloom, A. & Ireland, J. (with revisions by Watkins, P.J.) (1992) *A Colour Atlas of Diabetes*, 2nd edn. Wolfe Publishing, London.

Boulton, A.J.M., Connor, H. & Cavanagh, P.R., eds. (2000) *The Foot in Diabetes*, 3rd edn. John Wiley & Sons, Chichester.

Bowker, J.H. & Pfeifer, M.A., eds. (2001) Levin and O'Neals: the Diabetic Foot. Mosby, St Louis.

Day, J.L. (2001) *Living with Diabetes*, 2nd edn. John Wiley & Sons, Chichester.

Dornhorst, A. & Hadden, D.R., eds. (1996) *Diabetes and Pregnancy*. John Wiley & Sons, Chichester.

Dyck, P.J. & Thomas, P.K., eds. (1999) *Diabetic Neuropathy*, 2nd edn. W.B. Saunders, Philadelphia.

Edmonds, M.E. & Foster, A.V.M. (2000) *Managing the Diabetic Foot*. Blackwell Science, Oxford.

Ekoe, J.M., Zimmet, P. & Williams, R. (2001) *Epidemiology of Diabetes Mellitus*. John Wiley & Sons, Chichester.

Fox, C. & Pickering, A. (1995) *Diabetes in the Real World*. Class Publishing, London. [A practical handbook advising on the needs of diabetic patients in general practice.]

Frier, B.M. & Fisher, M., eds. (1993) *Hypoglycaemia*. Edward Arnold, London. [The most authoritative reference book on the subject at present.]

Frier, B.M. & Fisher, M., eds. (1999) *Hypoglycaemia in Clinical Diabetes*. John Wiley & Sons, Chichester.

Gill, G., Pickup, J. & Williams, G., eds. (2001) *Difficult Diabetes*. Blackwell Science, Oxford.

Gill, G., Mbanya, J-C. & Alberti, G., eds. (1997) *Diabetes in Africa*. FSG Communications, Reach, Cambridge.

Hasslacher, C. (2001) *Diabetic Nephropathy*. John Wiley & Sons, Chichester.

Heller, S.R. (2000) Sudden cardiac death in young people with diabetes. *CME Bulletin of Endocrinology and Diabetes* 3, 4–7.

Hollingsworth, D.R. (1991) *Pregnancy, Diabetes and Birth: a Management Guide*, 2nd edn. Williams & Wilkins, London.

Jeffcoate, W. & MacFarlane, R. (1995) *The Diabetic Foot: An Illustrated Guide to Management*. Chapman & Hall, London.

Kahn, C.R. & Weir, G.C., eds. (1995) *Joslin's Diabetes Mellitus*. Leonard Febiger, Philadelphia.

Kelmark, C.J.H. (1994) *Childhood and Adolescent Diabetes*. Chapman & Hall, London.

Kirby, R., Holmes, S. & Carson, C. (1999) *Erectile Dysfunction*, 2nd edn. Health Press, Oxford.

Krentz, A.J. & Bailey, C.J. (2001) *Type 2 Diabetes in Practice*. Royal Society of Medicine Press, London.

Leslie, R.D.G. & Robbins, D.C., eds. (1995) *Diabetes: Clinical Science in Practice*. Cambridge University Press, Cambridge.

MacKinnon, M. (2002) *Providing Diabetes Care in General Practice*. 4th edn. Class Publishing, London.

Malins, J.M. (1968) *Clinical Diabetes Mellitus*. Eyre and Spottiswoode, London. [A splendid clinical description of diabetes.]

Mathias, C.J. & Bannister, R., eds. (1999) *Autonomic Failure*, 4th edn. Oxford University Press, Oxford.

Mogensen, C.E., ed. (2000) *The Kidney and Hypertension in Diabetes Mellitus*, 5th edn. Kluwer Academic Publishing, USA.

Nattrass, M. (1994) *Malins' Clinical Diabetes*, 2nd edn. Chapman & Hall, London.

Owens, D.R., Zinman, B. & Bolli, G.B. (2001) Insulins today and beyond. *Lancet* **358**, 739–746.

Pickup, J.C. & Williams, G., eds. (2003) *Textbook of Diabetes*, 3rd edn. Blackwell Science , Oxford. [A substantial account in two volumes; beautifully illustrated.]

Pickup, J.C. & Williams, G. (1994) *Chronic Complications of Diabetes*. Blackwell Scientific Publications, Oxford. [A one-volume updated version taken from the authors' two-volume textbook.]

Ritz, R. & Rychlik, I., eds. (1999) *Nephropathy in Type 2 Diabetes*. Oxford University Press, Oxford.

Shaw, K.M., ed. (1996) *Diabetic Complications*. John Wiley & Sons, Chichester.

Sinclair, A. & Finucane, P. (2000) *Diabetes in Old Age*, 2nd edn. John Wiley & Sons, Chichester.

Tooke, J., ed. (1999) *Diabetic Angiopathy*. Arnold, London.

Warren, S., Le Compte, P.M. & Legg, M.A. (1966) *The Pathology of Diabetes Mellitus*. Henry Kimpton, London. [A classic account.]

Watkins, P.J. (2002) *ABC of Diabetes*, 5th edn. BMJ Publishing Group, London. [A short, illustrated, very practical small book.]

Watkins, P.J. (2002) The diabetic traveller. In: *Travelers' Health* (ed. R. Dawood), 4th edn, pp. 509–515. Random House, New York.

West, K.M. (1978) *Epidemiology of Diabetes and its Vascular Lesions*. Elsevier, New York. [A classic review of diabetes in a world setting.]

Williams, R., Wareham, N., Kinmonth, A.M. & Herman, W.H. (2002) *Evidence Base for Diabetes Care*. John Wiley & Sons, Chichester.

Young, A. & Harries, M., eds. (2001) *Physical Activity for Patients: An Exercise Prescription*. Royal College of Physicians, London.

IMPORTANT PUBLICATIONS AND REVIEWS

Atkinson, M.A. & Eisenbarth, G.S. (2001) Type 1 diabetes: new perspectives on disease pathogenesis and treatment. *Lancet* **358**, 221–229.

Barnett, A.H., Eff, C., Leslie, R.D.G. & Pyke, D.A. (1981) Diabetes in identical twins: a study of 200 pairs. *Diabetologia* **20**, 87–93.

Barrett, T. (1999) Inherited diabetic disorders. *CME Bulletin of Endocrinology and Diabetes* **2**, 47–50.

Carron Brown, S., Kyne-Grzebalski, D., Mwangi, B. & Taylor, R. (1999) Effect of management policy upon 120 Type 1 diabetic pregnancies: policy decisions in practice. *Diabetic Medicine* **16**, 573–578.

Diabetes Control and Complications Research Group (DCCT) (1993) The effect of diabetes on the development and progression of long-term complications in insulin dependent diabetes. *New England Journal of Medicine* **329**, 977–986.

DIGAMI Study Group. (1997) Prospective randomised study of intensive insulin treatment of long-term survival after acute myocardial infarction in patients with diabetes mellitus. *British Medical Journal* **314**, 1512–1515.

Euclid Study Group (1997) Randomised placebo-controlled trial of lisinopril in normotensive patients with insulin dependent diabetes and normoalbuminuria or microalbuminuria. *Lancet* **349**, 1787–1792.

Expert Committee on the Diagnosis and Classification of Diabetes Mellitus (1997) Report of the Expert Committee on the Diagnosis and Classification of Diabetes. *Diabetes Care* **20**, 1183–1197.

Groop, L.C. & Tuomi, T. (1997) Non-insulin-dependent diabetes mellitus: a collision between thrifty genes and an affluent society. *Annals of Medicine* **29**, 37–53.

Halban, P., Kahn, S.E., Lernmark, A. & Rhodes, C. (2001) Gene and cell replacement therapy in the treatment of Type 1 diabetes. *Diabetes* **50**, 2181–2191.

Henquin, J.C. (2000) Triggering and amplifying pathways of regulation of insulin secretion by glucose. *Diabetes* **49**, 1751–1760.

HOPE study: Heart Outcomes Prevention Evaluation Study Investigators (2000) Effects of ramipril on cardiovascular and microvascular outcomes in people with diabetes mellitus. *Lancet* **355**, 253–259.

Hoppener, J.W.M., Ahren, B. & Lips, C.J.M. (2000) Islet amyloid and Type 2 diabetes. *New England Journal of Medicine* **343**, 411–419.

Jovanovic, L. (1998) American Diabetes Association's Fourth International Workshop Conference on Gestational Diabetes Mellitus: summary and discussion. Therapeutic interventions. *Diabetes Care* **21** (Suppl 2), 131–137.

Jovanovic-Peterson, L., Peterson, C.M., Reed, G.F., Metzger, B.E., Mills, J.L., Knopp, R.H. & Aarons, J.H. (1991) Maternal postprandial glucose levels and infant birth weight: the Diabetes in Early Pregnancy Study. National Institute of Child Health and Human Development – Diabetes in Early Pregnancy Study. *American Journal of Obstetrics and Gynecology* **164**, 103–111.

King, G.L. & Brownlee, M. (1996) The cellular and molecular mechanisms of diabetic complications. *Endocrinology and Metabolism Clinics of North America* **25**, 255–270.

MRC/BHF Heart Protection Study of cholesterol lowering

with simvastatin in 20 536 high risk individuals: a randomised trial. (2002) *Lancet* **360**, 7–22.

Redondo, M.J. & Eisenbarth, G.S. (2002) Genetic control of autoimmunity in Type 1 diabetes and associated disorders. *Diabetologia* **45**, 605–622.

Ritz, E. & Orth, S.R. (1999) Nephropathy in patients with Type 2 diabetes. *New England Journal of Medicine* **341**, 1127–1133.

UK Prospective Diabetes Survey (UK PDS): several papers in the *Lancet* and *British Medical Journal*, 12 September 1998, and many subsequently.

Ulrich, P. & Cerami, A. (2001) Protein glycation, diabetes and aging. *Recent Progress in Hormone Research* **56**, 1–21.

MAJOR DIABETES JOURNALS

The major journals reporting on diabetic research and care are as follows.

Diabetes, American Diabetes Association.

Diabetes Care, American Diabetes Association.

Diabetic Medicine, Diabetes UK.

Diabetologia, European Association for Study of Diabetes.

All are issued monthly. *Diabetes* and *Diabetologia* are the more orientated towards basic research, while *Diabetic Medicine* and *Diabetes Care* are more clinical in orientation.

Index

Page numbers in **bold** represent tables, those in *italics* represent figures.